WINNING THE AGE GAME

WINNING
THE AGE GAME

GLORIA HEIDI

A & W Visual Library

Excerpt from "Vogue's Point of View," May 1973 issue of Vogue; excerpt from "Vogue's Point of View," July 1974 issue of Vogue. Reprinted courtesy of Vogue.

Library of Congress Catalog Card Number: 76-39705
ISBN 0-89104-061-7
Printed in the United States of America
Published by arrangement with
Doubleday & Company, Inc.
Garden City, New York

This book is dedicated to
Ageless Women everywhere

ACKNOWLEDGMENTS

Many people helped me bring together the diverse information in this book. I want to take this opportunity to thank Dr. Gaylord Whitlock, extension nutritionist at the University of California at Davis; Brinkley Long, chief marriage counselor for the Superior Court of Sacramento; psychologist Dr. Arthur Sherman, of California State University, Sacramento; nutrition consultant Gladys Lindberg; Linda Canfield Scott, a most knowledgeable fashion and merchandising expert; Al Baeta, track coach at American River College in Sacramento; Dr. Joan Ullyot, of the Institute for Health Research in San Francisco; and Beth De Seelhorst, whose competent secretarial skills put the manuscript into shape. I am indebted to the late Adelle Davis, whose diet theories have had such a positive influence on my well-being, and whose writings are referred to extensively in the chapters on diet.

I also want to thank my good friends Duane Newcomb, who started it all, and Luther Nichols, West Coast editor of Doubleday & Co., whose constant support and enthusiasm encouraged me to finish it. And finally, special thanks are due my husband, who laughed at all my jokes.

CONTENTS

WINNING THE AGE GAME

ONE

The Mature Woman Strikes Back!

"You're not getting older, you're getting better!" That's the punch line for one of the most effective ad campaigns around. But how can you believe it, when for the last decade society has been on a youth kick that is unique in the world's history? Well, it's time for you to kick back. You *aren't* getting older; you *are* getting better!

That's the purpose of this book: to prove to you that it's really true. And to show you how to express this truth in the way you look, the way you feel, the way you act. Moreover, this book will help you change your attitude about yourself as a mature woman, with the bonus that when you change what you think about yourself you change what other people think of you. In the eyes of husbands, children, friends, employers, you can change your image from that of middle-aged matron to that inspiring figure, the Ageless Woman.

"YES, BUT . . . THIS TALK OF 'IMAGE'
DISTURBS ME. IT SEEMS SO FALSE AND
AFFECTED. I JUST WANT TO BE MYSELF."

But that's the heart of the matter, isn't it? The mature years do
present us with an identity crisis that might be summed up this way:

"Mirror, mirror, on the wall, I don't know myself at all. I know
I'm not the young girl I once was, yet I'm certainly not an old
woman. So . . . who am I? Isn't there a place in between that
expresses the real me?"

You'll find the answer to this question in the portraits of three
women. Do they sound like anyone you know?

1. *The Professional Middle-aged Matron.* (Let's call her the Professional M.A.M. for short.) Her life style represents the least creative answer, since it is based upon the safe, conservative, tried and
true life style of her grandmother. There is at least one Professional
M.A.M. in everyone's life, so you must learn to recognize her for
what she is and be aware of the negative influence she can exert on
you. The best way to sum up her influence is to say, "With friends
like this, who needs enemies?"

Her solution to the identity crisis of middle age represents a "giving up," a lack of growth; so she is almost inevitably unhappy and
frustrated, as all human beings are frustrated when they cease their
God-given assignment of perpetual inner growth and development.
Since she is devoted to maintaining the status quo, she is always the
first to ridicule any attempts at growth or change by her contemporaries. She seeks to herd her friends and relatives into a closely knit
group that exists in a dreary, self-righteous limbo. She is the first to
complain to her children, "Wait until you're my age. You'll see that
life isn't a bed of roses." She's the first to sigh to her contemporaries,
"Well, none of us is getting any younger, are we?"

And her most powerful weapon is ridicule. I wonder how many
lives have been blighted by this unhappy woman, with her caustic
comments: "Did you see Millie in her new blonde wig? Absolutely
ridiculous, at her age." Or, at her helpful best, "Good Lord, Helen,
you're not *really* going to wear your skirts that short, are you?" And
her final coup de grâce, "Why don't you just grow old gracefully?"

I wish I could advise you to avoid this woman like the plague. Unfortunately, it isn't always that easy, since she is often a member of
your family group. But you can be aware of her negative presence.

You can understand her for what she is, an unhappy, frustrated person . . . and go your own way.

2. *The Unwilling Middle-aged Matron.* In many ways she's the real heroine of this book. Instinctively, she rebels against the settled, stolid matron's role of thirty years ago. Whether she knows it or not, her rebellion is a reaction to the new reality facing today's woman.

An amazing thing is happening to women in today's world. We are all getting younger—every year. I don't mean in the sense of the tired old joke about the ten best years of a woman's life—those between thirty-eight and thirty-nine. I mean we actually are getting *younger.*

In 1900 the average life span of a woman was forty-eight. At thirty, the average woman in 1900 was middle-aged and could only expect to live another eighteen or twenty years.

Today the average woman can expect to live for seventy-five or eighty years. And by the year 2000 a woman's life expectancy will be a hundred.

So our heroine, the Unwilling M.A.M., has a unique problem to solve. When she reaches forty her life isn't over. On the contrary, she can expect an equally long life ahead of her. Modern science has given her the priceless gift of a second lifetime.

And what will she do with this new lifetime? Not much—if she clings to gloomy, outmoded ideas about growing old gracefully. Plenty if she is willing to shape up (literally), sharpen up (fashionably), and join the twentieth century.

However, this isn't as easy as it sounds, because this new reality has created a dilemma for our heroine. She may be at the mid-point of her life, but she is definitely not middle-aged. She isn't old . . . and she isn't young. It's an in-between period, much like adolescence. So much so that Dr. Robert Lee and Marjorie Casebier, in their book *The Spouse Gap,* term this period middlescence, ". . . a new stage in life that has long gone unrecognized." As in adolescence, the mature woman's quest for a new identity can result in uncertainty, lack of confidence, and then sometimes a burst of sudden bravado, symbolized by Millie's purchase of the new blonde wig.

Now there was nothing wrong with Millie's wig. Mature women wear blonde wigs effectively every day. But Millie's burst of bravado was premature. She had not yet acquired the confidence needed to wear that wig. So when her "friends" sweetly suggested that she "looked like a retread Mae West," she was discouraged and depressed. Feeling, "What's the use?" she abandoned her brave new resolutions, her wig, *and* her successful diet program and gained ten matronly pounds.

So we see another characteristic of the Unwilling M.A.M. Like the adolescent, she becomes so supersensitive to ridicule that she hinders both her growth and the development of a new self-image. Her sensitivity puts her right under the thumb of the Professional M.A.M.—and doesn't M.A.M. love it.

Adding to her uncertainty is the specter of her changing sexual identity. She's learning that in our culture the mature woman loses her identity as a *woman*, and she doesn't quite know what to do about it. Much of society is still forcing the mature women into a negative, limited role. Instead of passing from the role of young person to that of mature person (as men do and, most important, as her husband does), she has had to trade her identity as a woman, an exciting female woman, for the neuter image of that slightly ridiculous non-person, the Middle-Aged Matron. Unless she's aware of this threat to her sexual identity, little by little she gives up.

What are the symptoms of this "giving up?" I see them every day, in the attitudes of students who come to me for help. As you might expect, depression is one of the first symptoms. Many of the so-called unexplainable depressions of the menopause can be traced to this apparent loss of sexual identity.

Uncertainty about her role as a mature woman is also reflected in unfeminine dress. She feels as feminine as ever, but she thinks, "At my age, I don't want to make a fool of myself." Her tailored suit, classic shoes, and short, serviceable hair style all proclaim, "I'm a sensible, settled matron, through with sex, the chase, and all that nonsense."

This growing uncertainty as to her role is revealed, inevitably, in her body. Fatigue and a general run-down condition go hand in hand with inactivity and overweight. And we all know what *that* does to our morale. Convinced that she is no longer a desirable woman, our unhappy and unwilling heroine begins to express this neuter personality in her body language. Every movement telegraphs the message that she is no longer *woman*. Eventually, her negative attitude about herself is reflected in the attitude that others have toward her, creating a self-defeating vicious circle.

Well, is there an answer to her problems? Yes, yes, YES! She has another identity choice. She can decide to become . . .

3. *The Ageless Woman.* She is, quite literally, Ageless. Neither old nor young, she is her vital self. She has learned to shift her consciousness from the passing of time to the realization that time is a concept, not a reality. You won't catch *her* saying, "None of us are getting any younger, are we?" She knows better. Snapshots taken of her ten years ago prove that she looks better now than she ever did. And she feels better, too. Why? Because she has embraced all the new knowledge that makes her agelessness possible: exercise, diet, vitamins, hormones—all have a place in her dynamic life style.

She is especially aware of the growing body of knowledge about the power of mind over matter; she has adopted certain attitudes that create agelessness and rejected those that make age a reality. She has learned from both scientists and seers that bodily changes can actually be prevented or postponed by our mental attitudes. (What are these attitudes? We'll be discussing them in this book.) She also knows that scientific advances make her years younger than any mature woman in the history of the world. She is conscious of her unique position and her importance as an example to those younger women who will follow her Ageless image.

And so, because she has knowledge, she has *confidence*, a confidence that is expressed in many ways. Foremost among these is her refusal to accept society's outmoded attitudes about mature women. She knows that she stops being a woman when she stops thinking of herself as a woman, and so she expresses her femininity in a thousand subtle ways. The way she dresses, the way she moves, the way she feels, all reinforce her identity as the Ageless Woman. And we'll be learning, in detail, just how she does it!

MEET THE AGELESS WOMAN

We all know the famous ones, those legendary creatures whose fabulous faces grace the pages of the fashion magazines and Sunday supplements. But let me introduce you to some friends of mine who are real women, with real lives, who have decided to become Ageless Women.

First, there's Carol. When she first enrolled in my classes several years ago she was a rather doughy matron with a ho-hum job, a ho-hum marriage, and the prospect of an empty future when the youngest of her five children left for college. Today she is a beautiful blonde with the figure of a teen-ager and a glamorous part-time career as a model and fashion co-ordinator. Yes, she's still married to the husband, who's fallen in love with her all over again. Not only is she a stunning woman he can be proud of ("Makes Him Feel Younger Just to Look at You") but her enthusiasm and unlimited outlook have changed his life too.

Then there's another student, Liz. Within a year she progressed from an Unwilling M.A.M. to an Ageless Woman. This fabulous grandmother has a sound reason for pursuing the Ageless image. "After all," she says, "my youngest daughter, Tracy, is just ten. I have to minimize the generation gap in every way possible." And she does. She and Tracy swim eighteen laps a day, winter and summer. They ride, and Liz is completing her second year of ice-skating lessons, an interest that Tracy doesn't share. But Liz sees no reason why a grandmother shouldn't be out on the ice, perfecting those figure eights, maintaining her perfect size ten, and feeling a bit smug about showing off her brief skating costumes.

Laura is one of my oldest and dearest friends. Frankly, I never thought she'd become an Ageless Woman, although she was completely familiar with my work. Because of her delightful flair for words, I had often called on her in emergencies to help script fashion shows, and I had used her as a sounding board for new lecture ideas.

However, she remained the total matron, immersed in her home-making—cooking, sewing, knitting, and gardening. She lamented the change from a size fourteen to a size sixteen, but I can remember her saying, "Oh well, face it. Something happens to a woman's figure when she passes forty. I'm not going to kill myself dieting. Anyway, Ed likes me just the way I am."

Everyone was shocked when that twenty-five-year marriage suddenly fell apart—Laura most of all. I didn't see her for two years, but she wrote frequently. I was worried by letters describing her grim financial predicament. She had to go back to work—a middle-aged woman without recent working experience. Descriptions of her desperate search for a job read like a Russian novel. Unlike Russian novels, this story has a happy ending.

Recently I met Laura for lunch, partly to catch up on our friendship, partly to celebrate her recent promotion to ad executive in one of Los Angeles' leading agencies. The woman who greeted me in the restaurant simply bowled me over. I couldn't believe it was Laura. She had lost thirty pounds at least, and her new hair style and make-up reflected the latest trends. But it wasn't fashion alone that turned her into a beautiful woman. Her confident stride, the way she carried herself, and most of all her vital facial expression all combined to make her a fascinating woman—a fact that wasn't lost on the men lunching nearby. We talked of her career, her new apartment, and (at great length) about the new man in her life. Here was the perfect example of a mature woman who refused to take the back seat that society has saved for the woman of "a certain age."

She had learned slowly and painfully, but she had learned well.

HOW DO THEY DO IT?

Carol, Liz, and Laura had several things in common: they had knowledge, determination, and a genuine desire to beat the middle-aged blahs and become Ageless Women. And they were open-minded. They were willing to try new ways of looking, new ways of acting, new ways of thinking about themselves and the world around them. Finally, they had the wisdom to start on first things first.

And what comes first in winning the age game? Updating your physical appearance comes first, and that's the way this book is organized. The first chapters deal with the outer you because, "when you look ageless, you *feel* ageless." The Ageless Woman understands the psychological importance of living in and reflecting the current picture—the contemporary fashion scene. She knows that, when you look *great* and know it, you feel great and show it; and somehow when your morale zooms, other, more serious problems become manageable.

The Ageless Woman vehemently rejects the puritanical concept that fashion and beauty are frivolous and, somehow, even sinful. She knows that psychiatrists' notebooks are filled with examples of the beneficial effects of improved physical appearance on the depressed and insecure.

She also rejects the smug statements of the very young that make-up and hair styling are artificial, because she knows that twenty years from now these young girls will be mature women and will have learned better. Or, instead, they may still be smugly looking "natural" but wondering, secretly, why the world (and perhaps their man) seems to have passed them by.

The Ageless Woman also rejects the puritanical concept that the body is sinful, a thing to keep covered and fed, but to be thought about as little as possible. She respects her body. She diets to keep it healthy and slim. She exercises to build up a buoyant excess of strength and energy. She knows that her care of her body will determine what kind of mature woman she will be. She knows that she can choose to be a healthy, vigorous woman who literally climbs mountains if that pleases her: she refuses to give up, as so many women do, and spend her mature years trapped in a prison of weak and flabby flesh.

So this book will describe the unique diet and exercise programs that can rapidly change you from middle-aged to ageless, and it will describe the body language that gets this message across to your public. Further, it will tell you how the healthy, well-nourished, well-adjusted Ageless Woman can sail easily and painlessly through those needlessly dreaded years of menopause.

And then there are the mental attitudes that characterize that fascinating creature, the Ageless Woman. Much of the book will deal with winning attitudes: what they are, how to develop them, what they can do for you . . . and for your relationship with the man in your life.

But before we begin our first winning move in the age game—updating the outer *you*—what about some winning attitudes to start you on your way? What about . . .

1. *Courage.* You've taken the most important step toward becoming the Ageless Woman when you decide that you have the *courage* to be bigger than the opinion of your next-door neighbor or the outmoded opinion of society in general. The Ageless Woman has the courage to turn her back on yesterday. She's the woman of today.

2. *Knowledge.* You've taken another important step toward your goal when you know the truth about your age. You *aren't* getting older. Science tells us that you're actually younger than your chronological years. But your potential goes far beyond the goal of simply being younger. You're getting *better*, because, as the Ageless Woman, you can take the best of both worlds—maturity and youth. Therefore, your potential is unlimited. *Agelessness is maturity without limitations.* Use this knowledge to take a mental accounting.

Analyze your attitudes toward yourself as a woman. Have you allowed negative attitudes to develop? Have you become accustomed to thinking of yourself in limited terms? Oh, oh. That's bad! Instead, consciously start building a positive attitude about yourself and your life. The material in this book will give you knowledge to build on. Your future *is* unlimited. Claim it.

3. *Watch your language.* Never use such negative M.A.M. words and phrases as, "I'm not as young as I used to be"; "None of us is getting any younger"; "At *my* age—"; "When I was a girl—" The spoken word has a powerful effect on the subconscious. In her book, *The Dynamic Laws of Healing,* Catherine Ponder says, "When a word is spoken, a chemical change takes place in the body. Because of this, the body may be renewed, even transformed, through the spoken word." And of course the reverse is true. So build yourself up. There are others who will try to tear you down. Why help them? Which brings me to the next point.

4. *Take an inventory.* Look at the middle-aged women in your circle. See if you can recognize the Professional M.A.M.s and the Unwilling M.A.M.s. Is there an Ageless Woman in your group? Can you spot the attitudes that make her so special?

When you have pinpointed the Professional M.A.M.s in your life —and, baby, they'll be there—carefully analyze what they do to make you feel uncomfortable. Chances are, you have become so accustomed to their needles that you don't recognize them for what they are. You just know that you hurt. Now that you understand the situation, repress that urge to *kill.* Just learn to recognize those needles. They will become totally ineffective as knowledge creates self-confidence.

5. *Action.* You've taken perhaps the most important step toward becoming the Ageless Woman when you put into action the guidelines that follow. Did I say action? Come on. Let's get started.

TWO

Fashion: Friend or Foe?

Many women seem to feel that fashion is out to get them.

"They'll never get *me* into those new longer . . . or shorter . . . or narrower styles."

"Thank heaven, I've found my own 'look,' so I just ignore the crazy new things 'they' come up with."

"Fashion? Everyone knows it's dominated by a group of people who hate women and just want to make us look ridiculous."

These are just a few of the negative comments you'll hear if you eavesdrop a bit at that next fashion show luncheon you attend. And if you look closely at the women making these comments, I'm sure you'll agree with my observation: *the more completely a woman has succumbed to middle age, the more belligerent she becomes toward fashion.*

Our friend, the Professional M.A.M., is a walking example of this negative attitude. As she joins the "girls" at the next table, we can get a close look at what she's wearing.

It's her favorite style, almost a uniform by now. A jacket dress with three-quarter sleeves because "a woman of my age shouldn't show her elbows" and a hemline that stubbornly fights the current trends (it's either too short or too long) because, "I don't care what the designers say, the new hemlines are ugly."

This particular outfit is in her favorite shade of muted soldier blue, a color that hasn't been in style since the Civil War. However, our Professional M.A.M. shops doggedly until she finds her "uniform." It isn't easy. She has trouble shopping for everything: clothes, shoes, handbags, accessories. "They" keep changing things, you see, just to annoy her. She has to hunt and hunt to find the out-of-fashion things she's used to, a sure sign of creeping M.A.M.-ism. The Ageless Woman simply walks into a store and asks, "What's new?"

Getting back to M.A.M., the "Best-Dressed Woman of 1955," she completes this wildly becoming costume with the addition of a cameo pin and—What's that she's wearing on her head? Good Lord! It's one of those horrid little net thingamajigs called a whimsey. (About as whimsical as Saturday night at the Old Folks' Home.)

Our matron is only forty-four years *young*—but in this outfit she could fool anyone into thinking that she's many years older. The sad thing is, she's fooled herself too.

That's what happens when the mature woman carries on a running battle with the fashion industry. She can only lose. And it's too bad. Because, if she stopped fighting long enough to look around, she'd see that fashion could be her best friend.

FASHION: IS IT REALLY YOUR WORST ENEMY?

Not at all. New, exciting on-the-spot fashion is the quickest, most effective way to change your image, and with a minimum of effort on your part. Diets take weeks, new hair styles take hours, but you can change your dress in a minute. What's more, "The way you dress— or package yourself—is the one thing over which you have absolute control." That's the expert observation of Academy Award-winning designer Edith Head, in her book, *Dressing for Success*. She goes on to say, "What you wear, more than any other factor, can improve the type you are or *change your type* completely."

That's why our first winning move in the age game is designed to show you how you can change from age to ageless by putting yourself into today's fashion picture.

There are three reasons why wearing current fashion is important in winning the age game.

    1. Looking current keeps you looking young and *feeling* ageless.

    2. Fashionable clothes tell the world you're not living in the past.

    3. Wearing today's fashions has a stimulating effect, forcing you to look at yourself and the world around you with new awareness.

Sounds great, doesn't it? But what if you don't feel comfortable in the latest styles? What if you're unsure of what's appropriate for you now that you've passed that forties milestone? If this describes your feelings, you can do one of two things. You can give up or you can fight back.

If you decide to fight back, knowledge is your weapon. You *can* wear the latest styles with confidence. It's all a matter of understanding fashion and how it works. Mainbocher, one of America's greatest designers, put it this way: "A woman can wear anything with authority, if she understands it."

UNDERSTANDING: THE BASIS OF MAKING FASHION WORK FOR YOU

Maybe women get emotional about the changing face of fashion because they just don't understand the situation. If they realized that the fashion world operates on two levels, perhaps it wouldn't be such an enigma to them.

On one level, admittedly, fashion is motivated by profit. How the fashion czars manipulate you and your image to get to your pocketbook is something we'll discuss later in detail. But first, let's look at the other level of fashion . . . the level that is so significant to you.

True fashion is not shallow, meaningless, arbitrary. On the contrary, it is the visual essence of any civilization. Anatole France once said that if one really wants to understand a civilization he should study its fashions rather than its statesmen. Since fashion reflects the society you live in, it's essential that you use fashion to make you part of your society, part of today. I must emphasize that I am not urging you to leap aboard every fad bandwagon that comes along— chandelier earrings tinkling in time to the "clump-clump" of your one-inch platform shoes. That's not the idea at all. Fad must be used carefully, as we will discuss later in detail. True fashion, together with its brash relative fad, can be used creatively and selectively to express your personality. But if you completely ignore fashion's dictums you'll appear to be an inflexible bystander, a relic of yesteryear, watching the parade go by.

How does fashion become the mirror that reflects our civilization? It all starts with the mysterious creatures commonly called "they." As in, "Why are 'they' making skirts longer?" "Why are 'they' bringing back the padded shoulder?" And so forth.

"WHO ARE 'THEY' AND WHY ARE 'THEY' DOING THOSE TERRIBLE THINGS TO MY HEMLINE?"

"They" are the gifted designers in Paris, London, Rome, and New York who have the ability to tune in on the mass subconscious of our society. They are doing those terrible things to your hemline as one way to express the hopes, fears, sex lives, and even financial climate of our era.

Does this sound as if I'm overstating the case? Not according to James Laver, the eminent British fashion historian. This authority on fashion's social and psychological implications says that fashion is never arbitrary and meaningless. Rather, it reflects each era in some fascinating ways.

For example, there is a relationship between headdress and architecture. The dome of the mosque repeats the rounded shape of Moslem turbans. Soaring Gothic cathedrals were reflected in the exaggerated, pointed headdress worn by medieval ladies. Throughout modern history there has been a relationship between dress length and the health of the economy. The most famous instance occurred in the twenties. Where were hems in 1929? Up. And where were they in 1932? Down. You *know* what was happening to the economy.

Even industrial developments have their effect on fashion. The steel hoop of the mid-nineteenth century could be termed a triumph of the machine age. What's more, it symbolized a society in which the male was dominant and the female totally helpless. And who can deny the comment of another fashion historian that, "next to the Pill, pantyhose are the greatest contribution to women's liberation?" Remember girdles? You've come a long way, baby.

And, speaking of women's lib, how long has it been since you've worn a hat? Years, probably. Hats have long been out of style in this country because they are a symbol of male domination. We do see purely functional hats—sun hats, rain hats, fur hoods—but the truly feminine "hatty" hat (complete with veils, flowers, and/or fruit) is a thing of the past. Yet, on a recent trip to England I noticed that many women still wear hats. What's more, the larger cities that we visited had thriving millinery shops—a real anachronism to American eyes. I also noted that, except for a few swinging types in London (hatless, by the way) the Englishwoman's role seems more submissive than ours.

So you can see that fashion is much more than a superficial exercise in planned obsolescence. It is rather the designers' reaction to the subconscious needs and desires working within the society.

However, to become the Ageless Woman, you don't need to psychoanalyze the latest fashions. Instead, you simply study current fashion trends and make fashion an expressive part of your life.

FASHION TRENDS AND HOW TO SPOT THEM

Women become irritated with fashion's seemingly erratic changes because they aren't paying attention. These changes are never arbitrary and they're never sudden. They occur slowly, subtly, and predictably. If you're aware of the basic elements that reflect fashion's changes, you'll always have time to adjust your wardrobe without any traumatic shocks to your eye or pocketbook.

Basic fashion trends are always concerned with proportion. Everyone is aware of skirt lengths, for instance. But changing the length of a skirt is only a small part of a fashion trend. Equally important factors can be:

1. The width of the shoulder—natural or exaggerated
2. The placement of the belt—high, low, or at the natural waistline
3. The shape of the silhouette—flared, straight, voluminous, or body-hugging
4. Sleeve shape and armhole fit

All are proportions that indicate fashion trends. In turn, these proportions add up to a mood: elegant and formal in the fifties, iconoclastic and radical in the sixties, casual and dégagé in the seventies.

That's why merely shortening that ten-year-old cashmere coat doesn't put it back in fashion. Chances are the proportion of shoulder, sleeve shape, and even silhouette are hopelessly out of style and clash with the current mood of fashion.

You don't have to be a dedicated clothes horse to follow the trends. Just read two magazines a year. Trends of the coming season are discussed in the early spring and late summer issues of *Vogue* and *Harper's Bazaar*. Their editorial pages will spell it out for you. But you won't get the message unless you *read* those editorials. No fair just looking at the pictures and poking fun at the kooky models. Enjoy the elaborate put-ons (toss this sable jacket over your jeans and T-shirt . . .) or take-offs (. . . for a totally casual effect, wear your shirt dress unbuttoned to the navel . . .) for the fun spoofs that they are. But while you're laughing, look for gems like these:

"First, let's talk about the new skirt. It is as sleek and as straight as a pair of . . . trousers. It is often pleated to give movement and sometimes, it is in very lightweight fabrics, slightly flared."

"Now, let's get down to the silhouettes. The first is the seven-eighths coat, cardigan, or sweater. . . . The second silhouette we'd like you to know about is a bulky outsize one that gives a new soft width across the shoulders. . . . It gets its width easily with raglan and caftan sleeves, and dropped shoulder lines."

"*The New Breeze in Fashion*—proportioning is the key—*balance*—both in the cutting of clothes and how they're worn. It means that when you see a coat with more roominess on the shoulder, it will have more length on the body as well; and that with this scale of coat, you will find yourself wanting—you will find your eye wanting: a skirt that's a little longer than last year's (2 to 3 inches below the knee) and full enough to swing but not to bulk . . . a shoe with a higher heel . . ."

Now, if you study these editorials carefully, you won't get stung the next time you're trying to decide between two fashions that are equally appealing to you. You will always choose the coming style in preference to one that's on its way out. For instance, if you had been shopping for a coat back in 1973, you'd have learned that the bulky one with raglan sleeves and a dropped shoulder line was a better buy than the fitted princess style. According to the fashion trends for 1973, the fitted coat was already a bit out of fashion. The loosely fitted, wide-shouldered coat was part of a new trend, and since basic trends change slowly, it would be fashionable for years.

IT'S STRICTLY BUSINESS

If one aspect of the fashion industry is concerned with reflecting the world we live in, the other is just what you've suspected all along —a high-powered business whose sole business is to *sell.* And the fashion czars do this by creating fads. "Pastels for fall" means that you are supposed to rush out breathlessly and buy a lot of new clothes, because last autumn "the tawny shades" were the thing.

Fads can be "in" colors, a certain shoe style (clogs, for example, or the exaggerated platform style), costume jewelry (bangle bracelets in bright colors or exotic materials, American Indian themes in mock silver and turquoise).

Even a specific dress can be a fad. The tennis syndrome is a good case in point. A few seasons ago there were red and blue tennis stripes on everything from pajamas to evening dress. But the next season the tennis look was out and the shirt dress was in. Sad news for the woman who spent $150 on a white crepe "tennis" dress for evening wear.

How do you spot a fad? It's easy. Put on your walking shoes and visit four or five stores. The fad items are the ones that are featured in every store. Magnin's, Macy's, Penney's, and Lerner's . . . they'll all have their version of the tennis look. Magazines and newspaper ads will also help you pinpoint the current fads. Here's an example from Vogue: ". . . with a little cotton lisle T-shirt for example, you can stripe your arm with bangles of green, purple, red, orange, yellow, black—all the same width—click-clacking up to the elbow. Next year, who knows?—right now, it sounds wonderful."

Since fads are strictly business, doesn't the smart money ignore them? No, because in spite of their mercenary background fads have a certain charm. They're fun, amusing, and ageless. Vogue says, "Don't forget that fad has a place in fashion; it has wit and it gives pleasure." What's more, if fashion gives you the look of today, fads make you look "right this minute."

If you ignore fads completely, you'll have less fun and run more risk of looking matronly. At best you'll create the look that I call "Behind every Successful Man there's a 'Tasteful' Woman" or "My dear, we've had scads of money for generations. . . ." Many mature women affect this totally classic and conservative way of dressing. You know, the understated little suit or dress, the heirloom jewelry, the elegant tailored pump, and the unobtrusive handbag. Although this look does spell "old money," it spells "old lady," too.

Selena "PooPoo" Radcliffe is an example of this fashion approach. She attended my classes in Pasadena for seventeen weeks, yet I never saw her wear anything but a gray flannel suit and a matching cashmere sweater. Her most daring accessories were a discreet string of beautifully matched pearls ("Mumsy gave them to me on my twenty-first birthday") and her sorority pin. Her hair style was a holdover from college days too. She wore her now graying locks in a short pageboy, parted on the side and held in place with a girlish barrette—solid gold, of course, but who could care? Certainly not Mr. Radcliffe, who hadn't really looked at "PooPoo" for years. By the way, his private secretary displays a vulgarly fashionable armload of solid gold bangle bracelets as she slips into her faddish fox polo coat.

Poor Selena, so smug and inflexible. It doesn't pay to say "PooPoo" to the changing scene. *Everything* changes—as she found out.

So let's not complain about the changeability of fads, which are only a bad choice when women mistake them for fashion. Instead, let's see how to use them to accent your ageless look . . . and to save money, too. (Aha, Mr. Fashion Czar. Gotcha!)

HOW YOU CAN USE FADS FOR FUN AND PROFIT

Should you add The Look, that is, the current fad outfit, to your wardrobe? That depends on how startling it is and how daring you are. Going back to that tennis dress fad, a white crepe dinner dress with tennis stripes of red and blue bugle beads was never startling. After all, a tennis dress never scared anyone except Bobby Riggs. But suppose the current fad is a total gypsy rig complete with beads and feathers? That takes guts. And in all the right places.

However, it isn't necessary to submerge yourself in the total look, that is, the fad dress, coat, shoes, bag, and jewelry. A more economical approach is to use short-lived fashion accessories to accent the enduring fashion items in your wardrobe. Although specific fad accessories change from season to season, you can choose from these basic elements: costume jewelry, scarves, separates, shoes and bags, color, fabric, and fabric treatment.

Specialty shops can be another guide to the fashion trends. Because they are small, they specialize, rather than try to be all things to all people (as the department stores do). They try to develop their own fashion philosophy in relation to the current trends and offer only those fashion items and fad looks that express the philosophy of their store.

This eclectic approach just proves that following fashion doesn't mean that women have to be like so many docile sheep. You can choose from the various elements that contribute to current fad and fashion, and create your own look. And often a good specialty shop can help you do just that. So go in. Browse. Look and listen. The salespeople in a really good specialty shop can be top-notch teachers.

Another source of information are the display artists of local stores. When you're out window-shopping, train your eye to be aware of the placement of a pin, the combination of colors and textures in a flow of necklaces, how separates are combined in new and unusual ways.

As long as you're window-shopping, go to the very best stores and see how they put together a look when price is no object. But suppose that price is a consideration? That's when knowing how to play the fad game can stretch your fashion dollar.

My friend Kate is an expert player. She has to be. She's public relations director for an elegant shopping mall in a San Francisco suburb. Her job means that she's representing one of the most fashionable shopping centers in the West. And she looks it. Every five feet five inches of her. Walking up and down that mall twenty times a day helps to keep her a trim size ten. And weekend bicycle riding gives her complexion a vital glow. The total impression is one of energy and health, saved from looking too bucolic by her aristocratic nose and high cheekbones. The duchess effect is heightened by blonde hair ("I just have it touched up once a month, now that I'm getting so gray") which she wears shoulder length, pulled back and tied with a ribbon. The style that *Women's Wear Daily* calls the "Status Pull."

Kate is such a picture of blonde perfection, always dressed at the peak of fashion, you'd never know that she does it on a shoestring. Her salary has to stretch to help a daughter in a special school for retarded children and a husband who's recovering from a heart attack. Yet, to look at her, you'd think she hadn't a care in the world.

HOW KATE PLAYS THE FAD GAME . . .

1. Kate buys the most expensive *fashion* she can afford. Why? Because true fashion changes slowly and predictably. A well-designed coat, for instance, should be fashion-right for at least four years. Well-tailored slacks, a cashmere sweater, an expensive and beautifully made handbag, all are good fashion investments. There's an added bonus. Expensive, well-made fashion has as much status old as new. Gloria Guinness, who has been called the world's most elegant woman, says that she never wears clothes that are obviously "new."

2. Kate buys inexpensive *fads*. During their short fashion life, fads are copied by many stores on all price levels. The most exclusive stores are first with the current fads, then the medium-priced stores pick them up, and finally those on the bottom of the fashion totem pole climb on the bandwagon. However, these myriad versions of one theme often have no obvious difference in quality. Kate says, "Since I don't care if fad items are made to last, why pay more for quality I can't see?"

3. Kate spends time, not money, and is a compulsive comparison shopper. This is how she shops for the total fad look. Suppose that "the" dress for this season is the "Gigi" dress, a two-piece charmer with a navy-blue pleated skirt, white top, and sailor collar. I. Magnin showed their version first for $79.95. Now Macy's has it for $45. Penney's sells theirs for $29.95. Lerner's has it for $15. Often, the $29 version looks *almost* as good as the one for $79. Kate knows that she'll see the dress coming and going anyway, and since she's not buying anything exclusive, why pay more?

4. Kate shops the sales of the most exclusive stores. The best stores have a high-fashion image to maintain. They can't afford to have a fad item in their store a moment after it's lost its first bloom. While the jet set may have tired of the Gigi dress early in the season (or even last season, since they're always a couple

of jumps ahead of everyone else), it still has a lot of fashion mileage. This is where it pays to be aware of current fads. Kate often buys a high-quality fad dress at the height of its popularity, and at less than half price.

No matter what the price, clothes are just clothes . . . until you put them together to create a look. This is how Kate combines fashion and fad, expensive and inexpensive, to create a whole new outfit.

MORE ON THE PROFIT MOTIF

Let's go back to the season when the tennis look was the current fad. This was Kate's recipe for mixing fad and fashion.

She started with these currently fashionable items from her wardrobe:

1. Navy-blue pants from a three-year-old I. Magnin pant suit ($69.95).

2. A navy-blue calf shoulder bag. She's had it so long she doesn't remember *where* she bought it, but it's the best quality —and looks it.

3. White calf sandals with a single wide strap across the instep (therefore, not too delicate to wear with pants), a slight platform sole, and a heavy wooden heel. These are a holdover from the previous summer ($25.00 at the local bootery).

She added these fad items;

1. A tennis sweater set in polyester knit from Sears ($12.95).

2. Two chunky white plastic bracelets from the dime store ($.69 each).

Kate has the confidence to mix old and new, expensive and inexpensive, because she understands the underlying principles of fashion (proportion) and fad (accent). This frees her from what I call "the Tyranny of the Label."

To be even more specific, the proportion of the slacks was still in the current trend; that is, cut wide, fairly straight, and long enough to almost cover her shoes. A tapered, ankle-length slack would have been the wrong proportion, even if the color would co-ordinate. Again, with an eye to proportion, she chose the platform sandals to offset the extra-long cut of the slacks. The inexpensive sweater set was *almost* identical to Magnin's $45 version. True, theirs was softer and made of *virgin* wool, but, as Kate said, "For a difference of $35, I should care what the lambs were doing."

WHEN IT'S A MISTAKE TO FOLLOW FASHION

The mature woman must also realize that, though fashion is almost always her best friend, there are times when it can become her worst enemy. Sometimes the current fashion mood is all wrong for her.

Nostalgic styles are one example. Recently the designers have been looking backward . . . to the fashions of the thirties, forties, and fifties. Should you take this trip down Memory Lane? Not if you've already been there. If you were old enough to wear the original fashions of the forties, you'll look like a female Rip Van Winkle in a rerun of ankle-strap shoes, deep red nails and lipstick, or crepe dresses with peplums and sweetheart necklines. *You should avoid fads and fashions that are a literal translation of clothes from your youth.*

Instead, choose a very subtle adaptation of styles from your past. For example, Halston, who dresses Jackie Onassis and other Beautiful People, recently revived that appealing style of the 1940s, the sweater set. If Halston had shown the classic cardigan and pullover in its original setting, with a string of pearls and a straight long skirt, it would have been a disaster for the mature woman. But Halston added his own timely flair. The classic pullover was paired with a swinging knee-length pleated skirt. The cardigan part of the sweater set was tied casually around the shoulders. It was a look inspired by the past, but with a totally current viewpoint, making it an excellent choice for the Ageless Woman.

"YES, BUT . . . I'M STILL WORRIED ABOUT WEARING FASHIONS THAT MAY BE TOO YOUNG FOR ME. BESIDES NOSTALGIC FASHIONS, WHAT OTHER STYLES MAY BE TOO YOUNG FOR THE GROWN WOMAN?"

According to that same designer, Halston, "There are no older women in America today." (What have I been *telling* you?) "Women are all young in mind, young in spirit; they can wear any kind of clothes." While this is basically true, there are a few no-no's that you should be aware of.

Avoid anything girlish. That is, pinafores, Peter Pan collars, dainty little blouses with ruffles or lace edging, ruffles in general unless big-girl ruffles (that means dramatic and sexy), puffed sleeves, little-girl shoes like Mary Janes or those baby sandals we used to wear to the beach.

Avoid fabrics such as dotted swiss, organdy, gingham. Also to be shunned are pastel colors: pale pink, pale green, pale yellow. Pastels are too blah. They are for the very young—or the very old.

I think peasant things come into this category too. You know, dirndl skirts, laced bodices, kerchiefs, the Lanz look. Playing Heidi is for *young* girls. The mature woman is apt to look like a stolid hausfrau. Gypsies? That's a different story. A gypsy is the essence of woman, worldly and mysterious, no matter what her age.

Oddly enough, clothes with a little-boy look are marvelous on a mature woman. They seem to accent her femininity, where little-girl looks accent her age. The distinction here is that it must be a *little-boy* style. Anything too masculine is definitely out. Some good examples are knickers, Lord Fauntleroy suits in velvet or flannel—add a lace-trimmed shirt and a bow at the neck . . . terrific! A tailored jacket, long shorts, and knee socks, like a little boy's first suit, can be charming, but naturally for the petite woman only; the Dandy Look—velvet vest accented with a heavy gold watch chain, satin shirt, and tartan pants—is another charmer.

TOO OLD FOR YOU?

I've described fashions that are too young for the mature woman, but a much more important consideration is this: "Is it too old for me?" An overwhelming majority of mature women wear clothes that make them look older than their years—clothes that accent the negative rather than the positive, clothes whose style, color, and over-all mood create a matronly, settled, and stodgy look. Take Diane, for example, a student of mine who looked years older than she should have, simply because of her choice in clothes.

She was thirty-eight when I first knew her and had a pixy face, slightly tilted green eyes, and luxuriant auburn hair. With her wow figure and impish personality she should have been a stunning woman, but her appeal was overshadowed by her matronly clothes. Perhaps her taste was excessively conservative because she made all her own clothes. She sewed beautifully, always using the most expensive fabrics, and I suppose that cutting into a piece of wool that cost $35 a yard could make anyone conservative. However, the colors and patterns that she chose were also strictly English governess, which is what I told her when we got together after one class. Since Diane was recently divorced and trying to rebuild her social life at this time, the image of an English governess was the last thing she wanted to project. I made a list for her of all the styles, fabrics, colors, and accessories that I call "Sure Losers in the Age Game." She was appalled when she realized that she used them all. I also gave her a list of "Winners," and with the help of my guidelines, she began to study fashion from the viewpoint of the Ageless Woman. And did she learn?

Well, I saw her recently, and she looked terrific. Her clothes created a vital, exciting image. She was wearing a copper-toned jersey dress and matching plaid cape, an outfit that dramatized her red hair. She had accented this costume with the ultimate ageless accessory—a good-looking man. When she introduced us, I discovered that he was not only her new husband but also the owner of a chain of fabric stores. (Now that's what I call planning.)

Diane is still an ardent "home sewer," and she's still using the most expensive fabrics. But now she gets them wholesale. All the signs point to a long and compatible relationship.

Here is the list I gave Diane:

WINNERS (YOUNG LOOKS)	LOSERS (OLD LOOKS)
JEWELRY	JEWELRY
Pearls—lots and lots	Pearls—one graduated strand
Gold or silver chains	Chokers or dog-collars
Jet, Rhinestones, Crystal } in dramatic contemporary setting	Jet, Rhinestones, Crystal } in conventional setting
Geometric pins	Poodle pins
Maltese crosses	Owl pins
Enamel wear	Pins and earrings in curved leafy shapes
Ivory	Matched sets . . . earrings, pins, necklaces all part of a set
Tortoise shell	
Amber	Dainty, ladylike antique jewelry, cameos
Large, bold antique jewelry	
Turquoise	

WINNERS (YOUNG LOOKS)	LOSERS (OLD LOOKS)
JEWELRY	**JEWELRY**
Coral	Ivory roses
Jade	Real leaves, dipped in gold
Brass buttons	Jeweled buttons
Eyeglasses—like lamps and TV sets, the uglier the better. *Functional*.	*Eyeglasses*
	Discreet blue or lavender plastic frames
"Aunt Polly" nose-perchers for reading	Jeweled frames
Super-studious tortoise-shell frames	Wild harlequin shapes in plaid, leopard print, etc.
Benjamin Franklin steel frames . . . (Look at what the young people are wearing)	Frames that are 10 or 15 years old. Keep them up-to-date.
COLORS	**COLORS**
Bright, definite colors	Muted, drab colors
Fad colors	Classic, conservative colors, without accent
Black (see color combinations)	Black (see color combinations)
White	That damned soldier blue
Beige	Royal blue
Camel	Wine and burgundy shades
Navy blue	Pale pink ⎫ Pastels are for
Bright red	Pale blue ⎬ the very young or
Yellow	Pale yellow ⎭ very old
Orange	Purple
Coral	
Bright green	
Turquoise	
Shocking pink	
Color Combinations	*Color Combinations*
Black and white	Black with any pastel
Brown and white	Brown with soft green
Navy blue and white	Navy blue with pale pink
Black and white plus bright yellow or red	Navy blue with pale blue
	Beige and white
Navy blue and white plus yellow or red or parrot green	Camel and brown
Lavender or lilac and turquoise and shocking pink	Camel and gray
Camel and black	Beige and brown
Beige and black	

More:

WINNERS (AGELESS)
Chanel suits in bright colors with
  pleated skirts

Pant suits with current jacket
Tailored shirt dresses in bright or
  dramatic colors, unexpected
  fabrics
Jumpers

Separates

Long sleeves, full
Long sleeves, loose, with cuffs
Short sleeves (see "The All-
  Important Inch")
Shirts: silk, cotton, tailored jersey
  (especially buttoned high with
  pussycat bow under the collar)
Trench coats
Polo coats (wrap and tie)
Sensible coats in bright colors

Capes—plaid, red, yellow
Hair ribbons (yes!), head bands,
  scarves, hoods

FABRICS (YOUNG)
Crepe in beige, white, red, black,
  navy
Denim
Understated evening fabrics
Knits with body
Currently fashionable fabrics if
  not one of those listed opposite
Polyester knits in rich colors—no
  prints (stripes, checks OK)

LOSERS (OLD)
Chanel suits with straight skirts
  in dark, conservative colors . . .
  or beige or gray polyester knit
Pant suits with chanel jacket
Tailored shirt dresses in menswear
  tweeds, dark and drab plaid,
  seersucker, pastel cottons,
  menswear shirting
Jacket dresses, coat dresses
Ladylike suits with fitted
  "dressmaker" jackets
Wrap dresses
Anything with a soft drape
Anything with ¾ sleeves

Blouses (especially with tucks,
  lace embroidery)

The sensible coat with ranch
  mink collar
The sensible camel coat
The sensible black coat
Capes—black, navy, gray (Here
  comes that governess again!)
Hats!

FABRICS (OLD)
Crepe in drab colors—wine, dark
  green, gray
Seersucker
Metallic brocades, lace
Menswear wools (drab, heavy
  tweeds, glen-plaids) These are
  too masculine
Soft, droopy fabrics
Polyester double-knits in weird
  prints (the woods are full of
  'em)

PRINTS

Checks (medium to large)

Houndstooth

Bright plaids—only for the young and slender? Not necessarily. Picture a bright red blanket plaid stole. Zing!

Geometric prints

Dramatic flowers

Abstract prints

PRINTS

Itty-bitty checks ⎫

Pin-stripes   ⎬ too

Glen-plaid,   ⎭ masculine

  shadow plaid

"Cute" prints . . . "I Love You" printed in seven languages

"Sweet" flowers

Dainty, old-fashioned flowers

Small, timid prints

Since my specific list of "Winners" and "Losers" for Diane might not work for all (tastes, appearances, budgets, and fashions do vary), let me offer in addition three general rules to guide you toward that ageless image.

THREE WAYS TO AVOID LOOKING MATRONLY

1. *Avoid the too-timid look.* Add a bit of drama. Any totally classic style (the shirt dress, the Chanel suit) in a conventional color and fabric will look matronly. Especially if deadened by the wrong accessories. For example:

Matronly is a beige polyester knit Chanel suit worn with a beige blouse with tucks and lace, a small gold pin, classic beige pumps, and small handbag.

This costume is so conservative, so *safe,* you'll fade into the wallpaper. (And you don't want to do that, do you?) On the other hand . . .

Ageless is the same beige Chanel suit, worn with a black silk *shirt* (blouses are *old,* no matter what the current fashion or fad). Add a red and beige silk scarf at the neck and several gold chains. Use a large gold pin in a geometric shape for a final accent, and get rid of that itty-bitty gold pin. It's grand-mother stuff.

Finally, the purse and shoes must be a subtle adaptation of the current fad. Classic purses in medium size with double handles are what the fashion trade calls "mama" bags. Con-servative pumps with sensible heels carry the aura of bunions and tired old feet. They've *got* to go. To complete the ageless look, choose shoes and bag with a little pezazz. How about a black patent shoulder bag and black and beige sling pumps?

2. *Accent your femininity.* In every subtle, ladylike way, let your clothes stress that you are a woman. Remember, this is the big hangup of the middle years. "Am I still a woman? Am I still appealing?" See that your clothes proclaim, "I am the Ageless Woman." You can't get this message across if you're wearing severely tailored, figure-concealing styles in dark, drab colors and heavy or rough fabrics. Of course, extremely mannish styles in menswear fabrics will completely submerge your femininity. For example:

Neuter is a gray and brown herringbone tweed coat dress worn without any accent except for a large man's type watch on a heavy leather band. The shoes are brown calf oxfords with heavy heel and sole. (They've been in style, but would be a terrible choice for the mature woman.) The purse is brown leather, totally unadorned, such as might be issued by the Women's Army Corps. Though we haven't mentioned hair styles yet, I must add that this look is usually accompanied by a very short, no-nonsense hair style. The total effect is: "Ve haff wayss of making you talk!"

Remember, a totally classic style in a drab color and masculine fabric is *impossible* for the mature woman. Tailored clothes are fine but should be chosen in bright, vivid colors and worn with dramatic accessories. Let's see how that same coat dress could become more feminine.

Feminine is a red double-knit coat dress worn over a camel and red checked silk shirt. The collar and cuffs of the shirt dress are turned back to show the silk shirt underneath. The large wrist watch has a tortoise-shell plastic band and is accented by two gold chain bracelets. Shoes are wedge-heeled pumps in camel-colored leather, accented with a small gold buckle. With this, a *non-matching* shoulder bag in camel-colored leather with a gold chain shoulder strap. (Doggedly matching all accessories is another approach that creates a matronly, behind-the-times mood.)

3. *Follow the fashion trends.* I can't stress this enough. You must follow the current trend of fashion to become the Ageless Woman.

Although these three points are essential to your new image, there is still another way that your clothes can contribute that Ageless Look.

CHANGING PROPORTIONS CAN CREATE
A YOUNG IMAGE

Sometimes the difference between "young-smashing" and "matronly-dowdy" is just a matter of changing proportions. Everyone knows that certain fool-the eye tricks can create the impression of figure perfection. Maybe you don't know that there are ways to camouflage signs of age, too.

YOUR FIGURE IS ONLY AS YOUNG AS:

Your bustline
Your waistline
Your back
Your buttocks
Your arms
. . . in that order.

YOUR BUSTLINE. THE ALL-IMPORTANT INCH

I'm not talking about inches *around* for a change, but inches up and down. The high point of a youthful bust is midway between the shoulder and the elbow. If your bustline is an inch or more below this mid-point, you'll look dumpy. If it's higher than the mid-point, be sure it's no more than an inch higher, or you'll look like a pouter pigeon. In addition to a good bra, there are several design elements that will visually lift the bust.

1. *Yokes*—the placement of a yoke can either lift or lower the bustline. The yoke should begin at the armhole, or higher.
2. *Sleeve endings*—short sleeves should end at the high point of the bust—or higher, for a real lift. Sleeves that end below the mid-point create a sagging look.
3. *Pockets*—the placement of pockets not only affects the up-and-down proportion of the bust (high pockets-high bust, low pockets-sagging bust) but also the width of the chest. Pockets

placed far from the center of the body will create the impression of a broad chest and perhps make you look heavy. Pockets too close to the center create a narrow effect and may accent wide hips. Pockets placed below the bust in the midriff area (a style that has been popular recently) are very unflattering. They create both width and bulkiness in the midriff.

4. *Darts*—as you know, darts should end at the high point of the bust. Be sure that the darts on your clothes do not end *above* your high point. The high dart will make your bust appear to sag by contrast. Darts that come from the waist *up*, rather than from the armhole *down*, will create a more lifted effect. Darts coming from the waist up to the bustline should start directly under the center of the bust or toward the center of the body. If waistline darts are placed closer to the side seams, rather than directly under the center of the bust, they will create the illusion of width in the midriff area and accent a "spare tire." The closer these darts are placed to the center front, the more slenderizing they become. The most flattering dart for the mature figure is the French dart, the one that starts from the side seam, near the waist, and angles up to the high point of the bust.

5. *Accessories*—be sure that pins, flowers, or bows are not positioned below the highest point of the bust. Necklaces and pendants should be short enough to end at the high point of the bust.

YOUR WAISTLINE. THE LONG AND THE SHORT OF IT

Many women haven't any idea whether they are long- or short-waisted, yet awareness of this proportion can help you create a more pleasing silhouette. One way to find out is to *look*. Wearing a leotard or matching slacks and top in a dark color, stand in front of a full-length mirror. You'll need three pieces of string. Tie one directly under the arms, one around the base of the hips (just where the thigh starts), and one around your true waistline. The ideal proportion is for the waist to be halfway between the underarm string and the one at the base of the hips. Ignore a slight variation. (After all, nobody's perfect.) However, as you can see, an extreme imbalance affects the whole visual impression you make.

Being short-waisted is probably the most matronly of the two extremes, because short-waisted figures can look very dumpy if clothes are not chosen with care. Women with this figure type usually have short bodies, sturdy waistlines, and long legs. We want to lengthen the waist visually and make it appear smaller, at the same time correcting the impression that the body is "all legs."

Long-waisted figures usually have very long torsos and shorter legs. At least the legs appear short in contrast to the long body. If you have this figure type you're probably proud of your slender waist. Our camouflage problem here is to make the waist look higher, thereby camouflaging the length of the body and making the legs look longer.

DESIGN ELEMENTS THAT WILL LENGTHEN
A SHORT WAIST

1. By-pass the waist.

Choose clothes that don't have a waistline at all. Or that have a dropped waist. Or that lift the waist to just under the bust (Empire).

2. Choose the one-color look.

Color contrast between tops and skirts will cut you in half and make your body seem shorter than ever. If you must have color contrast, be sure your top is the overblouse type that will come at least two inches below your natural waistline. Remember, the longer jacket or blouse will also make those long legs appear shorter by reducing the visible expanse of skirt.

3. Choose belts and waistbands with care. You'll look best in skirts and pants that have no band at all. These can sometimes be cut to ride one inch below your natural waistline to make your waist look that much longer. If the garment does have a waistband, it should be as narrow as possible—three fourths to one inch is best. Contour belts can also make your waist look longer.

DESIGN ELEMENTS THAT WILL SHORTEN
A LONG WAIST

1. Accent the waist. Choose styles that have a wide waistband or belt. If you are slender, you can wear belts up to three inches wide. Always choose a straight belt, not a contour style. The

straight belt, riding at the waist, lifts the eye and makes your torso seem shorter.

2. Avoid styles with a dropped waistline or long overblouse. Sometimes shortening an overblouse just one inch can do wonders to correct the body's proportions. The shorter jacket or blouse will break the long line of the torso and make short legs seem longer because you see a longer expanse of skirt. However, don't try to extend the skirt at the hemline, only at the top, by raising the waist. *Skirts that are too long will make your legs seem short.* Show as much leg as you can, fashionably. The more leg that is visible the longer the legs will seem.

3. Choose color contrast. The two-color look will "cut you in two." Just what you want to make your body appear shorter. Choose shirts and skirts in contrasting colors.

IS YOUR FIGURE GOING TO WAIST?

Long or short, the mature figure often has a less than slender waist. It's sometimes termed midriff bulge. If this describes you, avoid eye-catching belts, wide belts, and light-colored, reflectant belts (patent leather, metal, satin). Dark-colored belts will make your waist appear to be smaller.

For that midriff bulge, avoid clothes that cling to your mid-section. Even a slight bloused effect will fool the eye.

YOUR BACK: HOW TO FIGHT
THE BATTLE OF THE BULGE

Just because you can't see it doesn't mean it isn't there. I mean that unsightly roll of flesh that lolls just above the top of your bra. You don't have one? Good for you. But I'll bet you know someone who does, because it's one of the first signs of a matronly figure. The muscles in this area don't get much exercise in the ordinary course of events and so they quickly turn to flab. Diet and exercise can permanently cure the problem, but meanwhile, why not pass along some of these camouflage tricks to your friend with the bad back?

1. *The bra's the thing.* Does it fit front *and* back? A bra that is not suited to your figure can create or madly accent bra bulge. Maybe the back strap is too narrow, so that it doesn't control the soft flesh in this area. Or perhaps it doesn't come low enough on your back, or is it really too small for you so that it

creates unsightly bulges under the arms, both back and front? Always remember, a brassiere that really fits can do wonders in helping with the battle of the bulges.

2. *The cling's the thing.* Fabric that has too much cling will tell the world you have a bra bulge. When you try on that arnel jersey blouse, check it front *and* back for fit. Perhaps you'll decide to choose one in a less clinging fabric, one that can keep a secret!

YOUR BUTTOCKS: LET'S GET TO THE BOTTOM OF THIS DISCUSSION

High, rounded contours spell young, feminine figures. Droopy busts and sagging rears spell age. A good bra can give you a lift in more ways than one, but what about the rear action? Lots of panty girdles are available with a definite lifting action, so it's really just a matter of asking for one. But avoid garments that create that awful slab effect formed by a single strong panel of elastic straight across the fanny.

Since your buttocks are formed by the two largest muscles in the body, the gluteus maximus (and some of us are more maximus than others), their contour responds readily to exercise. (More about this in Chapter Six.) However, there are several ways to disguise this figure problem while you're working to eliminate it.

1. Obviously, long jackets, tunics, or overblouses will effectively camouflage a low-slung rear, especially if they hang straight from the waist (or from above it, depending on the style) to the fullest part of the buttocks' contour. If you have a tendency to be sway-backed, avoid styles that are form-fitting in the upper hip area.

2. Check skirts and slacks to be sure they don't cup under the lower part of the buttocks' contour. These garments should hang straight down from the fullest point of the buttocks.

3. Avoid styles that have a hip yoke at the back. Such styles will make the buttocks look low-slung.

ARMS AND THE WOMAN

I think beautiful arms are overestimated as a mark of beauty. After all, Venus de Milo has done all right for herself. So don't go to extremes in trying to camouflage wrinkled elbows, *slight* flabbiness or fleshiness.

If you find a dress that makes you look and feel sensational, even though it shows your aging elbows . . . buy it. What's so bad about having someone say, "Wow! What a gorgeous creature! Too bad she has such wrinkled elbows."

There *is* an area that bears watching (or hiding, as the case may be). Check that spot at the front of your underarm, just above your bust. The muscles here get very little exercise and as a result the skin often becomes crepy, with that awful "turkey-wattle" look. Sleeveless dresses usually cover this area, but cut-in armholes, halters, and strapless styles do not. So watch it.

FASHION AND YOU, THE AGELESS WOMAN

I hope I've been a successful matchmaker, and that you and Fashion really understand each other now. Remember, your friend Fashion can help make you the Ageless Woman in the following ways:

1. The A.W. looks contemporary because her clothes reflect a knowledgeable combination of fashion and fad.

2. The A.W. looks like a *woman*, not a *matron*, because she chooses clothes that stress her femininity, avoiding styles, colors, and fabrics that create a neuter effect.

3. The A.W. knows how to camouflage the subtle figure changes that will make her look older than she feels.

4. Finally, she doesn't commit the most aging blunder of all . . . which we'll discuss in the next chapter.

THREE

Put Your Best Face Forward

You've seen her. The woman who just misses being the Ageless Woman. Her figure is good, slender and youthful. And her clothes project that timeless blend of taste, fashion, and a bit of fun. Then she turns around, and you see she's committed the greatest fashion blunder. Her make-up is years behind the times. Does she look older than her years? You'd better believe it!

LET'S FACE IT

Nothing creates the illusion of age more effectively than out-of-date make-up. Nothing, that is, except the mature face with no make-up at all. If fashion is the mature woman's best friend, make-up (used correctly) is her very own fairy godmother. Yet the majority of women don't take advantage of the miracles modern make-up can accomplish.

How do I know? It becomes obvious whenever I study the hundreds of faces looking back at me as I lecture. Most of these faces are hopelessly out of fashion. In fact, as I look at my audience, I can usually trace the history of make-up fashions for the past thirty years.

There will always be lots of June Allysons, with scrubbed faces and little bippity-boo hair styles. Even June Allyson, who's graduated to a glamorous and sophisticated image, doesn't look like this any more. Then there are the Joan Crawford types. See all those 1950s eyebrows? There's so much pencil on those brows that I always feel like rushing out to call my stockbroker. "Quick, I've got a hot tip. Buy Maybelline."

The ones I just can't believe are the Kay Francis group. Their brows droop down at the end, giving a sad, "Oh, God, how I've suffered" expression. Wait, there's more. Bette Davis is there too, with that deep red, tortured mouth turned down at the corners, the lipstick slightly smeared. A few avant-garde types represent Elizabeth Taylor in her role as Cleopatra. That disaster of a movie was a bomb back in 1963. But serpent or no, Cleo dies hard. She's still around, eyes rimmed with black liner and topped with a gob of turquoise and silver eyeshadow.

And then, of course, there's Jimmy Stewart. Really! How else to describe the outdoor enthusiast with her short-cropped, graying hair and leathery skin? "I never wear anything on my face," she says proudly. We know, dear, we know.

I look at their faces and I wonder where these women have been for the past thirty years. Lost in the Twilight Zone? Or have they been trapped in the Hollywood Wax Museum?

If this description sounds catty and unkind, like a slap in the face, I hope some of you will say, as so many of my students have, "Thanks. I needed that." It's been my experience that most women are strangely inflexible when it comes to changing make-up and hair styles. They're so deeply mired in their rut that only shock treatment can blast them out. I'm not alone in this opinion. Eleanor Fait, state supervisor of the older worker program in the California Department of Human Resources Development, has this to say about women over forty-five who are trying to re-enter the labor market: "They're used to being around home in floppy dresses. Their make-up is dated —like what women were wearing twenty-five years ago. . . ."

THE GREAT ESCAPE

If you want to avoid the stereotypes that I've described you must come to terms with these two truths.

1. The mature face *needs* make-up.
2. The mature face needs a *fashionable* make-up.

Understanding the importance of make-up and its relationship to the complete fashion picture will allow you to analyze your own make-up needs confidently—and escape from the Hollywood Wax Museum forever.

THE NAKED TRUTH ABOUT THE NATURAL LOOK

The mature face *needs* make-up and if you want to look like the Ageless Woman (and not Jimmy Stewart) *you* need make-up. And when I say make-up, I mean *the works.* Foundation, rouge, blushers, glosses, the whole eye number. The mature woman who lets nature take its course is in for a downhill ride, all the way.

Celebrity hair stylist and beauty consultant Kenneth Battelle, who numbers among his clients many glamorous women including Paulette Goddard, has this to say about natural beauty: "As for natural beauty, I don't really think that this much exists today. Everyone uses lipstick, plucks her eyebrows, manicures her nails, at the very least. Most people help beauty along a good deal more than that. I know many glamorous women whose many artifices are used in such subtle ways and applied so wisely that while it's complete artifice, it's so beautiful that everyone would like to do it. I have rarely seen a frankly natural beauty. I'm sure a good many natural beauties exist, *but I don't think they're much past twelve years old.*" (Emphasis added.)

The totally natural look is charming on a twelve-year-old, enchanting on a sixteen-year-old. However, when a mature woman attempts the guileless, completely barefaced beauty of the very young, it's as inappropriate for her as the latest in teeny bopper fashions. You've *lived*, my friend, and after a "certain age" it's time to create a sophisticated, *womanly* face through the knowledgeable application of make-up.

Does this advice turn you off? Perhaps it's because you're picturing all the terrible make-up jobs you've ever seen. But make-up needn't be like that. The unaffected "natural look" that you admire is *not* created by letting nature take its course but rather by a knowledgeable use of a few simple make-up techniques.

Later, I'm going to give you a step-by-step plan that will spell out these techniques. But, as we've already found out, make-up alone isn't the answer. (Right, Cleo?) You must learn to use cosmetics to put your face in fashion.

MAKE-UP: THE FASHION YOU WEAR
ON YOUR FACE

We've already learned that fashion changes are made up of changing proportions, which in turn create a total mood. Make-up and hair styles are part of this total concept. So much so that most top designers recommend specific make-up effects that complement their designs.

The elements involved in creating make-up fashion are:

1. *Colors*—They can be pale and subtle or bright and dramatic.

2. *Finish*—Make-up elements can be opaque, translucent, matte, pearly, shiny.

3. *Proportion*—The size and shape of eyebrow and mouth may change subtly. Examples are the "bee-stung" mouth of the twenties, the thin round brow of the thirties, the square Joan Crawford mouth of the forties, the heavy brow of the fifties.

4. *Emphasis*—When the eye is superaccented, the lipstick is toned down and understated. When lips are brighter, eye make-up is less prominent. See how it works?

You can become aware of these changes of face by turning once again to the fashion magazines. The editorial pages often have excellent step-by-step descriptions of how to update your make-up. As you look through the magazine, study the *faces*, not just the clothes. In this way you will become aware of the color, finish, proportion, and emphasis that are currently fashionable.

But what if the editorial you read is superdramatic and unreal? Something like this: "The Peacock Eye (complete with gold paint and feathers) is the NOW look." Forget it! Turn to the advertising pages. The large close-ups used by the cosmetic, hair-coloring, and wig companies are usually instructive examples of current trends.

And the ongoing trends are what you're looking for, because make-up fashions, like clothing fashions, operate on two levels—fashion and fad.

Make-up fashions change slowly and are part of the over-all fashion picture. Make-up fads like the "Peacock Eye" are here-today, gone-tomorrow gimmicks.

How can you separate make-up fad from fashion? Ask yourself this question. How far does this effect differ from nature in color, proportion, and emphasis? If the effect deviates wildly from nature, it won't be around long and is, therefore, a fad.

TRICKS ARE FOR KIDS

Although fad is an important part of the Ageless Woman's wardrobe, *the mature woman must avoid make-up fads of all kinds.*

Pablo Manzoni, creative director of Elizabeth Arden cosmetics, says, "When you know yourself, you're not attracted to . . . fads for shock. Shock is for newcomers."

Some examples of recent fads are: foundation (make-up) and powder with iridescent gold highlights; yellow or pink eyeshadow; a ring of white "shadow" around the eye (like a baby raccoon?); silver pearl eyeliner; mascara in *bright* tones of green, blue, lavender; lipstick in weird shades of brown or pink or fuschia.

Whatever the fashion magazines may say, the rule is this: the mature woman must avoid make-up fads. Tricks are for kids.

Now I want to give you a little exercise that will show you how to analyze your own make-up in relation to current fashion trends. Is *your* face in fashion? Let's find out.

SEEING IS BELIEVING

Choose a time of day when you are wearing what you consider your basic make-up, when your make-up is fresh, and when no one is in the house who tends to giggle.

Now look through your current fashion magazines. Look for ads and articles illustrated by large, full-face close-ups. (The closer they are to life size, the better.) Every issue will have at least one. Choose one that represents fashion, not fad, and fold it in half, vertically. Look in the mirror and hold the photo so it covers half your face, lining it up with your features. Remember, you aren't expecting to look like the model in the photo. You are analyzing the color, finish, proportion, and emphasis of the make-up accents in an objective way.

1. Start at the eyebrow. How does yours compare with the photo? Is yours darker? Thicker? Is yours messy and unkempt compared to the model's? Compare shape and placement. Is your eyebrow right on top of your eye? The model's isn't. See? If you have chosen your photograph with care (that is, one that represents fashion, not fad) you'll also note that the shape of the model's brow is rounded with a slight arch. Is yours?

2. Now the eyeshadow. If you can find a photo where the model is glancing down, you'll get a clear view of this technique. Where is the shadow placed? In a thick, goopy line along the eyelashes? No. Clear up to the eyebrows? No. If you've chosen your picture correctly, you'll see that the shadow is concentrated in the fold of the eyelid, then fans up and out toward the temples. Yours does too? Smart girl.

3. The eyeliner is next. You probably won't be able to see the model's, because the trend is toward a subtle liner. Believe me, it's there. Yours should be subtle too. Is it?

4. Is the model wearing rouge—or face color, as I prefer to call it? In any color photo you'll see that face color has been used to round and accent the cheekbone contours. I'm going to tell you how to do this in a minute. But first, check *your* face color. You're not wearing any? That's what I thought. Now I want you to really *look* at that photograph and see what the color does for the over-all effect. Now look at your pale face. Get the message?

5. Finally, check the lip shape in the photo. Is the curve of the cupid's bow full and rounded? Or is it pointed, with the cupid's bow accented? See how the lip color comes out to the corners of the mouth? Does yours? Or does it stop short of the corners—a common error? How does your mouth compare in over-all shape? Is it just a thin slash, instead of curved and feminine? Is it messy?

6. Unfold the picture and look at the complete photograph. Does the mouth dominate the face? Or do the eyes? Now look at *your* face and check for make-up accent. How does it compare? Do we just see heavy, overpowering eyebrows and nothing

else? Or is it a face dominated by deep red lipstick, put on any old way because "I don't have time."

After a few run-throughs with this exercise, you should begin to really see your own face in relation to the current look. At this stage, it is possible to carry this exercise even further. To get a clearer picture, you might ask yourself a few questions.

"Have I changed my hair color and/or hair style in the last five years?"

"Have I tried a new lip color? Or am I still wearing Revlon's Fire and Ice?"

"Have I experimented with a new lip shape, new eyebrow line, new make-up techniques in the last five years? The last ten years? Or—good grief!—has it been twenty years?"

"Have I tried any of these contemporary make-up products: face gleamers, lip glosses, artificial eyelashes?"

If the answer to several of these questions is no, your face is probably dated and you're looking older than you should.

Always remember, the purpose of the exercise is not to compare your face to that of the model. Rather, the purpose is to train your eye so that you can look at your face objectively, in its relationship to current fashion.

When you've mastered this trick, you'll never again suffer from make-up myopia.

THE TWO FACES OF EVE

This is what I tried to tell Eve, a student who was forced to enter the job market after her husband was killed in a tragic auto accident. Her doctor had suggested my classes as part of her rehabilitation program, and she was an enthusiastic student. She made great progress in everything but make-up. In these classes she was pleasant but stubbornly devoted to her out-of-fashion face.

Stubborn she was, all right, but maybe that's the quality that helped her bounce back from the shock of her husband's death. Soon she was getting on her feet emotionally and was able to go on job interviews.

She called me shortly after completing her course, and her excited conversation seesawed from joy to depression at a dizzying pace.

"I got the job. Can you believe it? I got it! I'm going to be social director on that cruise ship. But listen. They kept stressing that it was a younger group I'd be dealing with. I think they were trying to tell me something—just like you were trying to tell me something in class. I promise not to be so stubborn this time. Can I have an appointment to review some of my lessons?"

When Eve came into my studio I could see that she hadn't changed a bit. Damn it! Still clinging to the "Italian" look of the early 1960s, which consisted of heavily accented eyes and a pale mouth. Eve's eyes were heavily lined, topped with lashes like *visors*, and framed with heavy brows. Her pale mouth looked chalky and lined because of the opaque pink lipstick she wore.

No wonder her new employers were concerned. The whole effect, which at one time had been fashionable, now gave the impression of jaded age. In spite of all this, her warm personality had impressed them, and I knew that, once we could whip her looks into shape, they'd be delighted with this charming and outgoing woman.

With all this at stake, you'd think it would be fairly easy to bring this look up to date, wouldn't you?

Ah, but that doesn't take into account the inflexibility of women when it comes to changing their make-up. However, I convinced Eve by using this simple teaching technique—an arm lock and handcuffs.

Well, actually, this is what I did. I changed the make-up on just one side of her face, toning down those heavy eyebrows which are not only out of style but also extremely aging. I used a light brown pencil and then powdered over her brows to soften them even more. Next, that black eyeliner was replaced by a muted plum brown, making her eyes look larger.

Artificial eyelashes are the greatest gift to mature women since the surgical face lift, but they must be subtle. I replaced one "visor" with a delicate, feathery lash. The kind that looks *almost* natural. (If it looks completely natural, why bother?) That chalky pink "I'm overdrawn at the blood bank" mouth was exchanged for a vibrant coral one. I outlined her mouth with lipliner and then filled in with a translucent, creamy lipstick (this doesn't accent lip lines).

For the final touch, a shimmery, copper-gold gleamer added color. I used this as cheek color and also as a highlight on her chin and across her forehead. Instant health. And how much more effective than the opaque, powdered blusher that gave her other cheek a flat, slablike contour.

Not until this half-and-half make-up job was finished did I let her near a mirror. When Eve could actually *see* the difference between Old Hat and Fashionable Face, she was finally convinced to change her ten-year-old face dress.

And her job? She's still cruising between New York and Bermuda and loving *almost* every minute of it. Her last letter told me that she was seasick only three days out of seven on her latest jaunt.

HOW TO PUT YOUR BEST FACE FORWARD

Just *knowing* what's in fashion isn't enough. Obviously, you have to know *how* to apply that new gleamer or that eyeliner. You have to know *how* to modify that eyebrow shape and lip line. What's more you must be aware of the make-up clichés that can make you look older than your years. In other words, there are sure losers and winning tickets in the make-up game, too.

The following make-up plan spells out those winners and losers and takes you step by step from the beginning—moisturizer and foundation—to the triumphant end—artificial eyelashes. Yes, they're definitely for you. Let's get started.

Dressing your face is a lot like dressing your body. Underwear protects the body by creating a silky surface for our clothes to glide over. Bras and pantyhose smooth and lift the body contours. Our first two make-up elements do the same things for your face.

MAKE-UP BASE

Never apply make-up directly to the skin. Always start with a lotion designed to protect the skin and give the actual make-up an ideal surface to glide over. Choose a product that has a moisturizing quality.

What is a moisturizer? A leading dermatologist has described it as any product that increases the water content of the outer layer of the skin. A moisturizer is especially important for the mature face because, according to *Vogue* magazine, "it smooths and plumps the skin surface by equalizing its parts." They go on to explain, "Most moisturizing emulsions put a film of oil on the skin that obscures minute textural flaws, fills in the gaps, stops the scattering of light." Translated in terms of the mature face, this means that a moisturizer will smooth those dry flaky patches so common after forty, fill in expression lines and wrinkles (shudder), and lighten up dull and sallow areas. So you can see why they're a boon to the Ageless Woman.

I recommend a moisturizing base that is made from natural oils. There is a special reason why mature women should avoid synthetic products. I'll be explaining why in a later chapter, but now, take my word for it. Natural is better. Health food stores have many products with natural oil bases. I like a commercial one that is based on avocado oil.

Apply moisturizer by smoothing it on with a few drops of water. Be sure to cover the entire face and neck area, paying special attention to eyelids and under-eye area—it fills in those tiny wrinkles. Let it soak in for a few moments and then—apply shadow cover.

SHADOW COVER

WINNING TICKETS	SURE LOSERS
You'll look younger if you have:	You'll look older if you have:
An even skin tone in the under-eye area	Dark shadows or circles under the eyes
Lifted contours, firm skin in the eye area	Heavy make-up in the eye area
Even skin tone in nostril area	Reddened skin, broken blood vessels in the nostril area
	Deep-set, "sunken" eyes

Shadows and circles under the eyes can make you look tired and old. Yet it's easy to camouflage these and other problems with a shadow cover. Just be sure to choose a product that will be flattering to the mature face.

Many popular shadow covers—generally flesh-colored—that come in a tube like lipstick are much too heavy, as you may have discovered. When you apply them to those under-eye circles you look great. Until you smile. Then that heavy paste turns into a thousand little lines and cracks.

Choose, instead, a light translucent cream or liquid. My favorite is a fluffy cream that comes in a pale shade of turquoise blue. This bit of color magic effectively blots out shadows because it is the color opposite of those violet shadows under the eye. Also effective is a light pink cream.

Apply this way: pat cream delicately with one fingertip just under the eye and toward the nose. This creamy cover-up can be used to camouflage other signs of age, too.

1. For bags under the eyes: apply cream cover-up to the indented area at the bottom of eye bag. Do not apply to entire under-eye area, as this will make the bag more prominent. By filling in the indentation with your light, bright cream, you'll make the entire under-eye area look lifted, and the eye bag will appear to vanish. Hooray!

2. For eyes that are too deep-set, giving you an aged, hollow-eyed look: apply cream cover-up to inner corners of the eye and onto eyelids. Do not apply cream up onto prominent brow bone.

3. For reddened nostril area (and incidentally to make a wide nose appear narrower) pat cream cover-up onto cheek area next to nostrils in a circular shape about one fourth inch wide. Bring cream cover-up around base of nostrils and into nostril opening, about one eighth inch.

4. The Five-second Face Lift. (Through the magic of optical illusion, of course.) After applying shadow cover over your dark circles—or under eye bags—continue to apply it in a line *up* from the corner of the eye to the hairline. This *really* gives your face a lift. Try it.

When applying your cover-up, be sure to pat, pat, pat. Don't rub. You're not trying to rub this cream *into* the skin but to smooth it onto the surface of the skin in a thin film. Remember this too when you are applying make-up *over* the cream cover-up. Pat, don't rub. Or you'll undo all our efforts.

MAKE-UP (FOUNDATION)

WINNING TICKETS	SURE LOSERS
You'll look younger if you use:	You'll look older if you use:
Make-up in beige tones to match your skin or one shade *lighter* (reflects light, minimizes lines)	Make-up base that's too tan, too pink, too dark (often worn in an attempt to create a healthy look and add color). These shades accent age lines
Moisturizing liquid base	
Make-up that's translucent, but with coverage	Make-up that has an opaque finish

Make-up that's too heavy (cream bases)

Make-up that's too light (lotion types)

"The most important trick for the over-thirty skin is to give the *impression* of color without coverage." That's what make-up artist Way Bandy of Charles of the Ritz advises. Yet it's difficult to find a foundation that is neither too heavy nor so light that it's a waste of money. I mean, why spend $7.50 for a bottle of Invisible Veiled Illusion if it goes on like a dab of hand lotion and totally disappears? I've found that the most effective solution is to mix my own goo.

Buy one bottle that's too opaque, one that's too translucent, and then mix 'em up. Since almost all liquid make-ups are compatible, this works beautifully.

Mixing is the solution to the color problem, too. Have several bottles—light, dark, pink, tan. In the summer, add more tan. When you'll be seen under fluorescent lights, at the office for example, add more pink tones. (But keep it subtle.) At night, wear your lightest shades; choose beigey-tan for daylight.

Use a slightly damp, not *wet*, make-up sponge to smooth the foundation over your shadow cover-up. Carefully blend it around the nostril area, just under the chin, and back to the ears. To avoid that mask effect, be sure to apply make-up to earlobes and to skin under and behind ears. It's quick and easy to do a professional job if you use a sponge, which is *the* technique of all professional make-up artists.

Jet-set beauty and star model Betsy Theodoracopulos uses a sponge which she splits in half like an English muffin, using the rough side to blend her make-up. She says that the uneven surface grabs the make-up more efficiently yet doesn't smear it. She also uses it to blend her rouge . . . which is our next step.

ROUGE (FACE COLOR)

WINNING TICKETS	SURE LOSERS
You'll look younger if you use:	You'll look older if you use:
Liquid or gel face color in tawny bronze shades	Any opaque rouge. This means most creams and all powders
Translucent gleamers, glossers and	Rouge in tones of pink or red

highlighters. These come in stick, liquid, or gel form
Pearlized products that lift the contours—in gold or beige

Blushers. All powder blushers are too opaque for the mature skin
No color at all—makes you look tired and old

Face color is the indispensable cosmetic for the mature face. I've seen hundreds of faces change from aged to ageless with the application of this single product. However, the majority of women still don't wear rouge. And I think this is the reason: they've been turned off by the sight of those old gals who wear two livid spots of opaque rouge from eyebrow to jowl. But face color needn't look like that. The new products, in case you haven't tried them, are aeons away from those heavy-handed creams and powders.

Translucent is the key word here. According to Hollywood's Mont Westmore, "In Nature—fruit, flowers, and the human complexion—color comes from beneath the surface. It is not spread, like a cookie's thick frosting, upon the top." To achieve this natural effect, choose a face color that allows your skin texture to shine through. In other words, one that is *translucent*. As an added bonus, you'll find that translucent colors are so subtle, it's almost impossible to wear too much. The coppery bronze shade that I've recommended creates a healthy, sun-kissed look on all complexions. Avoid any product in a red or pink shade, *especially those that have a blue undertone*.

High, rounded cheeks are part of nature's pattern for youth. You can give your face those apple cheeks again if you apply face color this way.

1. Smile a little so that you lift the cheek contour.

2. Apply tawny color on the high point of the cheek. Pat it into a circle about the size of a half dollar. Use *enough* color. A little dab won't do it.

3. The apple trick. Leave the highest intensity of color on the high point of the cheek, while you blend the edges of your "half dollar" up, up toward the temple and down toward the center of the cheek.

4. Highlight the very highest point of the cheek contour with a dot of your pearlized highlighter, just as if you were painting the highlight on an apple. Very gently, blend the edges of this highlight with your sponge.

Now, if you've been following directions, you will have created a three-dimensional effect of highlight and shadow which will give the illusion of a lifted, rounded contour. Just the opposite, thank heaven, of that flat and flabby effect created by applying rouge in a slab of color that covers the entire cheek with the same intensity of color.

You'll truly appreciate the magic of those iridescent glossers and transparent gleamers if you try this next technique. It's a favorite of international beauties Baroness Nina van Pallandt and Vicomtesse Harriet de Rosière. (There! Isn't that impressive?)

Simply dab a few spots of color across your forehead, close to the hairline, and blend with your make-up sponge. You should have a glow of color about one inch wide. To round the forehead contour, I suggest that you place a dot of your pearlized highlight in the center of your forehead (like an Indian caste mark) and blend into a half-dollar-sized circle. Notice that this little trick seems to lift all the facial contours and give your face a vital glow.

POWDER

WINNING TICKETS	SURE LOSERS
You'll look younger if:	You'll look older if:
Your face has the healthy *glow* of youth	You wear powder. Period

How do theatrical make-up artists create the effect of age? They use lots of powder to accent every line and wrinkle. *That* should convince you to say by-by to that compact of yours. Nose too shiny? Use those little blotters called Face Savers (available at any drugstore) to soak up excess oil.

If you keep dabbing powder on your nose you'll accent it and make it look larger and more prominent. You didn't really want to do that, did you? That's what I thought.

Wait. There *is* one place that we need to use powder. That's when we apply eye make-up.

EYESHADOW

WINNING TICKETS	SURE LOSERS
You'll look younger if you wear:	You'll look older if you wear:
Eyeshadow in subtle, shadow-colored tones. (Your eye color will look brighter by comparison)	Eyeshadow in bright shades (makes the eye color drab by comparison)
Eyeshadow in the fold of the eyelid, which opens and enlarges the eye	Eyeshadow in the wrong place—on the eyelid or blended up to the eyebrow

Most women misunderstand the purpose of eyeshadow. It should not be used in an attempt to add color to the eyes but rather as a means of shadowing the eye area to create a more pleasing contour. That's why bright eyeshadow colors are all wrong, especially for the mature face. Bright colors come forward, making the eye look puffy. They also accent any crepiness in the eyelid area.

Choose instead subtle, smoky colors. George Masters, Hollywood make-up whiz who numbers among his clients Elizabeth Taylor and Raquel Welch, suggests, "Do not match your eye color necessarily. The whole idea is to flatter it. Try light or deeper gray, muted green, or blue. Choose the color that most seems to open your eye. Don't reach for a bright blue shadow just because you have blue eyes." He suggests using shadows "in some tone of violet, regardless of your eye or skin color." Caution here. Be sure to choose a shadow that's *shadow*-colored. That is, basically a grayed tone with just a hint of the color you prefer. He also suggests using cake eyeshadows, applied with a moistened brush. I disagree. These are great if you're an accomplished make-up artist, a disaster if you're a bit fumble-fingered. Instead, use cream eyeshadow in a tube. It's easier to control than any other kind, and stays put, too.

Here's how: simply apply a band of tube shadow in the circular hollow just above your eyeball. Blend it in a soft crescent shape up and out, toward the outer tip of the eyebrow. Do not blend it onto the eyelid. The effect is a soft blurred line outlining the eyelid and fanning out toward the outer edge of the eye. Notice how the eyeshadow reduces the appearance of any puffiness in the area under the brow. If your eyes are extremely deep set (a characteristic which can create an aged, hollow-eyed look) bring the shadow over that prominent brow bone, but not up to the eyebrow. Isn't it amazing how this simple trick opens the eye and makes it look wider and younger?

Your final step in applying eyeshadow is to powder the eyelids *lightly*. Hey! Don't just plop that powder puff over the entire eye area. The eyelids *only*, please. This sets the eyeshadow and it will last all day. By avoiding the under-eye area, you haven't accented any little expression lines. See?

Now here's a tip that will help you in applying all types of eye make-up, as well as artificial lashes. Instead of trying to see what you're doing to that eyelid by squinting through half-closed eyes, try this instead. Hold the fingers of the left hand in the old V for Victory sign—or the Peace sign, if you don't want to date yourself.

Next, hold the left eye closed by gently placing the second finger at the inner corner of the eye, the index finger at the outer corner. If your eyelids are crepy, stretch the skin *very* slightly. Now, you should be able to see what you're doing very clearly by looking in the mirror with your unfettered right eye. Got it? To work on the right eye, you'll naturally reverse fingers, using the index finger in the eye corner, the second finger at the outer edge. Still can't see? That's because you aren't using a magnifying mirror. Every Ageless Woman has one. But you knew that, didn't you?

EYEBROWS: THEIR PLACEMENT

WINNING TICKETS	SURE LOSERS
You'll look younger if your eyebrows are:	You'll look older if your eyebrows are:
The width of an eye from the eye. Start directly above the tear duct (directions follow). Gives you an appealing, wide-eyed expression	Too close to the eye
	Too close to the nose (makes your nose look larger, gives a stern, disapproving expression; old!)
Flare up and out at the outer tip (lifts the entire facial contour)	Slipping down at outer tip (creates a sad, martyred expression)
	Too far from the nose (gives a shallow, vapid expression)

EYEBROWS: THEIR SHAPE

You'll look younger if your brows:	You'll look older if your brows:
Follow the classic, bird-wing shape. Never mind fashion. This is the line that follows nature's pattern for Agelessness. Fashion comes into the picture by influencing the color and thickness of your brows.	Are too straight. Remember, that arch gives your face a lift.
	Are too narrow. The thin, pencil-line brow is a nostalgia trip—circa 1935. So is—the silly circle. That round, surprised brow line gives you a foolish, clown expression.
	Are a totally natural, "I don't do a thing to my brows" shape

EYEBROWS: THEIR COLOR

You'll look younger if your brows:	You'll look older if your brows:
Are just dark enough to be seen if your hair is blonde or silver	Are too dark. Black eyebrow pencil

Are several shades lighter than your   is the ultimate vulgarity. *Always*
hair if you are a brunette. How   use shades of grayed brown.
to make them appear lighter?
There are two ways, powder or
bleach (directions follow)

Want to look younger in the blink of an eye? Then *learn* to perfect those eyebrows. I say learn because eyebrow make-up seems to
be the most difficult for women to master. Often, this is their solution: "I'm not sure of how to shape my brows, so I don't do anything at all." But that's not the solution, because they're still there,
those two expressive lines that can make you look older, younger,
happy, sad, intelligent, foolish. Wow! Are they important.

HOW TO HAVE THE PERFECT BROW

First keep in mind the three elements as I've discussed them
above: placement, shape, and color. To place your brow correctly,
you'll need a short ruler and a sharpened eyebrow pencil. Powder
over your own brows (this will help you to look at your face objectively). Hold the ruler vertically, lining it up with the tear duct.
With the eyebrow pencil, mark the spot where the ruler crosses your
brow line. This is point A. Now, look straight ahead into your mirror. Place the ruler at the outer edge of the iris. Hold it in a straight
line up to the eyebrow and make a mark where the eyebrow arches.
(Check. Did you use the pupil instead of the iris as a measuring
point? I don't know why, but half of my students make this error.)
This is point B, the highest point of the brow. Finally, place the
ruler in a line running from the nostril to the outer corner of the eye
and on through the brow line. Your eyebrow should end where the
ruler crosses the brow line. Mark this spot. It is point C *and should
always be higher than point* A. Do not let the end of the eyebrow
droop. Look. Does yours slip lower than point A? Get the tweezers.
Let's remove those slipshod offenders. Come on. While you have
your tweezers out, let's be sure that your brow isn't too close to your
eye. We can correct this effect by tweezing the offending brows.
Which ones? Here's how to find out. Look straight ahead into the
mirror. Take your ruler vertically and measure the width of your eye
—from top to bottom at the widest point. It will probably be an
inch wide, more or less.

Next, simply check to make sure that points A, B, and C are an eye width from your eye. If in doubt about this measurement, fudge a little and make the eyebrow even higher than an eye width. If this correction makes your eyebrow too narrow, add width at the top with tiny strokes of eyebrow pencil. And you'll use those tiny pencil strokes to connect points A, B, and C. Remember, point A should start just above the tear duct. This placement makes your eyes appear larger, more open. Point B should be the high point of the eyebrow arch—and that lifted arch gives your contours a lift. Point C should also lift the facial contours by angling *up*, toward the temple.

The color of your eyebrow should be very subtle. This is a fashion era when eyebrows are light and do not dominate the face. (If you can find a 1950s fashion magazine, you'll see that the dominant brow is the most obvious and dated element in the entire fashion picture. Heavens, we all looked like John L. Lewis.) If your brows are dark, you can powder them or you can bleach them, an exciting change of face. I bleach mine myself, but it is tricky, and I suggest you have your beautician do it, at least the first few times. The shops charge very little, and the beauty dividends are instant. (And, yes, they do grow back in your natural color. So you really have very little to lose.)

About those eyebrow pencils. Less is better. Don't use any at all if your brows are naturally full and well shaped. (Not too full, by the way. Delicate brows are *in*. That's another fashion trademark of the seventies.) Use short, hairlike strokes to fill in the places where your brow doesn't fit our ideal shape. And always use the lightest shade of pencil possible. And here's a tip: lightly powder the brow when you're finished. It softens the penciled accent and "sets" your eyebrow line. Try it. You'll like it.

EYELINER

WINNING TICKETS	SURE LOSERS
You'll look younger if you:	You'll look older if you:
Wear eyeliner in subtle shades to match mascara	Wear black eyeliner
Use a water-color cake-type eyeliner	Continue the line up past the end of the eye in a little "up" line (the
Keep the line soft	doe eye, circa 1950)
Use eyeliner to draw a few delicate lines among lower lashes	Don't wear eyeliner at all (never mind what the fashion magazines

to make them appear thicker. A   say)
real eye opener   Line upper and lower lids

We've all seen basically nice and attractive women who look cheap and hard because of obvious eyeliner. Don't let their mistakes prevent you from using this simple method of making your eyes look more appealing. The key word here is *soft*. A woman's eyes should look soft and gentle. Anything that is harsh in either color or line will give you the appearance of a beady-eyed wench, and an old one at that. Not exactly the effect we're striving for.

The easiest way to get the soft line that is a must for the Ageless Woman is to use cake eyeliner. Like water colors, this product can be made darker or lighter, depending on how moist your brush is. And for the best brush available, go to an artists' supply store and get a long-handled sable-hair brush.

What colors will you use? Brown, charcoal, dark blue, or green. In fact, any subtle color that is darker than your shadow can be becoming. Remember, the color should be so subdued that the over-all effect is one of a grayed no-color. What you should *not* use is a black liner or a bright blue liner or a bright green liner or a bright lavender liner. Okay?

To apply eyeliner, moisten the brush and test the intensity of the liner color by dabbing it on your wrist. Our *first* line will be almost transparent, so dilute the eyeliner quite a bit. Now, holding the eyelid closed (as we've already learned), draw a transparent line, about one eighth inch thick, right next to the lashes. Keep your eye closed for a minute to allow this to dry, then do the other eye. Your *second* eyeliner will be much darker. Test the color again on your wrist. Now draw a very fine line over the first line and almost *into* the lashes.

The first line softens the eyes and minimizes a puffy eyelid. The second, darker line gives the eyes definition and accents the eyelashes. If your eyelid is crepy and droops over your lashes, omit the second, dark line. You'll find that the soft line alone will still be very effective for you.

One final suggestion. If you have difficulty controlling eyebrow pencils, lip brushes, lipliners, and eyeliner brushes, here is the infallible method which will give you an artist's control over these beauty tools.

Using the eyeliner brush as an example, hold it as if you were holding a pen and going to sit down and write a love letter. (I thought that would get your attention.)

Now bring the brush up to the eye and steady your hand by extending the little finger and resting it against your upper cheek. You can control your hand by swiveling it from this little-finger base. You will also have more control if you are able to support your elbow while you're painting your masterpiece. This is why it's advisable to do your make-up at a dressing table, rather than standing at a mirror.

MASCARA

WINNING TICKETS	SURE LOSERS
You'll look younger if you:	You'll look older if you:
Use mascara in subtle shades of brown, grayed blues or greens	Wear black mascara
Wear mascara on lower lashes too. (This balances the eye make-up, makes the eyes look larger)	Don't wear mascara (Allergic to the stuff? Try old-fashioned cake mascara. Liquid and wand types can cause irritation, red, watery eyes)

Keep your chin up. That's the best advice I can give you to make mascara application a breeze. It's when you tuck your chin in and look up as you apply mascara that it gets messy. When you lift your chin and look *down* into your mirror you are able to brush on that lash magic without getting it all over your upper lids.

What does mascara do for the mature face? It widens the eyes and tends to camouflage crepiness in the eyelid area. You'll get the best results if you brush lashes straight out. Don't brush to the side, a technique that many of my students have carried over from the 1940s. Another holdover from the past is the eyelash curler. Get rid of this antique if you're using one. The effect is terribly dated and, what's more, no matter how carefully you use it, a curler will break your lashes and pretty soon you don't have any more. Take the word of your old teacher (that's me!) who has seen hundreds of bald eyes surrounded by stumpy little lashes all belonging to curler enthusiasts. You can get a more natural effect by using milk to moisten your cake mascara. This gives it a thicker consistency. After two applications, use your fingertips to gently push lashes up, a trick that gives them a natural-looking sweep.

Don't forget lower lashes. They should also have a generous

application of mascara. Be sure the brush is just slightly moist and apply color by gently brushing lower lashes.

ABOUT THOSE PASSES

If you wear glasses, forget Dorothy Parker's famous little poem about the lack of men in your life. You'll look sensational if you don't let your eyes disappear behind those glasses. The message is: wear *enough* eye make-up to accent your eyes. The subtle effects that enhance the eyes of non-eyeglass wearers will be totally lost behind your specs. Wear plenty of mascara, a heavier liner, and more eye-shadow than you're used to. Don't go overboard on this, of course. Use the ageless techniques we've discussed, but try to think of your eye make-up in terms of evening make-up rather than subtle daytime effects. You'll see. Your eyes will look large and expressive in spite of your glasses.

In spite of? Actually, the Ageless Woman uses her glasses to enhance her fashion image. They can be an exciting fashion accessory, so review the winning and losing styles in eyeglass frames listed in the last chapter.

LIP TIPS

WINNING TICKETS
You'll look younger if you:
Wear a bright, translucent lipstick
Avoid blue-toned lipstick
Keep your lip line distinct. (Use a lipliner pencil. Much easier than a brush and it keeps lipstick from running into lip lines)
Have a relaxed mouth, with full, curved lips.

SURE LOSERS
You'll look older if you:
Wear an opaque or matte-finish lipstick in a dark shade
Allow your lip line to be indistinct. (The lipstick then runs into those tiny lines on the upper lip)
Have a mouth that looks pinched, small, and disapproving

Your mouth tells just how feminine you are, and that's why it's especially important at this stage of the game to avoid any suggestion of a small, pinched mouth with thin, disapproving lips. (Do your lips seem to be getting thinner? This can be caused by an easily corrected vitamin deficiency that we'll talk about in Chapter Five.) Meanwhile, we can correct this condition visually with a little make-up sleight of hand.

The feminine mouth expresses a woman's emotional nature. It

should be soft and vulnerable-looking (whether she really is or not). Here is how to achieve this effect.

1. Be sure you have applied foundation make-up over the entire lip area. This will give your lipstick a lasting base, help the lipstick color to remain "true," and effectively mask your own lip line in case you want to make corrections.

2. Use a lip *pencil* to outline your mouth. These are much easier to use than brushes and have this added advantage for grownups: because the pencil is not as creamy as lipstick, it forms a little fence around your mouth outline, keeping the lipstick in line and preventing it from running into those tiny wrinkles that sometimes appear on the upper lip. Now, before you use that pencil, I want you to . . .

3. *Look at your mouth.* Decide where corrections, if any, must be made. If your reflection is telegraphing bad news, this may make you feel better. Almost all mouths, all features, for that matter, are lopsided. The trick is to decide which side of your upper lip and which side of your lower lip are most attractive. Got it? Good.

4. Next step. Keep your mouth closed (yes, it's hard for me too), lips relaxed, and smile slightly. Do *not* do a "monkey see, monkey do" number with your lips twisted from side to side as you apply your lipstick. How can you possibly follow a true outline if your mouth is twisted out of shape? Remember. *Relax.* Now, hold the lip pencil as I've suggested and steady your hand by resting your little finger on your chin. Draw five dots on the top edge of your upper lip as follows: one directly under the center of your nose, one directly under the center of each nostril, one in line with outer curve of each nostril.

5. Which side of your upper lip was fuller and prettier? Use that side as a model and follow the natural outline, using the dots to guide you. Start from the *outer* corner and draw a line with your lip pencil to the first dot. Then continue the line up to the dot directly under your nostril. This should be the high point of your cupid's bow. Next, round the line down to the center dot, which is the center of your mouth. Ah, ah! I saw you. You were twisting your mouth out of shape again. Keep it in a relaxed, natural position. There.

6. This is where those guidelines really help. Do the same thing to the other side of your upper lip, but this time correct

the shape to match the prettier side. See? It's much easier to match sides drawing short lines from dot to dot. To create a "smiling mouth," extend the lip line a fraction beyond the mouth corner, giving the line a tiny tilt.

To outline the lower lip, start at the mouth corner again, on the prettier side of your mouth, and follow the outline. Now correct the other side, making the lip fuller, narrower, or whatever is indicated.

About corrections: if you keep them subtle, no one will ever know. Enlarging the lips a quarter of an inch would create a grotesque, clown look. But changing the shape of your mouth by about the width of a pencil line will subtly make your lips seem fuller.

Once you have outlined your mouth to your new specifications, fill in with lipstick, using the tube to bring color right up to the pencil line.

What lipstick will you choose? Delicately frosted lipstick is best since it reflects the light and so makes the lips seem fuller. As a final touch, use a lip gloss to smooth the skin of the lips and give a shiny, moist look. The matte-finish mouth is definitely old. Translucent, shimmery, pearly . . . these are the qualities that are both young and in fashion. Lipstick color? Keep it light, keep it bright, keep it golden —and you can't go wrong.

However, you may be one of the many women who buys a lipstick called "Touch of Coral" and, after she applies it, finds that it turns a deep purple that could be called "Vampira's Kiss." This is easily corrected. Simply use an undercoat of green (yes, I said *green*) or yellow (yes, I said *yellow*) lipstick base to keep lipstick from turning dark. Many of the large cosmetic companies have these bases in their lipstick lines. You've probably seen them and wondered, "Who in the world would wear a green or a yellow lipstick?" Now you know.

A final word for those of you who find your lips getting smaller as the years tiptoe by. You can contour your mouth and create the impression of fullness by using this model's trick. Apply a gold or pearl lip glosser over your regular lipstick, but, instead of smoothing it over your lips in one continuous smear, highlight the fullest part of your lips by placing two highlights on the lower lip, two on the upper lip (just under the curves of the cupid's bow). Blend these highlights slightly with your fingertip but to do not blend the dots together. You should have four distinct highlights. You'll be amazed at how this little bit of magic creates the effect of full, curvaceous lips.

And *that's* how to put your best face forward.

"YES, BUT . . . WHO HAS TIME? *YOU* MAY BE ABLE TO SPEND TWO HOURS A DAY MAKING UP YOUR FACE, BUT I CAN'T"

I've heard variations of this comment since the very first make-up class I conducted. And the answer, then as now, is this. *No one* has time to spend hours on make-up . . . and *no one* who really knows what she's doing spends more than fifteen minutes to do a complete, razzle-dazzle make-up. Well, okay, say twenty-five minutes for a *big* evening.

I know this time schedule is possible because I have used it as a test for my make-up classes. All students not only have to learn to apply their own Ageless make-up plan but must do it within fifteen minutes. If they can do it, you can too.

They also learn another bit of make-up magic that adds just two extra minutes to that schedule. Can you devote two minutes to looking ten years younger? That's what I thought.

HOW TO APPLY ARTIFICIAL EYELASHES QUICK AS A WINK

If you've never worn artificial eyelashes you're in for a delightful surprise. The youthful effect they have on the mature face is nothing short of miraculous.

I remember one rather forebidding socialite whose face turned from grim to great with the simple addition of a pair of eyelashes. She was so thrilled, she literally danced around my studio like a little girl. She became a confirmed Lash Lady, and discovered this helpful tip for eyeglass wearers:

"If you can't see a bloody thing when you try to apply eyelashes (or any eye make-up) just put your glasses on *upside down.* They will perch on the end of your nose, allowing you to *see* and still get at the eye area."

Success starts in the store. If you know what to look for in buying those lashes, you'll save yourself a lot of trouble later.

1. Choose eyelashes with a delicate "strip." That's the thread to which the eyelash hairs have been tied. If lashes have a coarse strip, it will be stiff and will not conform to the curve of the eyelid.

2. Be daring. Choose lashes that are longer than you think

you'd *dare* to wear. You can always trim them, you know. And if you're like the majority of women I've worked with, you'll be surprised at how great these "longies" make you look. Lashes should be long and feathery. Buy length rather than thickness.

3. Choose brown, never black lashes.

4. Real hair lashes are the most natural and last the longest. Dynel lashes frizzle up if they get anywhere near heat—a fireplace, an oven.

5. *Most important.* Use Duo eyelash glue. It's the only kind I have found that really works. If you've had trouble with artificial eyelashes, it's probably because you're using that funny glue that comes with the lashes.

6. Don't be a sucker. Never spend more than $5.00 for lashes. I buy mine on sale for $1.00 to $1.95. Now that you know what to look for, you can too.

You'll find that lashes look more natural and go on easily if they fit. Don't expect to take them right out of the box and—zap!—glue them on your eyelid. They have to be tailored to *your* specifications.

1. Trim the strip to conform to your eye by holding the lash up to your eyelid with tweezers. (No glue yet.) It should be one eighth inch shorter than your eyelid. Measure both eyes; they are not alike. Note that lashes aren't interchangeable. There's a right and left side. Trim strip length at the *outer* edge where the lashes are longest.

2. Thin the lashes to give a natural look. Use sharp nail scissors to cut uneven lengths. Leave some lashes uncut. You should have a feathery, slightly uneven effect when finished. And if you wear glasses, you'll naturally trim the longest lashes a tiny bit so they don't flutter against the lenses of your specs.

3. Apply Duo eyelash glue by holding the lash with tweezers, the strip pointing up. Apply a small line of glue, about the diameter of a straight pin, to the *top* of the strip. Don't put it along the side, where it will run into the lash hairs.

4. Now. Holding the right eye closed with the left hand (V for Victory, remember?), place the outer corner of the right eyelash at the outer corner of your right eye. Use tweezers to place it, not your fingers. Hold the eyelash at the outer corner of your right eye for a slow count of ten. By that time it should stick. (This is a terrible time to sneeze.)

5. Next, take the tweezers and, by holding the lashes, position the strip at the center of your eyelid and then at the inner corner of your eye. The strip should be right on your own eyelash line. MOST IMPORTANT! At this stage, do not open your eye to see how gorgeous you are. Instead, be certain that the lashes are really stuck by using the blunt end of the tweezers to tap and press the strip along the full length of the eyelid. A count of twenty should do it. Now the lashes are really yours and won't pop off.

6. Okay. Open your eye. See? You *are* gorgeous. (Now don't forget to take your Pill.)

THE AGELESS FACE:
YOU CAN MISS IT BY A WHISKER

I don't mean to split hairs, but I must tell you that those middle-aged bristly whiskers have got to *go!* You don't have any? Are you sure?

I see so many (too many) lovely faces sporting everything from a few long, Fu Manchu hairs to a full-fledged mustache. And there's no excuse for it, when they can be removed so easily. Of course, electrolysis is one method for correcting this condition, but it's expensive and often painful. If you'll try facial wax to remove that hair, you'll find that it's easy to use and almost completely painless. (You do feel a twinge when you pull it off . . . zip!) But be brave and smile at that smooth, totally feminine face looking back at you in the mirror. You can keep smiling, too, because this method removes the hair root and so minimizes regrowth.

THE AGELESS LOOK:
YOU CAN MISS IT BY A HAIR

If facial hair is the ultimate in matronly frumpery, that glorious head of hair can be the essence of ageless beauty. Is yours? Let's see.

FOUR

Whatever Happened
To Your Crowning Glory?

That glorious head of hair! Whatever happened to it? If you're like
the majority of mature women, you've probably sacrificed your most
feminine feature on the altar of some high priestess of Professional
M.A.M.ism whose golden rule is, "Women of a 'certain age' should
never wear their hair long. In fact, it should be short, neat, and controlled."

Nothing could be further from the truth. The proof is that the
world's most glamorous Ageless Women, with few exceptions, prefer
longer hair styles. Their hair is voluminous, luxuriant, a veritable
mane—in short, sexy. What's more, their hair styles have another
feature in common: they all have a quality of elegant disarray.

Hair stylist George Masters, that darling of Hollywood and the jet
set, put it this way: "I detest the very word 'hairdressing.' I'd like to
invent a word that means 'unhairdressing.' If I preached anything, it
would be a gospel of artistic disorder in hairdos."

However, you'll never sell the Professional M.A.M. on this approach. She's dedicated to her own commandment (and you've heard it often, haven't you?): "Long hair is fine for young girls, but at our age, dear, a woman needs a short, neat coiffure." And to prove her point she has ruthlessly browbeaten all her friends, cousins, in-laws, acquaintances (every female she knows who is over thirty-five) into wearing the same uniform style. You know the one I mean. The Menopause Bob. It's that short, teased, shellacked, and grouted helmet that's ground out every Saturday afternoon at the beauty salons like so many sausages. It looks starched and ironed. Not one hair would *dare* be out of place.

It's sad to remember that this style is the grimly repressed great granddaughter of that carefree Italian cut of the fifties. The original of this style was part of the tousled, sultry look that (with a couple of other obvious assets) made Gina Lollobrigida so spectacular more than twenty years ago. But today that highly feminine style has evolved into the overteased, rigid helmet of hair that clutches the head of every Professional M.A.M. you know, totally destroying the last bit of her feminine appeal—which is exactly what she wants.

But what about *you?* Is that *really* what you want?

SOME THINGS YOU MAY HAVE FORGOTTEN ABOUT HAIR STYLES AND SEX APPEAL

Adam probably said it first—"Hair is sexy." Helen Gurley Brown, the duenna of all those alluring *Cosmopolitan* girls, said it again, and I'll repeat it. Hair, and lots of it, is sexy. You simply can't project a feminine image without a feminine hair style. In fact, next to your rounded, female body, your soft, pretty, *touchable* hair is your most feminine physical quality.

In our Western civilization, a woman's hair is a symbol of her sexuality. There are many examples of this symbolism. In conservative religious orders a woman cuts off her hair as a sign of her renunciation of the worldly life and as a mark of her celibate vows. In wartime, when a woman is suspected of consorting with the enemy, she is often shorn of her hair, a symbolic gesture that destroys her femininity. Finally, throughout the world, the matron traditionally hides and controls her hair as a sign that her days of being attractive to the opposite sex are over. This is especially true in peasant communities, where an older woman often affects a severe headdress that completely covers and controls her hair.

Hair as a universal symbol of sexuality has not been lost on the theatrical world. It is a familiar gimmick in Hollywood where visual shorthand is used to speak volumes. We're all familiar with these scenes from the Late, Late Show.

"It is really you, Miss Grundage? Without your glasses, and with your hair all soft and loose like that . . . why, I wouldn't have recognized the girl who works at the library every day. Do you think you could be happy as the wife of the college president?"

"Esther, you may be just a little dancing teacher from Walnutville, but when we get your hair out of those braids and put you into some nifty costumes, why, you'll be the toast of Broadway."

And then there's the old favorite. It usually stars someone like Joan Fontaine. In the "hair" scene, she's striding across the moors. Her sensible oxfords, shapeless tweed suit, and severe hair style express her character perfectly. She is the repressed spinster daughter of the village squire. But Cary Grant knows that beneath that Donegal tweed beats a smoldering heart. He catches up with her, takes her in his arms, and says, "Cynthia, there's something about you . . ." He takes the pins out of her severe hair style, and her long hair comes tumbling down. He starts kissing her. Wow! What a great scene.

Now, where was I? Oh yes. To get back to the point, the change from a severe, completely controlled hair style to a flowing, free look is a classic visual symbol of awakened femininity and sex appeal. So, if you want to proclaim that you are still a woman, forget all that nonsense about short, neat hair styles.

However, this does bring us to another consideration. Since woman's hair is so definitely a sex symbol, she must be careful. In the process of proclaiming that she's a woman, she must take care that her appearance also says that she's a lady. How does the mature woman find the middle ground between the "flashy," flowing mane of a show girl and the short controlled styles that spell matron? And how can she answer such questions as, "Is this style too young for me?" or "Does this style make me look older than my years?" or . . .

"HOW CAN I FIND THAT AGELESS, FEMININE HAIR STYLE?"

The answer should be familiar by now. The Ageless Woman follows fashion and adapts it to her specific needs. However, following the fashion trends in hair styling isn't as easy as following fashion in clothing or make-up, which may explain why so many unwilling M.A.M.s have traded their crowning glory for that Menopause Bob.

FASHION: CAN IT GO TO YOUR HEAD?

Many mature women find that their search for a fashionable hair style that is also appropriate, feminine, and glamorous can be an almost impossible goal. But, once again, the difficulty lies not with fashion but with a misunderstanding of fashion and its evolution.

If you look to the fashion magazines for direction, it seems that they are totally inconsistent. Although the beauty editors may breathlessly tell us that "the new look in hair is the short, short, cut. Simply blow it dry, and wear it like a shiny cap," you will look in vain for another example of this style. All the other models in the magazine are generally wearing their hair long and wavy, bouffant and curly, or, in fact, in any other style you can imagine except the one the editors are touting.

The explanation, of course, is that today there is no single style—at least not in the sense that a "style" existed a few years ago. Remember when everyone wanted to wear The Hairdo? It might have been the Italian, the bubble, or the bouffant; but during that time *everyone* wore basically the same hair style. And that very philosophy is what dates the mature woman's look. She is still clinging to a version of The Hairdo from her past.

But today there is no single hair style that is *right*. Today the trend of fashion can be summed up in one word—*health*. In his *Complete Book on Hair*, Kenneth Battelle (the famed Kenneth whose clients have included Gloria Vanderbilt, Joanne Woodward, and Jacqueline Onassis) explains it this way: "The great new hair fashion of today is *health*. This is a time of beautiful hair, luxurious hair, shiny hair, healthy hair. It can be long to the waist, or an inch long all over the head. It can be curly. It can be bone straight."

This analysis is accurate on one level and has been followed by the world's most beautiful and fashionable women, as we shall see in a moment. However, the mature woman must realize that this approach, while original and totally effective when practiced by experts, can become a beauty disaster if it is oversimplified. And unfortunately, oversimplification is what we usually get from the corner beauty salon. By the time this "Health is Beauty" theory has trickled down from the hair-styling maestros of the haute couture to the

corner beauty salon, it has usually degenerated to something like
this!

"Now look, luv. All that teasing and curling is passé now. What
you need is the natural look—the 'little nothing' style—uncluttered,
easy-to-care-for hair. Let's just give you a divine little blower cut and
forget all those ghastly rollers, shall we?" So you're lulled into it,
with the promise that it's a style that's practical (bad vibes for the
mature face) and easy to care for (so are tennis shoes). Snip, snip,
snip. There goes your hair. And how do you look?

Quite possibly, you look like hell.

This is certainly what happened to Norma, a friend of mine who is
finally recovering from one of these "little nothing" hair styles. Everyone considered Norma a real beauty. Her pale olive skin and dark
eyes contrasted with her glorious hair, which was long, thick, and the
color of new wheat—she was a knockout.

Because her hair was quite long (about four inches below her
shoulders) she usually wore it in a soft swirl on top of her head. But
I remember informal occasions when she looked fabulous with all
that thick blonde hair twisted into a single braid, entwined with col-
ored yarn, and worn hanging down her back.

Then she had it cut. And suddenly Norma became a M.A.M.
Just as a magician uses sleight of hand to distract you from what he
doesn't want you to see, Norma's beautiful hair had distracted the
eye from wrinkles, a slight double chin, and heavens, even a rather
outsized nose.

There's a lesson here for all mature women. The older you get *the
more help you need from your hair.* That doesn't mean that every
woman should wear long, dramatic hair styles. Sometimes a short,
perky style is exactly right for a woman's features and hair, although
the odds are against it. However, the "little nothing" hair style is
definitely a beauty loser for the mature woman.

WINNING HAIR STYLES

The hair style of the Ageless Woman will always have three winning qualities:

1. *Volume.* A look of thickness. A luxuriant mane implies
health and vitality, definitely ageless qualities.

2. *"Artistic Disorder."* The hair style that is too neat, too con-

trolled, or totally severe in its effect is instantly aging. What's more, it creates the immediate impression of inflexibility, repression, and sexlessness.

But a bit of artistic disorder has been a woman's weapon for ages. Over three hundred and fifty years ago, an Ageless Woman inspired Ben Jonson to write:

> Give me a look, give me a face,
> That makes simplicity a grace;
> Robes loosely flowing, hair as free.
> Such sweet neglect more taketh me
> Than all the adulteries of art;
> They strike mine eyes, but not my heart.

3. *A Feminine Hairline.* The French writer Colette said that a woman's face, like a flower, needs to be framed by tendrils. A charming idea, and one that creates a totally feminine look.

Let's discuss these qualities in detail and see how you can create the three ageless effects.

VOLUME

WINNERS (AGELESS LOOKS)	LOSERS (OLD LOOKS)
You'll look ageless in hair styles that:	You'll look older in hair styles that:
Create height at the top of your head and fullness around the face (gives the contours a lift)	Are flat at top of the head, sparse around the face (emphasize drooping contours)
Have volume at the crown of your head (offsets a double chin and softened jawline)	Are flat at the crown (emphasize fullness at the jaw and double trouble at the chin line)
Have some length and volume (camouflage softened contours, distract from signs of age)	Are skimpy and head-hugging (reveal all facial defects, signs of age)

Hair that is thick and luxuriant implies health and vitality. Sparse, thin hair implies age and tired glands. Today, almost every woman can create the effect of thick, luxuriant hair. Many artificial methods for creating this volume look have been developed recently, which is one of the reasons that it has become the very basis of the current trend. There are three basic methods for creating this look of volume.

1. *Body-Building Products.* These fillers, usually with a protein base, penetrate the hair shaft and give more volume to fine, limp hair. If you haven't tried them, I think you'll be delighted with the results. But use caution, because prolonged use may cause breakage. Many experts suggest that you use them only two weeks at a time and then let your hair rest for a week.

The fillers will give you volume, but too many women neglect the next step—which is to achieve the healthy hair look. And it's sad, because it's such a simple step. All you have to do is treat your hair to an effective conditioner as part of your shampoo routine.

If you've gone year in and year out without a regular conditioning program, your hair's been neglected—and it inevitably looks it.

There are many products that actually repair damaged hair, so resolve now to embark on a regular conditioning program.

I suspect that many women don't condition their hair because they think it's too much trouble. It's true that really elaborate conditioning treatments can involve warmed oils, heatcaps, scalp message, and so on. But new conditioning products now on the market are completely simple. They involve two steps: buy them and apply them. A little conscientious label reading will guide you to these supersimple yet effective treatments.

2. *The "Blunt" Cut.* This technique in haircutting has become increasingly popular in recent years as another way to add thickness and body to your hair. It involves cutting straight across each hair, instead of feathering the ends. The blunt cut leaves the end of each hair as thick as the entire hair shaft. In the hands of true experts, this approach can indeed add body to your hair. But, for reasons that I'll discuss later, I think it's the least effective way to give your hair that desired body and thickness.

3. *Backcombing.* Every woman over twelve knows that you can add volume to your hair style with this old faithful technique. But a quick glance around will convince you that few women know how to use it effectively. Backcombing does not mean "teasing" your hair till it bites you. It does mean backcombing a "base" into your hair style, which will give the hair a *natural* appearance of thickness and body.

You may be very adept at doing your own hair, but are you *sure* you aren't backcombing and teasing an extra ten years onto your appearance every morning? Let's be sure you're subtracting, not adding, by reviewing this simple technique. This is how you do it.

Start by *brushing* your hair thoroughly from front to back. This pulls the set together and distributes the curl. Part off the area you want to backcomb. The crown of the head, for example. (And most of us should create volume and height at the crown.)

With your rattail comb, part off a small section of hair and hold it straight up from your scalp with your fingers. Starting about half an inch from the scalp, comb this strand of hair toward the scalp, bunching it down near the scalp and creating an effect of thickness in the strand. Comb each section this way four or five times, working up from half an inch to an inch and a half from the scalp. *Do not backcomb clear to the end of the strand.*

Keep parting off small sections, backcombing the base, and leaving the ends free. To add fullness at the sides of the face, part the hair vertically, pulling the strands slightly toward the face when you backcomb to create the maximun volume at the sides.

Now take your hairbrush and smooth the hair into its style, taking care not to brush down into the "base" you have created, except around the hairline. You'll see that this subtle form of backcombing gives your hair body and a gentle control without spoiling the effect of a natural, "real hair" coiffure.

You'll finish off with a light spritz of hair spray, but not until you've added this ageless effect.

THAT QUALITY OF ARTISTIC DISORDER

WINNERS (AGELESS LOOKS)	LOSERS (OLD LOOKS)
You'll look ageless in hairstyles that:	You'll look older in hair styles that:
Have movement—longer hair should be able to move and swing and shorter hair should have curls that bounce	Are too neat, totally controlled
	Are immobile—Hurricane Helen wouldn't budge them

| Invite a touch, because the hair looks *real* (even if it's your favorite hairpiece) | Are teased into a wad and then sprayed and lacquered—become totally untouchable |

Losers in the age game have the mistaken idea that facial contours that have been slightly blurred by age will be put back into focus by a neat and rigid hair style. Visually, this is exactly the wrong approach to offset the subtle signs of age, because by contrast the sharp outlines of a rigid hair style tend to contrast with and emphasize facial contours that have been softened by the years. Severe hair styles are only for those with flawless features and perfect bone structure—the line forms to the right.

Most of us need a hair style that will camouflage and complement softened facial contours. We must strive for an effect of softness and, yes, even a tousled look. Here's how to do it.

If your hair is short to medium long (anywhere between the earlobe and the shoulder line), backcomb a base into your hair, then brush it into its basic style shape. Now shake your head from side to side to put a little air into your set and to allow the hair to fall naturally into the waves and curls that the set has created. Use your hands to gently shape the line, fingertips to separate ends that may have become clumped together.

Next, take a large hairpin and gently lift some strands from the top layer of hair, flipping the ends out to create a tousled effect here and there. *Now* you spray the hair. Lightly.

If you have really long hair, like Mérle Oberon for example, be sure that your hair style isn't a production number, what Kenneth calls "pastry chef sculptures that you can't run your fingers through without breaking a fingernail."

Next to the Menopause Bob, the Wedding Cake Cascade is the most aging hair style you can wear. This familiar little number features a topknot of gleaming fake curls, sculptured and shellacked into a completely immobile concoction that sits incongruously atop the *real* hair.

If you like the look of long hair worn up on top, be sure that it looks as if it's all yours, whether it is or not. Then avoid the look of a construction job, with every hair nailed into place by a battery of bobby pins. The ideal to strive for is to look as if you've just given your flowing locks a single twist, then put in two pins to hold it in place. If you happened to meet Cary Grant on the moors, he would just have to remove those two pins and your glorious hair would come tumbling down. (No, Cary, no! This is madness. . . .)

A FEMININE HAIRLINE

WINNERS (AGELESS LOOKS)	LOSERS (OLD LOOKS)
You'll look ageless in hairstyles that:	You'll look older in hair styles that:
Are drawn *softly* back from the face	Pull hair severely away from the face, pulling the skin taut
Feature tendrils and little waves at the hairline	Create a forbiddingly neat back-of-the-neck. Long hair pulled tight at the back of the neck is
Create a soft and feminine look at the back of the neck. Long hair can be cut so there are tendrils at the back. Short hair should be long to have a little curl or wave	spinsterish. Short hair that is blunt cut straight across or (shudder) shaved is . . . unbelievable

A mature woman should never wear her hair pulled back severely. This is especially unattractive when the hair is pulled so tight that the skin is pulled too. Such a hair style creates the impression that the facial skin is wasted and flabby, but psychologically it projects the image of your spinster aunt. Instead, the hair should be drawn back from the face loosely. When you bring the hair back from the face, or pull it up at the neckline, it should always have enough "give" so that you can push it back toward the face or neck, creating a soft fullness at the hairline. A "Gibson" style is a perfect example of the effect I mean.

If your hair is short or if you wear it up on top, you must pay special attention to your exposed neckline. The back of the neck is one of a woman's most feminine features. It may be slender and vulnerable or rounded and appealing, but it should always be graced with softness at the hairline—a tiny wave, curl or delicate tendril.

The back of your neck should *not* look squat and forbiddingly neat and covered with stubble. Five o'clock shadow on the neckline is an impossible image for the Ageless Woman. Remember, you don't want a totally neat and controlled neckline. If you wear your hair short, the hair at the neck should be taper-cut and left long enough to wave or curl.

Delicate tendrils around the face are becoming to almost everyone, and you can cut them yourself, this way. Part off a tiny section of hair next to your face or at your neckline. With nail scissors, taper-cut this strand at about one and a half to two inches long. Taper-cut? That means seesaw the scissors back and forth as you cut, so that the ends of the strand are uneven.

When you set your hair, roll these tiny strands on small rollers turned *toward* the face. Now, when you brush your hair, prior to backcombing it, brush these small strands right in with the rest of your hair. After combing your hair, and before spraying, take your fingers and push the hair around your face, coaxing these short hairs into a subtle wave or curl right at your hairline.

When you use hair spray, use this simple trick that is a favorite of Alexandre of Paris (Elizabeth Taylor wouldn't make a move without him). Put your hand directly over your hairline, covering any tendrils or little curls so that the spray doesn't touch them. That way, the hairline will always have the soft, approachable look that's so femi-nine.

Alexandre also uses this technique in other ways. For hair that's worn on top, he'll often pull out several longer strands or tendrils and cover them when spraying the rest of the hair. These tendrils will then have a bouncy, natural look—and, again, create that qual-ity of artistic disarray. Or he may pull forward all the hair around the hairline, spray the rest of the hair, and then smooth the unsprayed portion back over the sprayed base. The front hair is then totally soft and free to fall over the side of the cheek or to be pushed back with a graceful feminine gesture. (You devil!)

BEWARE THE "ARTFUL CURL"

While curls around the face are becoming to the mature woman, they must be soft and indistinct. The corkscrew curl, so often the bumptious companion of that Wedding Cake Cascade, is totally aging . . . and a little sad. It comes under the heading of Trying Too Hard. However, if you'll use the techniques I've described, you'll instead give the casual impression that "I've been to a better party than this."

MORE WINNERS AND LOSERS

Just as optical illusion can camouflage signs of age in the body, fool-the-eye tricks in hair styles can make your face appear younger.

What signs are we talking about? Two of the most prevalent after-forty signs are a softened jawline (could that little pillow of flesh *really* be called a jowl?) and a chin line that, if not quite double, at least rates a one and a half. At this time, a woman's neck may lose its youthful roundness and start to look a bit scrawny, and of course some of the facial contours may tend to droop. Sounds a bit depressing, doesn't it? Never fear—

NOW YOU SEE IT, NOW YOU DON'T

Constructive diet and exercise can keep these conditions to a minimum (as you shall see). Meanwhile, use hair-styling tricks to minimize these conditions.

1. *Double Chin and Jowls.* To counteract this contour, it is essential to create fullness at the crown of the head at about a 45-degree angle from the point of the chin. This visually counterbalances the fullness in the chin and jaw area. If the hair is accented too far forward, there are all those chins, just hanging out for everyone to see. And if the accent is too far down, toward the neck, it makes the neck and jawline appear that much thicker.

You can create this counterbalancing fullness by wearing your hair up, with the volume of hair concentrated at the 45-degree spot. Or if you wear your hair loose, in a casual pageboy for example, be sure that you have backcombed a base at the crown of your head. Use your trusty hairpin to pull the lower hair up a little, creating the counterbalancing fullness in the necessary area.

If your hair is short, never wear it flat at the crown. Any curls should come far enough back on the head to create fullness at the crown. This hair-styling trick is almost magical. Try it. You'll like it.

2. *Scrawny Neck and Jowls.* Longer hair does wonders to soften these signs of age. Hair that is long enough to cover the sides of the cheeks and to shadow the neck will do a subtle job of distracting from these agemakers. But if long hair is to be flattering, the style must have the correct line direction. Lank hair, falling in a straight line down the sides of the face, will make any woman look like Haggard Harriet. Which brings us to point number 3.

3. *Drooping facial contours.* The magic of the up line can visually lift drooping contours to a surprising degree. This doesn't mean that your hair must always be pulled straight up on top of your head. It does mean that the dominant line of your coiffure has an upward direction. This sounds so obvious, but look at your "favorite" M.A.M.'s hair. Notice what happens when the sides of her hair are swept *back* from the face, rather than *up.* A subtle difference, but the effect on a mature face is far from subtle. Even if you wish to wear your hair down at the sides, be sure that there is an *up* line at the temples, before your hair sweeps down at the sides of your face. Finally, be sure that any *up* lines in your hair style follow the line of the 45-degree angle that leads to the crown of your head.

THE LONG AND THE SHORT OF IT

One final word about long and short hair. Many fashion experts kindly suggest that the "woman who is getting on in years" (they mean over forty—can you believe it?) should wear her hair up and away from her neck, because age tends to make the neck shorter and thicker. Pooh to that! Longer hair at the neckline, whether in the form of tendrils, tapered curls (as in a long "shag"), or just long swinging hair (with the "winning" up lines), will make every woman this side of seventy look younger, more feminine, and glamorous.

Of course, if you're five feet one and weigh 220 pounds, your neck will look short and thick anyway. So wear your hair up at the sides and down in back, covering the sides of that sturdy neck. And promise me you'll go on a diet.

"YES, BUT—I'M STILL UNCERTAIN ABOUT WHICH HAIR STYLES ARE APPROPRIATE FOR MY AGE"

"You keep recommending longer hair, little tendrils, sexy styles . . . won't I look like an old fool in these young hair styles? How can I be sure they're appropriate for me?"

This is a fair question, since we have pointed out that you can't depend on the fashion magazines to give concrete fashion information about hair styles. However, would you believe that I'm going to tell you how to answer that question?

There's a foolproof way to find the most appropriate hair fashions for women in our age group. We turn to the Ageless Women who are spotlighted on the fashion, beauty, and social pages of magazines and newspapers—who are seen on the movie and TV screens. We study the Beautiful People. And we copy them.

WILL THE REAL ANGIE DICKINSON PLEASE STAND UP?

Pick a model, actress, TV star, or celebrity whose facial contours and type are similar to yours, and imitate her. Of course you'll choose someone in your approximate age bracket. (And should you choose someone a little bit younger, could it hurt?) But do choose a woman who is known for her fashion and beauty know-how. Queen Elizabeth or performers on the Lawrence Welk show don't qualify.

Beauty authority Emily Wilkens tells how to copy your model. "Suppose, for instance, you've analyzed your looks and find you are the Audrey Hepburn type—tall, slim, narrow, longish nose, marvelous eyes. Play Sherlock Holmes and track down her every photograph." The idea is to see how she's wearing her hair in the current season . . . and then copy it.

But suppose you're not tall and slim and narrow? The curvacious Gabors have squarish faces, less than sharp jawlines, short necks. Blonde or not, you might choose to copy them if your face and figure are round, feminine, and slightly padded.

Don't laugh. It's really easy once you've tried it. It's good for you, too, to continue to think of yourself in terms of the most glamorous women in the world. (Anyone who hoots and says, "Who me? And Audrey Hepburn?" goes to the back of the class and sits with the other Professional M.A.M.s!)

This little trick turned one of my students into a real beauty . . . and a television performer besides.

Sally was raised with four brothers, so she was always treated like a tomboy by her family and friends. When her own marriage produced three boys, she continued this outdoor, no-nonsense image. She came to my classes almost by accident when the members of her club decided to take modeling lessons to prepare for their annual fashion show. As president, she had to participate.

What a Cinderella story! Sally started as the most awkward, unwilling student I can remember. But as we progressed through the

lessons it was a joy to see the galloping tomboy gradually transformed into a graceful woman. Apparently she had never wanted to
be a tomboy at all. But she didn't know what else to be—or how to
go about being it. Angie Dickinson changed all that.

At the fashion show fittings, I watched her happily posing before
the fitting-room mirror in white crepe evening pajamas—at last out
of her eternal shirtwaist dresses—and it dawned on me that, with the
right hair style, she'd be the image of TV star Angie Dickinson.

She had the same high cheekbones and smiling eyes. She had
another Dickinson trademark—a cleft in her chin. And to top it all
off, she even had that same thousand-watt smile.

However, it took a practiced eye to spot the glamorous creature
that was hidden under Sally's impossible old-maid hair style. She'd
been wearing her mousy brown hair in a tightly plaited braid,
wrapped sternly around her head. If she was to lose that sexless tomboy image, she needed an emergency trip to the hairdresser, which I
tactfully suggested. (You know how touchy women can be about
their hair.)

To my surprise, she immediately agreed to a total restyling, and astonished me further by asking, "Do you think my hair could be
bleached a little too?" Yes, Sally had really gotten into the spirit of
the transformation. I think we could have called in the plastic surgeon and she wouldn't have batted an eye.

But these drastic measures weren't necessary. Instead, we took several pictures of Angie Dickinson to my favorite hair stylist, Mario.

With a fine Italian hand, he trimmed off all those split ends and
prescribed a conditioner for Sally's hair, which had been pulled and
twisted into those damned braids for years. After his skillful cut, a
touch of bleach, a subtle golden rinse, and a superb conditioner,
Sally emerged from the salon with a carefree blonde mane. The
transformation was complete. She looked fantastic!

When the big day arrived, she was the hit of the show. But the
Cinderella story doesn't stop there. Sally enjoyed her new image so
much that she collected all the pictures of Angie Dickinson she
could find, copied her style exactly, and soon perfected that glamorous yet outdoorsy look.

One day, when she was having lunch with some friends, a man
came over to their table, introduced himself as a leading local car
dealer, and said, "We've been looking for an Angie Dickinson type
to do a series of commercials on a new station wagon we're introduc-
ing. Would you be interested in being our Town and Country Girl?"

Would she? What do you think? Sally had an exciting two weeks doing three commercials for this firm. And did she go on to bigger and better commercials, movies, Broadway? Well, no. But the ego-building results of this experience changed her whole attitude about herself as a woman. I know that she's more confident and outgoing than she was before . . . and I suspect it's put a little pezazz back into that twenty-year marriage. The last time I saw them, I noticed that he wasn't calling her Sal or Dutch, which had been her nicknames. No, now it was strictly Baby. Is that a good sign? I ask you!

WILL THE REAL YOU PLEASE STAND UP?

And what about being original? Fashion and beauty experts are always nagging you to be individual—"express your unique beauty image"—but unless you're a fashion pace setter, "original" usually translates to "weird." The *real* original is rare indeed. And her original and distinctive look is, more often than not, the result of long and careful analysis by a battery of skilled (and *very* expensive) beauty experts.

As Sally said, "I figure that Angie Dickinson (or her studio) must have spent thousands of dollars hiring experts to match a hair style to her features and type. Since we look alike, and are the same type, I'm able to take advantage of all that expert advice and find out exactly what's most becoming to me—and it's all free."

So remember Sally. Don't try to be original. Almost everybody looks a bit like some fabulous woman in the public eye. Everybody is a "type." So choose your model and copy her brazenly.

OLDIES BUT GOODIES FOR YOU TO COPY

You might find your double among the following list of famous beauties, women who can—and do—consult the leading hair-styling artists in the world to find the look that's most becoming to the Ageless Woman. I've included an approximate age with each name, just to prove to you that being forty or fifty (or even seventy) doesn't preclude a hair style that makes the most of your crowning glory.

There isn't a Menopause Bob in the bunch.

Jacqueline Onassis. (Mid-forties.) She has been called "Her Elegance," and her modified Kenneth coiffure is an essential part of her inimitable style. She wears her hair fairly long, anywhere from an inch below the ears to shoulder length. The ends may be turned under or flipped up, but the over-all effect is one of a long full mane of healthy hair.

Merle Oberon. (Mid-fifties.) Throughout the sixties and early 1970s the fashion and decorating magazines made a yearly pilgrimage to the unique Acapulco home of Merle Oberon. All of these stories featured photographs of Merle in a caftan or bathing suit, with her black, waist-length hair flowing free. She looked terrific, at once both exotic and feminine. On more formal occasions (remember her spectacular appearance at a recent Academy Awards telecast?) she wears her "mane" swirled into a *soft,* uncomplicated pouf at the crown of her head.

Countess de Romanones. (Fifty-plus.) This stunning American woman, married to one of Spain's most distinguished noblemen, was recently photographed for *Town and Country* magazine in a feature celebrating the joys of being fifty. The article was accompanied by a series of glamorous photographs showing her with her long dark hair flowing free over her shoulders in at-home clothes (white lace patio pajamas, for instance) or swirled up on top (just two pins, remember) in a simple pouf as an accent to her elegant leather riding costume.

Elizabeth Taylor. (Forty-plus.) The Ultimate Brunette, she wears her hair in a variety of styles. However, they all have the essential qualities of length, volume, and movement. In her film *Ash Wednesday,* she wears her shoulder-length hair up, in the swirl we should be familiar with by now. Or slightly puffed out with tendrils around the face, then casually drawn back with a ribbon.

Dina Merrill. (Mid-forties.) *Harper's Bazaar* describes her as "all the things an American woman aspires to be." An accomplished actress, businesswoman (Amaranthe cosmetics), wife (her husband is actor Cliff Robertson), and mother, she has the fine-boned blonde looks that are the essence of the American beauty. For years she has worn her sweep of blonde hair in a Kenneth hair style, the length and fullness modified according to the current fashion trends. Sometimes she wears it pulled back in the "Status Pull."

Zsa-zsa and Eva. (Age? Who knows? Young they're not. But ageless? Yes.) A different type of blonde, the Heavenly Hungarians have made a trademark of their spun-sugar hair styles. Elegant for evening wear, ideal for the boudoir (Dahling, vot could be more important?), this style is a bit much for everyday wear. However, the superfeminine Ageless Woman can modify this look by keeping the waves and tendrils around the face, and then simply pulling the hair back loosely, or giving it a twist and securing it in a *simple* knot at the crown of the head.

Marie-Hélène de Rothschild. (Early forties.) "Officially, she is the Baronesse Guy de Rothschild. But to friends and to France, she is simply Marie-Hélène . . . her country's extroverted answer to Jacqueline Onassis." That's how this spirited Dutch-Egyptian beauty was described by the New York *Times* on a recent visit to New York. For this interview, she was wearing a suede Dior cape over a rust-colored skirt and sweater set, a spectacular amber necklace at her throat. These tawny colors matched "her full mane of auburn hair," which she wears full, loose, and shoulder length—at least for daytime wear.

Mrs. Aileen Mehle—"SUZY." (Her age? A closely guarded secret. In 1963 she was quoted as saying, "Just say my son is twenty-one—and I'm thirty-one." Hmmm, let's see, that makes her over forty, at the *very* least.) Known to thirty million gossip-hungry readers as "Suzy," Aileen Mehle has been described by *Vogue* as "this petite, cat-eyed, toughly fragile, craftily tousle-topped blonde. . . ." Her hair is a long-short cut, about five to seven inches long around her face, worn in a tumble of waves and curls that is both youthful and seductive. She embodies that word "glamor." As Suzy says, "Glamor will never die. It is the whipped cream on top of everything."

Marlene Dietrich. (After seventy, we all stopped counting.) What can you say about this legend, except—what she doesn't know about being the Ageless Woman just isn't worth knowing. Now in her seventies, she is still glamorous, still beautiful, still a *woman.* And she still wears her blonde hair rather full, in loose waves around her face, then turned under in an above-the-shoulder-length pageboy.

Barbara Walters. (Forty-plus.) *Time* magazine recently put her on their cover and called her "Star of the morning . . . television's queen." Barbara not only proves that brains and beauty go together (has any woman ever doubted it?) but she also follows our A.W. formula. She wears her sun-streaked hair quite long, with width and fullness created by soft waves around her face.

A series of photographs in that *Time* article provide a graphic example of how the right hair style can contribute to the image of the Ageless Woman. Several current photos show long-haired Barbara as a glamorous celebrity—truly one of the Beautiful People. And then, in a photo taken in 1967, there's Barbara in a short-short skimpy little hair style. She looks years older (and far less attractive) than she does today.

There are a few Ageless Beauties who wear their hair short (though not many, which just proves my point). Two examples would be Audrey Hepburn and Polly Bergen. Though they're both over forty, they have a facial characteristic in common, one that makes short hair possible for them. They both have strong, well-defined jawlines and if your facial structure is similar to theirs, maybe—just maybe—a short haircut may be right for you. But the odds are against it.

However, finding the hair style that's right for you isn't your only consideration. What about color?

GRAY HAIR: IS IT A WINNER OR A LOSER?

A time will come, inevitably, when you'll ask yourself this question about your own silver threads. Leslie Blanchard, Manhattan's master hair colorist, gave this definitive answer: "One must be *young* to have gray hair." He went on to explain that a woman must have a young face to wear gray hair effectively. The older you are, the older your gray hair will make you look—and feel.

Kenneth (my favorite expert) feels that graying hair can be stunning when the original hair color is dramatic—deep black hair, strong red hair, or very blonde. However, going gray can be a real loser if your hair is an in-between shade. It makes the hair look drab and dull, and it's liable to make you *feel* drab and dull.

Another consideration is your skin tone. If your complexion is sallow or an in-between tone, the lack of contrast between your skin and your graying hair can make you look like a "before" model for Geritol. On the other hand, women with very pale or dark skin who find their hair turning gray often discover a brand-new beauty dimension. Latin types and black women can be stunning with a silver mane.

If you decide to stay on the silver standard, you still must beware of the "Mary Worth" image that is implied by your graying locks. You can do this by avoiding the safe, conservative hair styles we associate with graying hair. Young, dramatic, even girlish styles are highly effective on gray-haired women. Surprise? Let me give you some examples.

> *Seen at the Supermarket;* A tiny woman about five feet tall, with a well-proportioned figure and young face, was wearing her

totally silver shoulder-length hair pulled up at the sides, tied with a red ribbon, and swinging loose and free in the back. She looked absolutely sensational, and I told her so.

Seen at the Beach; A Katharine Hepburn type, thin and lanky. Her thick red hair, laced with silver strands, was worn in two pigtails. It was naturally curly, and the damp air turned every little wisp into a wave or ringlet. Did this style make her look twenty again? Hardly. But she looked casual, distinctive—like *somebody.* And I don't mean somebody's mother.

Seen at a Restaurant in San Francisco; The Lady in Red. Her scarlet dress was a perfect foil for deep olive skin and totally white hair. It was styled in a dramatic asymmetrical cut, very short on one side and swept back over the ear. The other side of her hair was chin-length and waved into a soft wing that curved over her cheek. A neat lesson in How to Look Fantastic at Fifty.

Another suggestion for those who are devoted to their gray hair is to have it highlighted around the face. Ask your beautician about this. It's a solution when hair is about fifty per cent gray yet hasn't developed the dramatic impact of totally light hair. What's involved? Selected strands around the face are treated with a lightener and then wrapped in foil for a timed period to bleach them to their lightest color. The total effect is finished with a platinum rinse.

Or suppose your hair is medium brown and laced with gray—just enough to make you look like That Nice Little Woman Next Door. Get out of that apron and into a blonde rinse.

A temporary rinse in a golden-blonde shade is an easy way to achieve a sun-streaked effect on graying brown or blonde hair. Redheads might try one of the pinkish-blonde shades. A blonde rinse won't work on all graying hair but is terribly effective on most. It's an easy and inexpensive way to lift yourself out of those gray-lady doldrums. And it will help you decide if you want to do something more permanent about your hair color.

DOES SHE OR DOESN'T SHE? SHOULD YOU?

Frankly, I think the decision to color your hair should be based on one consideration only—will it make you *feel* better? There's just no getting around it. Gray hair is a symbol of age—so if your hair is going mousily gray and it's getting you down, change the color—and join the club. It's estimated that over fifty per cent of the females in the United States use some hair-coloring product. So why shouldn't you?

Aside from graying hair, the mature woman finds she has two other physical reasons for giving her looks a lift via a color change.

1. *Drab Hair.* Although your hair may not be turning gray, it may be losing some of its natural color and brightness, framing your face in a sort of taupe brown—hardly the most becoming color in the world!

2. *Changing Skin Tone.* Sometimes your skin tone changes with age and becomes paler or yellower than it was. As one student said, "My hair isn't getting gray. *I* am." Although I'm sure it's not as bad as all that, you may find that brightening your hair color can effectively offset your changing complexion tones.

Once you decide to take the step, there's no question that you can find some hair-coloring shade that will be madly becoming. Just avoid these common errors that many mature women make, errors that can turn artificial color into a much more aging look than gray hair ever was.

That Old Black Magic—won't work for you if you're over thirty. Unless you are of oriental or Indian extraction, do *not* try to recapture the deep brunette shades of your youth. Jet-black and deep brown shades make pale skin look positively wan and give you a cheap, hard look. The same is true of intense red shades.

Shanghai Lil—Brassy, bright, all-one-color, doxy-blonde hair is bad news on everyone. The mature woman tends to look like the aging you-know-what-with-a-heart-of-gold to match her gleaming hair.

The Blahs—You'll look as if you've got them, if your hair-color change is too timid. This is the most common mistake of all, to change the hair just one or two shades, so that skin and hair are all one tone. If you're going to do it, *do it!*

You can avoid these three mistakes by following the advice of such experts as Kenneth Battelle and Leslie Blanchard.

Kenneth says, "Generally speaking, as you get older, make your hair lighter than its original natural shade." If you've been trying to do this, yet find that your hair color always comes out darker than you had intended, remember that color on color produces a darker color. The hair-coloring product you use, combined with the natural color still in your hair, combines to create a shade much darker than that indicated on the color chart of the product. So always choose a shade much lighter than the color you are striving for.

Brunettes, as well as blondes, will benefit from this suggestion by Leslie Blanchard. Observing that a child's hair is never just one solid shade, he strives for gradations of color. This tone-on-tone approach, which gives a natural, youthful hair color, is accomplished by first bleaching strands of hair, usually around the face. Then, when the toner or tint is applied (whether you're a brunette, blonde, or redhead), the result will be subtle gradations of color, rather than the "I dunked my head in a bucket of paint" look that is all too familiar. Often, a skilled colorist will use four or five toners to get the subtle effects he wants. The result is natural, young, becoming—and expensive.

A more inexpensive way to make a dramatic hair change is streaking. It's also a sure cure for the blahs. As Kenneth says, "It gives an exaggerated color change and yet has some relationship to one's own coloring." Streaking is done by bleaching fairly large strands of hair around the face and is much more effective for the mature woman than frosting.

You're probably familiar with frosting—it's the old tourniquet-on-the-head trick, with tiny strands of hair being pulled through holes in that tight rubber frosting cap. The strands are then saturated with bleach. At its best, the effect is so subtle that it's hardly worth the expense. At its worst, it can create the look of gray and silver threads among the gold.

So generally, you're better off to have your hair *streaked*. It's a bolder approach that creates a healthy, sun-kissed look that's dramatic, too—always an effective image for the Ageless Woman.

Should you do it yourself? That depends on the kind of person you are. I have friends who can cut, color, and permanent their hair (not all at the same time) with the skill of professionals. Other women can't even seem to get a comb through their hair without looking as if "loving hands at home" had designed their hair style. However, whether you're adept or addled, the best advice is to *start* by going to professionals. Observe what they do. Ask questions. Then try some of the simplest, one-step hair-coloring products to start.

Whether you are concerned with hair coloring or hair styling, it's a good idea to start with professional care. That is, it's usually a good idea. But sometimes professionals can be your biggest problem, if you let them.

WHY YOU AREN'T GETTING THE RESULTS YOU WANT FROM YOUR HAIRDRESSER, OR HOW TO COMMUNICATE WITH MR. BEVERLY

It's one thing to decide on a new, ageless, glamorous, exciting hair style—but can you get it? According to many of the women I've talked to, the chances are slim. In fact, the universal complaint seems to be, "My hairdresser doesn't do my hair the way I *really* want it."

Well, whose fault is it? Sorry, but it's basically yours. Because you and Mr. Beverly (or Margo or Suzette) just aren't communicating.

First of all, *you* must decide what you want. None of this, "I put myself completely in your hands. I want something different." Unless you're totally familiar with his work, the chances are excellent that you'll be unhappy with the results. You'll leave the salon feeling utterly miserable, unspeakably ugly, and ready to fling yourself under the wheels of the first passing car.

But suppose you're completely familiar with his work and you're still unhappy. Suppose you've been Mr. B's steady, Friday, 10 A.M. w/set for years—and you hate your hair. Then, chances are you've both gotten into a rut. And if you want to climb out, you must be *specific* about the changes you want.

Okay. What to do next?

No, the answer is not to storm into the salon and clobber Mr. B. with your umbrella. And usually you won't solve the problem by going to other hair stylists either. Because, if you can't give them better directions than you gave Mr. Beverly, you're going to need a lot of umbrellas.

The best way is to follow these three steps. (But don't throw away that umbrella yet.)

1. Do a little homework before you even go to the salon. Get out that collection of photographs of the glamorous Ageless Woman that is your model. (Remember Sally and Angie Dickinson?)

Fool around with your hair. Try parting it on a different side. Brush it all back smoothly, or fluff it forward, or give it an asymmetrical look with one side forward and one back. Try bangs or little curls brushed onto your cheeks. Incidentally, this is a good test for you. Are you really willing to be flexible and try something new? Or does your hairbrush automatically create the same "old faithful" effect that you've been wearing for years?

You might find additional styles that you like in the hair-coloring or wig ads in magazines. Sometimes the fashion magazines will have some detailed close-ups of a great new style that's not too kooky.

But never even consider copying those "nothing" hair styles that are "for the mature woman" or are called "styles for silver hair." (Too many of these are found in "housewife" or hair-styling magazines.) They're much too old for you. They're much too old for *anyone*—anyone living, that is.

2. Try on some wigs in the style and color you're contemplating. (Much more about wigs in a minute.) If the change would be a drastic one—if your model is a blonde, and you're a brunette—you might even buy that blonde wig, wear it for a while, and see how you like the effect.

3. When you are ready to confront Mr. Beverly, be prepared. Take the photographs that show what you want. Take the wigs. And don't forget to take the umbrella—just in case.

4. Talk length in inches. Be specific. "I want my hair to be three inches long at the sides, seven at the crown (remember that 45-degree angle) and five at the back." Or, "I want to be able to wear my hair back in a ribbon sometimes, or up on top, so allow for that when you trim it."

If your hair is longish and you want it trimmed, don't just say you want it shorter; but specify, "I want one inch off all around." (Shake the umbrella a bit here.) Or, if you're not exactly sure of the length needed to get the effect you want, discuss it before you allow those scissors anywhere near your hair. Don't just tune out and become engrossed in the latest movie magazine—"Liz tells why she did rr." Snip-snap. And it's too late to discuss anything.

"YES, BUT . . . MR. BEVERLY WON'T LET ME DISCUSS MY IDEAS"

Oh. Well, you do have a problem. If you're really content to play a meek Trilby to some hairdresser's Svengali, I can't help you. But think about this. Hairdressing is a *service*. And the hairdresser works for *you*.

It is sad to watch women being bullied by their hairdressers—but it happens all the time.

But not to you—at least, not any more. By now you should be getting some idea of what you need in order to achieve that ageless look.

You are becoming *the* expert on *you*, the Ageless Woman. You know what styles are best for you, and you can demand what you want. It's your hair, it's your money, and somewhere in town you can find a competent hairdresser who will be interested in both—and will listen.

Are you afraid to take charge? Don't be. So you make a few little mistakes. So do your hairdressers make mistakes unless you watch them—and don't you know it.

And what if you aren't completely happy with the new hairdo? So what have you lost? You weren't happy before.

But suppose you still aren't satisfied. Well then, back to the drawing board. Hmm. Let's see. Perhaps that new hair style is too old for you. . . .

MORE PLAIN TALK

There are two additional reasons why you may not be getting the results you want when you settle down in the salon chair. A common complaint is, "My hair just won't hold a set. It's lifeless." Or, "My hair is just like a brush now that it's gray. I can't do a thing with it." These are two valid reasons why many women turn, in desperation, to the Menopause Bob. At least, it *stays*. But there's a good chance that the problem is not with your hair but with what's being done to it at the salon.

1. *The Unkindest Cut of All is the Blunt Cut.* Yet it's used almost exclusively by hairdressers everywhere to "add body to the hair." It's become such a popular gimmick that many beauty schools seem to stress its value above all other haircutting techniques. As a result, almost anywhere you go for a haircut, you'll get a blunt cut. If the hairdresser is truly an expert you may—just *may*—have good results. But usually those with fine hair discover that after a blunt cut it has suddenly become lifeless and won't hold a set.

Those with gray hair (and they're getting blunt cuts on their coarse hair just as often as the baby-fine customers) will find that their hair becomes bristly, the ends flying every which way like a brush. Sound familiar? You bet. For either coarse or fine hair, the blunt cut can spell trouble.

Blunt cuts are so difficult to do well that even hair-styling maestros proceed with caution. Ara Gallant, who designs coiffures for the pages of the leading fashion magazines, says this: "I take a long time to do any haircut, and when the hair is fine, I take longer than anybody in the world—one mistake on fine hair can be disastrous. . . . Fine hair should be cut with scissors and 'effilated'—that is, holding the scissors in an upright position and lightly feathering the underneath hair so the outer layer turns under naturally. It looks like a blunt cut but isn't—the ends have more flexibility."

If you can find a hairdresser who effilates, you *are* in luck. However, if you ask Mr. B. what he thinks of effilation, and he says, "Well, it's okay, but only among consenting adults," then insist that he give you a classic, tapered cut or find a hairdresser who will.

How will you know if your hair is being blunt-cut or tapered? Watch him as he's cutting your hair. If he's using scissors to taper-cut, he'll be cutting the ends with a slithering, seesaw motion, with lots of wrist action. Not SNIP. Straight across.

If he's using a razor, you'll notice that up-and-down wrist motion as he slithers the ends of the hair into a taper cut.

Should he be using the razor at all? This is a controversial point among hairdressers. Some, like Kenneth, go so far as to say that a razor should never be used on the hair, that "you should get right up out of the chair and leave" if your hairdresser comes anywhere near you with a razor. However, a taper cut with scissors requires a very skilled hand and many stylists simply aren't up to it. If your hairdresser insists that, in order to do a taper cut, he must use a razor, go ahead and let him slice away. You'll still like a taper cut, even a bad one, better than a blunt cut any day. You'll see.

2. *Your Troubles May Come Out of a Bottle.* Be aware of the products used on your hair. Watch out for creme rinses unless your hair is extremely coarse and hard to manage. Creme rinses soften the hair and can take all the body out of it. Fine

hair especially becomes absolutely limp and lifeless after a creme rinse. But because a creme rinse takes the snarls out and makes the hair easy to comb, many salons automatically follow each shampoo with a creme rinse—it makes their job easier.

Some temporary hair colorings can also make your hair limp and lifeless. Some of them (not all) contain a softening agent. This is because most of these products are designed to cover gray, and usually as hair grows gray it also becomes coarser and more wiry. However, a little experimenting may reveal that the temporary rinse is softening your hair too much—to the point where it has no body at all. Add this revolting development to the possibility that a creme rinse has *also* been applied to your hair—which was blunt-cut in the first place—and you can see why anguished cries of "My hair, my hair . . . I can't do a thing with it" are heard throughout the land.

TWO HEADS ARE BETTER THAN ONE

Especially on those days when you have problem hair.

If you haven't discovered the convenient and becoming world of wigs, you just don't know what you're missing. For one thing, they allow you to experiment without ruining your hair. You can experiment with styling to your heart's content and never run the risk of having to wait six months for your hair to grow back out. Then, as we have mentioned before, you can take the styled wig (and the umbrella) to Mr. Beverly and show him exactly what he is about to do to your hair—or else.

Wigs also let you give your hair a rest (from sprays and rollers) and still look bandbox-beautiful every day. And if you put your own hair in pincurls under the wig, you'll also look appealing at night when you take the wig off.

Then too, wigs can be the salvation of the Unwilling M.A.M. who says, "I don't really like this Menopause Bob, but it's the only way I can keep my hair looking like anything at all between salon appointments." This Unwilling M.A.M. does have a genuine problem, because no hair style in the world excepting that lacquered Menopause Bob can be expected to last more than four days. But why succumb to the Menopause Bob when a couple of wigs will provide such a pleasant alternate solution to the problem?

Here's how it works. Once you have developed your soft, glamorous, natural hairdo, you can luxuriate in each beautiful salon styling for four whole days. Then you pin up your drooping hair, put on one of your soft, glamorous, natural-looking wigs, and you can smugly relax during days five, six and seven. Try it. It's fun.

If you don't like the idea of wearing a wig over hair that needs shampooing, that's easy to fix. A dry shampoo will keep your hair and scalp fresh until your next salon appointment. Or if you wash your own hair, just give it a quick shampoo in the shower, put in a few rollers around the hairline, and wrap the rest of your hair around your head. You'll find that you can wear a wig comfortably, even if the bulk of your hair is still damp.

COMFORTABLE—THE KEY WORD ON WIGS

If you haven't been wearing wigs, it is probably because you have found:

1. *Wigs are Uncomfortable.* Yes indeed, they are—if they are too tight. And salespeople so often insist on cramming your head into a wig that fits as tight as possible. Of course it's uncomfortable—so is a tight girdle or a tight shoe. So take the word of one who wears wigs constantly, comfortably, and happily. When you buy a wig, buy it *big.*

Don't worry about it falling off. You can pin it so securely that a tornado won't budge it. The secret is to make several big pin curls at the crown of your head and several at the nape of your neck. Then you can use large hairpins stuck right through the body of the wig and through those pin curls. Once the wig has been securely anchored at the crown and neckline, one hairpin at each temple will secure it at the hairline in front. (Don't use bobby pins for this. They are uncomfortable and even cause headaches.)

2. *"Wigs Give Me Claustrophobia"* . . . *"Wigs Are Too Hot"* . . . *"My Scalp Can't Breathe."* If this has been your reaction to wigs in the past, you haven't tried one on for several years. The new capless wigs are ingeniously designed so that the wig fiber is attached to strips of ribbon. These modern wigs are unbelievably cool and comfortable. (You can scratch your scalp right through them—and can't one good scratch cure a lot of claustrophobia?)

3. *"They Look Wiggy."* And that can be true. If you go into a department store, plop an unstyled wig on your head, and

then expect to look like anything but the Witch of Endor—well, you *are* an optimist. Wigs, just like your own hair, have to be carefully combed and styled before they will look like anything. Now here's the secret that will give your wig that totally natural look. *Always blend some of your own hair with it.* Before you put your wig on, part off about one inch of your own hair around the hairline; then pin the rest of your hair on top. Now put the wig on, leaving the hair around your face loose; then blend your hair in with the wig. Even if the wig features bangs put a few wisps of your own hair in with them, to create a natural effect.

HOW MUCH SHOULD YOU SPEND FOR A WIG?

Forget the expensive real-hair wigs and buy synthetics. Shop the sales, and you should be able to find a fabulous wig for under $30.

But more important than the price is what you do *after* you buy your wig. Plan to invest in a personalized salon styling. Have your hairdresser trim and thin the wig to suit your face and your needs. Almost every wig needs a little subtle shaping to make it just right for you. One of my friends has a wardrobe of wigs that she bought at the dime store. Really! She takes every one of these little $8.95 numbers to her hairdresser for a personalized styling, and they look great, natural, and just right for her. Of course, she has shopped carefully and chosen wigs that do not have the brassy, shiny fiber that you still see occasionally. Nothing can improve *them.*

Lyn Blair, wig expert at New York's Saks Fifth Avenue (and that's a long way from the dime store), suggests that you choose a wig in Kanekalon fiber for longer wig styles. He feels that shorter styles will be most effective in the slightly finer Elura fiber.

Though some of the new fibers allow you to cut, curl, and reshape your wig into countless styles and variations, I've always felt that the beauty of wigs is that you *don't* have to do much with them after that initial styling. You have to comb them, yes. But basically they should be *convenient.* That's why I recommend a wardrobe of wigs in a variety of styles, rather than one wig that can be styled many ways. This approach isn't extravagant because wigs are certainly inexpensive enough—even the ones at Saks.

You might have a short, tousled, Jill St. John type; a longer, smooth pageboy that you can tie back with a scarf or ribbon; and a medium length to flip up or under. Any style will look natural if you follow my suggestion to blend your own hair in at the hairline and, finally, if you resist the impulse to backcomb excessively.

Wigs can simplify your life, help you to look beautiful every day, and give you a chance to be versatile in your choice of hair styling. But most of all they are a boon companion to the Unwilling M.A.M. who decides to reject the Menopause Bob and grow into a feminine, Ageless Woman. A flattering wig will help you live through that awful growing-out stage. It will even cover up a little mistake or two. So stick with it and have faith.

Remember, any hair style that destroys your feminine image will make you look older—it's a loser in the Age Game. An ageless hair style, one that has volume, a touch of "artistic disorder," and a feminine hairline is the choice for the Ageless Woman. With the right hair style, you can win by a head.

FIVE

Diet Is a Four-Letter Word

If you're really determined to become the Ageless Woman, there's one fact that must be faced. Fat is old. With every overweight pound you add a year to your visual age! Not only do you look *older*, you look matronly. Excess weight is still another sure way of creating a neuter image. There's nothing like being fifteen pounds overweight to inspire people to call you "ma'am."

On the other hand, a slender, well-proportioned figure helps you win the age game because it implies many things—health, vitality, enthusiasm. A lithe and active body inspires the love game; but the dumpy, flabby player is usually doomed to sit on the bench.

Well, that's the bad news. Now for some good news. The majority of mature women think that they need to lose more weight than is actually necessary. They say, in desperation, "Oh, my God, I have to take off thirty pounds, at least." They strew ashes on their heads, rend their garments (size sixteen), and set this totally arbitrary and impractical goal—thirty pounds. That thirty pounds looms like Mount Everest, an overwhelming, frightening, impossible challenge.

Now, setting this impossible goal does have its advantages. If the goal is totally *impossible*, who can blame our hefty heroines if they rarely get past the foothills of that mountain before they become discouraged? How can they feel guilty if, in the face of this huge challenge, they go right on stuffing themselves while explaining to their luncheon companions, "Fat runs in my family"?

Actually, except in the case of extreme obesity, very few women really *need* to lose more than fifteen pounds to change their image from that of the dumpy matron to the Ageless Woman.

That is good news. But it's only good news if you are willing to be honest with yourself and give up that most insidious, self-defeating, and sneaky diet game of all—the one called All Talk and No Do. This game is enormously popular because it lets you talk endlessly (over a lasagne lunch) about the *impossible* task of losing thirty pounds, instead of shutting up, knuckling down, and really losing the realistic fifteen pounds that will make you look ten years younger.

Once you have set a realistic goal, you are being honest with yourself. You are setting a goal that is within reach—and with the slightest bit of determination and help (which is coming up in this chapter) you can accomplish that goal.

Naturally, when you do lose that extra weight, you must make a few sacrifices. You will have to give up those lasagne lunches, of course. But even worse, you can no longer participate in that other well-known diet game called "Why don't they make any stunning clothes in a size sixteen?" You'll just have to wear your size twelves and keep quiet.

Though many women do set impossible goals, there is, sadly, the other extreme. Some women never set any goal at all. They're convinced that they're terribly overweight, so they eternally mope about under a big fat cloud of gloom called diet—generally, a "starve today, stuff tomorrow" way of life. What a weigh to live! Miserably hungry while starving, miserably guilty while stuffing. DIET, a ghastly four-letter word, hovers like some malevolent demon over every meal.

Now, if you really want to break the spell and exorcise this diet demon, if you honestly want to get off the diet merry-go-round, your first move is to set a *realistic* goal. Here is how you do it.

HOW MUCH SHOULD YOU *REALLY* WEIGH?

It's supposed to be fairly easy to find out. Everyone says so. Simply look at one of those insurance tables, match up your height and your build (large frame, small frame) and *kazam!* The table gives your ideal weight. Right? Wrong!

These tables are usually so generalized and allow for such a variance in each category that they are only useful in the most superficial way. For instance, if you really are thirty-five to fifty pounds overweight, they'll tell you that you're in big trouble—as if you didn't know that already. (And, if this describes you, stick around. Big help is on the way.) For those who are only five, ten, or fifteen pounds overweight, these charts don't help at all.

Let's face it. For one thing, they allow you to cheat. In fact, they encourage it. A typical chart will say, "If you are 5'5", you should weigh 115 pounds if you have a small frame and 135 pounds if you have a large frame." Now, if you just happen to weigh 133 pounds, are you going to admit that you have a small frame? Are you going to admit that your brother called you "toothpick" all through high school? Or that you played Juliet because you were the only girl light enough to stand on that rickety balcony? Well, are you? Heavens, no! Any red-blooded American woman will mutter to herself, "I was always sturdy—and I've got two pounds coming."

But you want to be a red-blooded *Ageless* Woman, don't you? You want to stop playing these little diet games so that you can start winning the big games.

And this is the first move. First you need to know an honest way to calculate how much you should really weigh.

THE WRIST METHOD

By using your wrist measurement as a guideline, you can arrive at the ideal weight for your bone structure. Measure around the wrist immediately above the wrist bone on the least developed side (that is, your left wrist if you're right-handed).

If your wrist measures:

4 ½" to 5 ⅛"—you have a small frame, delicate bone structure
5 ⅜" to 6 ⅛"—you have a medium frame and bone structure
6 ¼" and up—you have a large frame and sturdy bone structure

If you have a small or large frame, start with 100 pounds for five feet of stature and add five pounds to your weight for each inch over five feet. For example, five feet five would give you a total of 125 pounds. But wait. You're not through yet. If you have a small frame —subtract five pounds from this total to obtain your ideal weight. If you have a large frame, add five pounds to the total.

If you have a medium frame—allow 100 pounds for five feet of stature, then add four pounds for each inch over five feet.

Using the wrist method can keep you from setting impossible goals. This was Dorothy's problem. In fact, we used to call her Diet Dora, because she always preceded every class session with the sad tale of her sins at supper. "I can lose easily until I get to that last ten pounds. They simply won't budge."

This would go on for weeks while her weight went up and down like a yo-yo. When her weight went down she kept trying for that last, impossible ten pounds, predictably becoming more and more hungry and discouraged. Then suddenly something would snap. She would go on a ferocious eating binge and her weight would balloon up. Remorse would set in and her weight would creep down during a period of stern starvation. This kind of dieting is not only mentally depressing but also physically devastating, as anyone could see by looking at Dorothy's ravaged face.

During one of her "thin" periods I commented that she looked well proportioned to me, but she said, "I'm still on my 900-calorie-a-day diet—I'm determined to get into a size eight. After all, I'm only five feet three—and here I am, wearing a size twelve. I hate it." However, after some discussion, she agreed to try the wrist method and it showed her that the weight she'd attained after moderate dieting was, indeed, her ideal weight. Here's how it broke down:

Wrist measurement—6¼", indicating a large frame,
sturdy bone structure

Height—	5'3"
Ideal weight—	100 pounds for 5'
plus—	15 pounds for additional 3"
plus—	5 pounds for large frame
	120 pounds—ideal weight

Dorothy wore a size twelve because, like it or not, she was a short woman with a very large and sturdy bone structure. All the dieting in the world wouldn't change that. And once she had a realistic picture of her own body structure, she was able to maintain her ideal weight without the seesawing weight changes that are so destructive to health—and beauty.

Her friend Sybil, on the other hand, illustrated a different problem. She had a delicate frame that should have been lean and streamlined. But she had worked hard to convince herself that all that padding around her tiny bones was "natural." She consoled herself over the loss of her trim figure by saying, "As a woman gets older, some weight is inevitable." Then, to prove her point comfortably, she scrambled around until she found the charts that are the real cheaters —you know the kind, don't you? They let you make an allowance for both your frame size *and* your age. Such charts encourage a very dangerous attitude, by the way, because as soon as you begin to make concessions to age you *are* old. (And you may be taking that first tottering step toward becoming a Professional M.A.M.)

But you can avoid the trap that caught both Sybil and Dorothy by developing a realistic picture of your ideal weight and working with rather than against your bone structure.

Now that you know how much you should weigh, how will you get there?

WHY YOU DON'T LOSE WEIGHT, OR EVERYTHING YOU KNOW PERFECTLY WELL ABOUT WEIGHT CONTROL BUT DON'T LIKE TO FACE

Have you been kidding yourself? If you can put yourself in the following scene, the answer is *yes*. Listen to the "girls" at lunch.

"I'll have the lobster thermidor, and would you please bring some more bread and butter?" Agnes says as she hungrily bites into the last piece of French bread. "I know I shouldn't. But I'm just starved. I started this new diet last week and I can't stay on it another minute. Anyway, I won't feel guilty today. I'll go back on the diet tomorrow."

"Oh, Agnes, you always say that. You just don't have any will power. You should do what I do. Limit yourself to just 8oo calories a day. The weight simply pours off." Lois toys with the tiny salad she's ordered, then stretches out a pale hand and covers her eyes. "Darn. I'm getting another one of my headaches. Do you mind if I skip the art exhibit? You and Phyllis go. Phyllis—Phyllis?"

But Phyllis has her own approach to the diet question. Being for the moment an enthusiastic follower of the drinking man's diet, she just finished her fourth martini and, with a dignified hiccup, slid quietly under the table. It looks as if Agnes will go to that art exhibit alone.

What's wrong with the diets of our three friends? Let's see.

THE ELEVATOR GAME

Up and down. Up and down. That's the story of Agnes' diet life. Energetic, outgoing, and impatient, she wants to see results *right now*. So she's perpetually embarking on a crash diet plan. You know. The kind that begins, "Breakfast—½ grapefrt, blk. coffee . . ." Because her energetic body needs enough of the *right* foods to keep her going, such a diet cannot possibly last. Her body rebels and demands food, food, *food*. She stuffs, she starves. She stuffs, she starves. Her weight seesaws up and down. Somehow, though, it always manages to be more up than down, so Agnes looks like a well-padded dowager in her size sixteens.

THE CARE-PACKAGE SYNDROME

Does slender Lois have a problem? You bet she has. But by now she has a health problem, not a weight problem. Lois has literally starved herself until she is sick. She is able to stay on her stringent diet because her whole system is run down, not because she has will power. She has no appetite because she's unhealthy.

True, she continues to wear a size eight. But what a price to pay. Lack of energy, circles under the eyes, and, most aging of all, flabby skin and wasted muscles caused by malnutrition. She has made the deadly mistake of equating starvation with diet. She eats too little. And she eats the wrong things, as we'll discuss later.

THE GIMMICK GAME

And what about Phyllis? She's a dreamer. She's just sure that there's a magic, instant way out of the diet dilemma. Consequently, she's a sucker for every fad diet that comes along. One week, it's the peanut butter and macaroni diet—or carrot tops and eggs, maybe. And next week, who knows? Perhaps pig knuckles and papaya seeds, "a centuries-old secret diet, stolen from a Hunza priest and smuggled down the mountain passes in a hand-carved teak yogurt pot."

True, she has been unusually loyal to the Drinking Man's Diet, of late. And is she losing much weight?

"Wheeeeee. Who cares?" (We've *got* to get Phyllis out from under that table.)

Actually, she *has* lost some weight on her fad diets, but again, at the expense of her health and physiological age.

The trouble is that these approaches to diet are old-fashioned, they don't work, and they can be dangerous. Certainly, they're not for the Ageless Woman, who demands a slender figure but who also cherishes the plus qualities of health, vitality, and energy to spare.

If fat is old, so is sick. I mean, how can you be that fascinating Ageless Woman when you're starving to death? There you are, at a cozy dinner for two. You're toying with your last shred of lettuce leaf, and he's looking deep into your eyes.

"What are you thinking about?" he murmurs.

"I was just wondering if you were going to eat all of your baked potato—" you whisper hungrily.

No, they won't do. These unhealthy reducing diets just won't do for the Ageless Woman.

What *is* needed is a new approach to the diet question. An approach that will help you establish and maintain normal weight, and at the same time build optimum health and energy reserves. Would you believe it? I just happen to have such a diet plan up my sleeve. But before I share it with you, I invite you to take a look at a startling new approach to the entire problem of excess weight.

OVERWEIGHT IS UNDERNOURISHED

Overweight is as much a symptom of malnutrition as underweight. This is the opinion of a growing number of doctors and nutritionists. Nutrition reporter Linda Clark states, "You may be overfed but still undernourished. Stout people, just as frequently as skinny people, are often victims of malnourishment. Frequently, obese people live on calorie-rich rather than vitamin- and mineral-rich foods." She adds, "Overweight not only can cause you to be a target for deficiency diseases, it can *be* a deficiency disease."

In her terrific book *Feel Like a Million*, Catharyn Elwood says,

"Overweight is as much a symptom of malnutrition as underweight. And just as soon as the missing food elements are supplied, the water and fat roll off."

This was also the opinion of that guru of all nutritionists, the late Adelle Davis. In a recent interview she stated, "At no time in the history of the world have there been so many overweight persons in a single nation as in America today. What causes so many people to be overweight today is that *too few nutrients are supplied in their diets to burn fat readily*." (Emphasis added.) She found that many of the obese people who came to her for reducing diets were too malnourished to be placed on such a program. Instead she advised, "Let's forget about reducing for a least three months and concentrate on building health." By concentrating on building health, rather than merely losing weight, the basal metabolism can be built up so that energy is produced and the weight normalizes.

After years of taking this approach (with thousands of clients) she concluded that this is the way every person should reduce. She found that these extremely obese clients who followed a super-energy diet (one that supplied all nutrients) might gain weight for a week or two, then steadily and inexorably the weight peeled off.

I can vouch for this, since many of my students have achieved the same results following the special, high-energy super diet that I devised. I remember one student in particular. She found that my diet plan enabled her to finally and permanently lose the extra thirty-five pounds she'd been carrying around since high school days. Not only did she find that she had a new figure, but she was also enjoying a new and successful life—a thrilling but not unusual result of building dynamic health. In fact, Faye was the one who named my diet for me.

"It's so *super* to be myself, finally—to be the person I've always wanted to be." And somehow in our conversations "super to be" became Super-B. And that's what we all called the diet from then on —the Super-B Diet.

Faye wasn't one of those women who had overestimated the amount of weight she had to lose. While not what you'd call obese, she was thirty-five hefty pounds overweight—and she knew it.

This excess weight was just one of the things that had made Faye an unwilling candidate for middle age as far back as her early thirties. Her futile attempts at dieting—you know, starve today and stuff tomorrow—kept her chronically tired, depressed, defeated, and yes, a bit dull—in addition to being fat.

She was about forty-five when she enrolled in my classes—a gray, doughy woman in a dreary maroon half-size dress—a woman who had obviously come to me as a last resort.

"Look, my husband Harry has just walked out after twenty-five years. I'm stuck in a poverty-wage, nowhere job at the insurance company. I feel a thousand years old—and look sixty. But I'm determined to be a new me." (When I heard that word "determined" I knew that Faye would make it.) "And I want to start by losing this excess weight. After all, now that I've lost Harry"—her eyes filled with tears—"what else have I got to lose?"

We both smiled at her feeble joke as I recorded her height (5′6″), weight (159 pounds) and wrist measurement (6″). Since she had a medium frame, we figured her ideal weight to be 124 pounds.

The following week, she brought in her doctor's approval card and started the Super-B Diet.

And it was not smooth sailing at all. First, I had to convince this confirmed diet-aholic that she had to eat the quantity of food indicated on the diet. She was used to those starvation diets that only allow three tiny meals a day. She was convinced that a weight loss could only be *earned* through prolonged suffering. Then, when she actually gained five pounds the first week, I almost lost her.

It took all my powers of persuasion to convince her to hang in there. I had to convince her that the Super-B Diet needs a little time to build health and energy—time to help the body normalize its metabolism and efficiently burn off unwanted pounds. Finally—a little grudgingly—she agreed to stay on the diet for three weeks.

Then things started to happen. Here's the breakdown on Faye's weight loss. Remember that her ideal weight was 124 pounds and her beginning weight was 159 pounds.

Weight at the end of the first week—164 lbs.	Gained	5 lbs. (!)
2nd week—162 lbs.	Lost	2 lbs.
3rd week—157 lbs.	Lost	5 lbs.
4th week—154 lbs.	Lost	3 lbs.
5th week—151 lbs.	Lost	3 lbs.
6th week—148 lbs.	Lost	3 lbs.
Total lost from beginning weight		16 lbs.

At the end of six weeks, a 16-pound weight loss—Faye, the
Super-B Diet, and I were friends again.

7th week—146 lbs.	Lost	2 lbs.
8th week—144 lbs.	Lost	2 lbs.
9th week—140 lbs.	Lost	4 lbs.
10th week—137 lbs.	Lost	3 lbs.
11th week—134 lbs.	Lost	3 lbs.
12th week—131 lbs.	Lost	3 lbs.
13th week—128 lbs.	Lost	2 lbs.
14th week—126 lbs.	Lost	2 lbs.
15th week—124 lbs.	Lost	2 lbs.

You can see that after the initial disaster of the five-pound weight
gain Faye slowly but steadily peeled the weight off. Being familiar
with those "magic" crash diets that allowed her to lose a dramatic
twenty pounds in a very short period of time, she was also familiar
with the depressing "here we are again" reappearance of those twenty
pounds. So she stuck with the Super-B Diet—which wasn't really
such a sacrifice. As she told everyone who would listen, "I haven't
had so much to eat in years."

But the Super-B Diet did more for Faye than help her lose weight.
As Adelle Davis said, "Fat is lost only when energy is produced." And
for the first time in years Faye was a *healthy* woman with energy to
spare. The change in her personality was dramatic. And as the weeks
went by this quiet, seemingly dull woman began to sparkle. She had
energy, she had enthusiasm, and she was fun to be around. Gone was
that tired, despondent (and I suspect nagging) matron who had
walked into my studio. She told everyone, "I've never felt better in
my life."

Because she was full of energy and enthusiasm (for the first time
in years), she aggressively went after a better job in the insurance
company—one that she could have had years before if she had had
confidence.

She's now one of the best insurance investigators in the country.
With a new figure, a revitalized personality, a new job, and an exciting new social life, formerly dowdy and half-sized Faye is sitting on
top of the world.

And if you ask her today about Heartbreaker Harry, the husband
who ran out on her, she's liable to say, "Harry? Harry who?"

So the ultimate solution to your weight problems (perhaps your marital problems as well) is to forget all those bleeping, four-letter-word reducing diets, and instead take the positive approach summed up in this nine-letter word—nutrition.

A diet based on satisfying your nutritional needs, rather than solely devoted to weight loss, will help you achieve your normal weight and will give the additional advantage of building beauty and vitality as well. What's more, you'll find it easy to stay on a nutritionally superior diet because it satisfies those hidden hungers that cause the overweights to stuff themselves.

Finally, and this is the clincher, there's increasing evidence to indicate that you can actually rejuvenate your body and reverse the aging process by giving your body all the elements it needs to rebuild aging tissues and tired blood.

RE-CREATE YOUR BODY THROUGH PLANNED NUTRITION

The Professional M.A.M. accepts the gradual deterioration of her youth and health as inevitable. It gives her a chance to go into her "we're not getting any younger" routine.

"Let's face it," she sighs with grim satisfaction, "a woman has to expect these lines and wrinkles as she gets on in years. As I tell my kids, there's a wrinkle for every heartache you've caused me. . . ." (How they *love* to have Mother come and visit.)

The Ageless Woman doesn't accept this situation. She *is* ageless because she bases her opinions and actions on the latest findings of the intellectual and scientific world. She isn't content to subsist on a stale diet of old wives' tales.

Just how important is diet in conquering those signs of age? Gloria Swanson is a shining example. Described as having a "near-fanatical enthusiasm for health foods," this is how she impressed writer Bob MacKenzie. "At the age of 75, Miss Swanson's beauty is striking. It isn't the mellow beauty of a serene old age, but the calculating beauty of a woman still full of sex and vinegar." (And all the right foods.)

Gladys Lindberg, the Los Angeles-based nutrition expert who plans dynamic diets for leading athletes and film stars, has this to say about nutrition and aging: "Our diet between the ages of fifteen and twenty-five lays the groundwork for our old age. . . . At forty or fifty we begin to deteriorate and we don't know what we've done wrong! Yes, most women have terrible diets in those young years, but fortunately you can reverse aging even after twenty-five, because every organ can renew itself. (You're making trillions of new cells with every breath you take, and your body changes completely every seven years.)"

Dr. Tom Spies, in an address to the American Medical Association, explained the importance of nutrition to the aging process: "As tissues become damaged because they lack the chemicals of good nutrition, they tend to become old. They lack what I call tissue integrity. There are people of forty whose brains are senile. If we can help the tissues repair themselves by correcting nutritional deficiencies, we can make old age wait."

Good Lord! Senile at forty? That makes it doubly important to plan your nutrition so that, for the rest of your life, you'll have a sound mind *and* a sound body. Only *you* know how your brain is chugging along, but let's see what state your body's in.

HOW OLD IS YOUR BODY? THE PINCH TEST GIVES THE ANSWER

If you want to know how old you *really* are, pinch the skin on the back of your hand. The elasticity of your skin will tell you if you're older than your years. If your skin is elastic, and snaps back, it means that you're physiological young. If the skin is flabby, if the pinch mark just crawls back—then you're crawling toward old age.

Now that I've ruined your day, check out these other signs of age and see how you rate:

1. Muscles lack tone—facial muscles, back of the arms, and breasts are flabby and tend to droop.
2. Hair and nails break easily and lack luster.
3. Facial expression is drawn and tired-looking—the result of fatigue and lack of endurance.
4. Skin has a gray or yellow tone—lacks color (often the result of anemia), tissues under the skin are wasted, creating wrinkles.
5. Eyes are puffy, ankles and hands tend to swell—especially noticeable in the morning after eight hours of sleep.

What was your score? That bad, eh? Well, don't despair.

Every one of these aging characteristics can be a common symptom of protein deficiency. If you are otherwise in good health, you can dramatically reverse these signs of age by supplying your body with all the protein it needs.

ADD PROTEINS AND SUBTRACT YEARS

Every schoolgirl learns that protein is an important element in human nutrition, every weight-conscious woman has heard of the benefits of a high-protein diet, and every television viewer has been treated to commercials touting a "high-protein breakfast food" or a quick-snack cake that has "as much protein as this eight-course dinner." Yes, everybody talks about protein, but unfortunately most people don't know enough about protein to reap the many benefits that can be derived from a protein-rich diet. So let's have a quick review.

1. "Every living cell in the body contains protein." (Gladys Lindberg, *Proteins and Amino Acids.*)

2. "Every cell must have a *continuous* supply of protein to maintain its life. Any limitation or irregularity of this supply causes changes in the normal composition of the body cells with the result that the entire body is affected." (Gladys Lindberg, *Proteins and Amino Acids.*)

3. If the body's protein needs are undersupplied, the body feeds on the protein stored in the less important body tissues in order to rebuild essential organs.

See? That's why short-changing your body on its protein needs results in the aging symptoms we've discussed. Those crepy eyelids, sagging facial muscles, and flabby arms are all results of this process of "robbing Peter to pay Paul." When protein needs are met, these aging symptoms tend to disappear, sometimes with dramatic swiftness. I've seen it happen countless times, when my students have jumped off the Reducing Diet Bandwagon and hopped aboard the Rejuvenating Jet. Take Trudy, for example.

Gertrude (Trudy) Cartwright had been my assistant for several years, and consequently was totally aware of all the beauty secrets that could make the most of her brunette beauty. However, because she was a "former fatty," she was obsessed with the idea of dieting—

and no amount of discussion would persuade her to give up her star-vation approach. Until the day she looked in the mirror and sighed, "You know, I'm beginning to look like a bloodhound. Look at the way my face is falling . . . like a cold soufflé. I'm going to have to have my face lifted—and soon."

"Look," I said, "I'm completely in favor of cosmetic surgery, but it won't be very successful on a face that's just starved for protein. You're not looking old, you know. Just hungry."

"You're always saying that," she said grumpily. "Really, I'm *on* a high-protein diet."

"Gotcha," I thought.

"Okay, Trudy, I dare you to prove it," I said. "And if you really are on a high-protein diet I'll never say another word about it. *And* I promise to bring you posies if you really decide to have your face done."

When we actually made a list of everything she'd eaten for the last couple of days she was shocked to learn that, far from being on a high-protein diet, she was only getting about one third of her daily age-defying requirement. When I left she was quite cross, somewhat red-faced, and leafing earnestly through my Super-B Diet.

Trudy had overestimated her protein intake for the same reasons that most people do:

  1. She didn't know how many grams of protein she needed to meet her youth-building requirements.

  2. She had never learned to count protein grams, a technique that instantly showed how much protein she had actually been getting each day.

  3. She considered such foods as gelatin (which is an in-complete protein) to be a valuable protein diet food.

How much do *you* need? How much *are* you getting? I'll go into this in detail, but first let me finish Trudy's story.

Shortly after this discussion I was booked out of town on a six-week lecture tour. When I returned Trudy met me at the airport. She looked marvelous and I thought, "Well, she's done it, she's re-ally had her face lifted—and what a superb job."

I could hardly wait to ask her about it. "Come on, Trudy, tell me everything. Who did your face . . . and when?"

"I do look pretty good," she admitted smugly. "But *you're* the doctor. I call this my Gloria Heidi, Handy-Dandy, Super-B Nutritional Face Lift because it's all come about since you nagged and hounded me into changing my diet."

What were the results of her improved nutrition? First, her skin was firmer with a finer texture than before. The tiny lines along her upper lip were gone. What's more, the muscles under the skin were firmer, lifted, strong. This gave her face a vital, rested look. Finally, her skin had that essential layer of padding under the surface. Old skin looks as if the face underneath were slowly dissolving. Young skin has an underlayer of supportive tissue—tissue made of protein.

And what happened to Trudy? I lost the best assistant I ever had, that's what happened.

Ironically, after all the times she had accused me of being a nag, she became a complete fanatic on the subject of nutrition. Like the reformed drunk, she lectured everyone she could corner on the importance of a superdiet. Finally she bought a health food store that is so successful she is now happily nagging hundreds of customers each week—healthy customers, too.

Of course, protein isn't the only answer to a beauty-full diet. Vitamins, minerals, and a totally balanced diet make up the complete answer. But protein is the foundation.

HOW MUCH DO YOU NEED?

The Food and Nutrition Board of the National Research Council recommends 65 grams of protein each day for men and 55 grams for women. However, most nutritionists would consider this amount much too low to *rebuild* a body that has been malnourished for years and that is showing the signs of deterioration that we've described. Catharyn Elwood suggests, "Fifty-five grams will do if you are a female in excellent health, rather small than large, and not very active. If you have been suffering from any of the protein deficiency symptoms, *double your protein content for a month.*" (Emphasis added.)

In her book, *Let's Eat Right to Keep Fit,* Adelle Davis said, "If you wish to maintain your attractiveness, vigor, and youthfulness as long as is humanly possible, it is probably wise to eat considerably more protein than the Board recommends and/or to count only the grams of adequate protein you eat. Whenever the diet has been deficient in protein for some time, an intake of 150 grams or more daily is probably advisable for a month or more."

Can you eat too much protein? Dr. G. C. Thosteson in his column in the San Francisco *Chronicle* says, "Protein is such an essential bodily need, that it is rare to hear of a person's getting too much." He adds that the system of a normally healthy person utilizes protein as the body needs it and expels the rest as waste. There are some systemic disorders—Bright's disease and gout are two—in which excess protein could cause trouble. But "generally speaking, there is a tendency not to get enough protein in the diet. Excess is rarely encountered."

Some experts suggest that an easy way to figure your protein needs is to base the total day's requirement on ½ gram for each pound of your ideal weight. Suppose you should weigh 120 pounds. Simply divide by two and you know that 60 grams of protein is what you need to *maintain* your body's needs. To rebuild protein-starved tissues, try to get 100 to 150 grams of protein daily for three months. At the end of that time you'll *see* what adequate protein can do for you. And you'll probably want to keep your protein intake at 80 to 100 grams per day after this three-month period.

WHO SAYS YOU'RE GETTING ENOUGH?

Now, how much protein are *you* getting? Unless you're one of the growing number of people who have become "turned on" to nutrition, you'll probably be shocked when you discover just how deficient your diet really is. Let's take a look at two daily menus, one an example of the "average" American diet, and one that was given to me by a student as an example of a "high-protein" reducing diet.

AVERAGE Breakfast			SO-CALLED HIGH-PROTEIN Breakfast		
FOOD	AM'T.	GRAMS PROTEIN	FOOD	AM'T.	GRAMS PROTEIN
Sweet roll	1	3	Egg	1	6
Juice	1 c.	0	Bacon	1½ sl.	2
Coffee	1 c.	0	Wh. wheat toast	1 sl.	2
			Coffee	1 c.	0
		3			10

AVERAGE *Lunch*			SO-CALLED HIGH-PROTEIN *Lunch*		
FOOD	AM'T	GRAMS PROTEIN	FOOD	AM'T	GRAMS PROTEIN
Liverwurst sandwich:			Yogurt	1 c.	8
White bread	2 sl.	4	Cheddar cheese	1" sq.	4
Liverwurst	1 oz.	4	Celery, carrot sticks		1
Carton milk	1 c.	9	Apple	1	0
		17			13

Dinner			*Dinner*		
FOOD	AM'T.	GRAMS PROTEIN	FOOD	AM'T	GRAMS PROTEIN
Spaghetti with meat sauce	1 c.	13	Hamburger patty	3 oz.	21
Salad—mixed green		1	Mixed vegs.	1 c.	2
Fruit	1 dish	1	½ grapefruit		1
		15			24

Isn't it easy to see why so many mature women show those aging signs brought on by a protein deficiency? Remember, the minimum protein intake suggested by the most conservative nutritionists is 55 grams. At 47 mingy little grams, that "high-protein" diet doesn't even measure up to those conservative estimates. When you realize that you really should be getting close to 100 grams to maintain health and youthful vigor, well, good grief! Is it any wonder that so many people are sick, tired, and just plain *old* before their time?

And how does your diet stack up next to these two examples? Chances are, Adelle Davis was describing you when she said, "Until a person knows enough about nutrition to estimate his daily intake by counting protein grams easily, and to distinguish between complete and incomplete proteins, he almost invariably believes he consumes a far better diet than he does. Thousands of persons think they get adequate protein from one egg at breakfast and meat at dinner; their actual intake may be 26 grams or less, although their requirement is perhaps many times that amount."

So the magic words are Protein Grams, and I've included a list of protein foods with their gram equivalents to help you become a gram counter rather than a calorie counter.

SOME HAVE IT—SOME DON'T

You'll notice that the proteins on the Gram Counter are divided into two groups, complete and incomplete. This classification is based on the amino acid content of protein foods. You remember, amino acids are the building blocks of proteins. Complete proteins contain the eight *essential* amino acids that the body cannot manufacture. Incomplete proteins, which are lacking one or more of those amino acids, will not by themselves support life, growth, or reproduction.

To put it another way, incomplete proteins are like your dotty Aunt Agatha—they don't have all their marbles. Complete proteins are like Paul Newman—they have everything that a red-blooded female needs. However, some incomplete proteins are so high in other essential nutrients that they have an important place in the Super-B Diet. (A *rich* dotty Aunt Agatha?) These are:

Brewers' yeast
Wheat germ
Soybeans
Millet
Nuts and seeds

YOUR PERSONAL PROTEIN GRAM COUNTER
COMPLETE PROTEINS

FOOD	PROTEIN GRAMS	CALORIES
1 egg	6	75
1 glass milk	8	165
1 tablespoon powdered milk	3.5	35
½ cup cottage cheese	20	100
1″ square Swiss or American cheese	8	100
1 cup commercial yogurt (plain)	11	148
(sweetened, with fruit)	11	280
4 ounces liver	23	140
4 ounces fish	25	140
4 ounces chuck roast	22	190
4 ounces hamburger	19	240
4 ounces sirloin steak	21	156
4 ounces chicken	18	125
4 ounces pork chops (lean)	23	240
1½ slices crisp bacon	2	53

COMPLETE PROTEINS

FOOD	PROTEIN GRAMS	CALORIES
½ can salmon	17	120
1 can sardines	22	175
½ can tuna	25	170
1 heaping tablespoon dried liver powder	15	22

INCOMPLETE PROTEINS

Brewers' (nutritional) yeast		
1 heaping tablespoon	7	22
thirty 7½-grain tablets	7	22
1 tablespoon wheat germ	3	25.5
½ cup kidney beans, cooked	8	115
½ cup lentils, cooked	7	97
4 ounces millet mush	10	93
½ cup soybeans, dried, cooked	20	108
½ cup lima beans, dried, cooked	8	130
½ cup broccoli, steamed	2.5	22.5
½ cup peas, fresh, steamed	2.5	35
10 medium almonds	2	65
¼ cup sunflower seeds	6	140
18 Peanuts	5	110
2 tablespoons peanut butter	9	203

The important thing to remember is that incomplete proteins must be eaten with complete proteins in order to get the protein value from these foods.

Be especially aware that a highly touted "beauty" food, gelatin, is an incomplete protein. The same student who gave me the example of the "high-protein" diet explained that she intended to increase her protein intake by taking gelatin in a glass of fruit juice three times a day. No way! Not only is gelatin an incomplete protein, but some nutritionists feel that taking large amounts can actually produce a dangerous imbalance in essential amino acids.

By now you may feel that you already know more about protein than you ever really wanted to know, so let's get on with the diet.

THE SUPER-B DIET: BE HEALTHY, BE SLIM, BE AGELESS

At first glance, the following menu plan may look like the usual high-protein, low-carbohydrate diet. Look again, you'll see some not so common foods mentioned there. Later I'll be explaining why these foods can help you create a fountain of youth right in your own kitchen. Meanwhile, if you want to start on the diet right away, remember these two sensible precautions.

If you have any specific allergies or medical problems, you should check this diet with your doctor. And it's always a good idea to start any change in diet gradually—even if, dietetically speaking, the change represents a shift over from a broken-down Edsel to a Rolls-Royce. You still must give your system time to adjust, so work into the diet over about a week's time.

THE SUPER-B DIET

Breakfast	PROTEIN GRAMS
1 orange	0
2 eggs, scrambled with 1 teaspoon soy oil,	12
1 tablespoon powdered skim milk, and	
1 tablespoon water	3
1-inch cube cheese	8
1 slice whole wheat or rye toast	3
	26

—OR—

3-ounce serving of meat: steak, hamburger, etc.	23
¼ cup cottage cheese with fruit	
(fresh or diet pack)	10
1 cup hot vegetable bouillon with 1 teaspoon	
soy oil, ½ teaspoon kelp added	trace
	33

—OR—

½ grapefruit	0
½ cup hulled millet mush with 1 teaspoon	10
soy butter. Sprinkle 1 tablespoon wheat germ	
on top and sweeten with honey if desired	3
8-ounce glass skim milk (fortified with 1	
tablespoon powdered skim milk)	11½
	24½

Midmorning	PROTEIN GRAMS
8-ounce glass skim milk	8
1 tablespoon soy-lecithin, stirred into milk	0
and	

PROTEIN GRAMS

24 dried liver tablets or
24 brewers' yeast tablets or
24 yeast tablets (start with 8, work up
    to 24)   approx. 8
                                                                                          16

—OR—

8-ounce glass Yeast for Beginners (recipe follows)   approx. 10

—OR—

8-ounce glass Liver Cocktail (for the Brave . . .
    and the Beautiful)
    (recipe follows)   approx. 15

Lunch   PROTEIN GRAMS
(This can be very light if you need to lose a lot
    of weight.)
A green salad with ½ cup cottage cheese, oil and
    vinegar dressing   20

—OR—

1 portion cheese (2"×1"×1")   12
Rabbit food (celery, carrots, etc.), as much as
    you want
10 almonds   2
                                                                 14

—OR—

¼ cup cottage cheese, ½ cup yogurt and fruit   15½

Midafternoon   PROTEIN GRAMS
Same three choices as midmorning

—OR—

1 cup vegetable bouillon with 1 teaspoon yeast
    and 1 teaspoon soy oil and ½ teaspoon kelp
    added   3½
1 portion cheese (2"×1"×1")   12
2 crackers   1
                                                                 16½

Dinner	PROTEIN GRAMS
4-ounce serving calf's or beef liver with	23
grilled onions	trace
½ cup broccoli with 1 teaspoon mayonnaise or	
soy butter	2½
½ cup yogurt (not commercially sweetened	
kind—too fattening) with fruit and 1 teaspoon	
honey	5½
	31

–OR–

½ cup (4 ounces) canned salmon	17
½ cup (frozen type) green peas	2½
½ cup beets	½
1 apple and	
5 raw pecans	1½
	21½

–OR–

Cheese omelet (2 eggs, 1-inch cube cheese)	14
1 slice fried millet mush	5
Lettuce and tomato salad with soy oil and lemon juice	
(⅛ head and ½ tomato)	1
¼ cup raisins and nuts and sunflower seeds, mixed approx.	1
	21

Nighttime Snack (You're still hungry?)	PROTEIN GRAMS
1 cup hot fortified milk with ¼ teaspoon butter and	
honey (if desired)	11

–OR–

1 cup hot vegetable bouillon with 1 teaspoon yeast	3½

The above menus are merely suggested combinations of high-protein foods along with the special superfoods that I will talk about later. Using the Gram Counter and the following food descriptions, you can work out endless combinations to create your own Super-B Diet menus.

Every Day Eat:
  1 piece of bread (whole wheat or rye or 14 grain)

1 orange (not the juice . . . the orange) or ½ grapefruit
2 green vegetables
½ baked potato or boiled-in-the-skin potato (if you do not eat the
   bread)
3 tablespoons vegetable oil
1 or 2 teaspoons kelp
1 tablespoon wheat germ
3 tablespoons lecithin

Avoid:
   Large amounts of fruit, especially canned, in syrup
   Pastas—macaroni, spaghetti
   Commercial sweets and pastries
   Oil and starch combinations—potato chips, etc.

ADDITIONAL NOTES:

All milk should be skim or, if you can't stand that, a half-and-half
mixture of low-fat and skim.

Drink one glass of water after every serving of protein food. Why?
Water is necessary in the digestion of protein and will help you
process it effectively and prevent constipation.

Salt substitute—if you've ever been on an extreme low-calorie diet
and find that the pounds just don't budge it may be because you
need potassium. Salt substitute contains potassium, which many nutritionists feel should be added to reducing diets to prevent waterlog-
ging. You can mix salt substitute (potassium chloride) half and half
with table salt (sodium chloride) in your shaker. Of course, salt
should be used moderately, but adding potassium to your diet in this
simple way can often work reducing wonders.

Soy butter is made by mixing one stick of butter with ⅔ cup soy
(or any other unsaturated vegetable) oil. This mixture retains the
flavor of butter but is lower in unsaturated fats than butter. I find
the taste superior to any margarine. (And, if you look at the labels,
you'll see that most margarines contain additives—colorings, flavor
enhancers, preservatives—which I avoid whenever possible.)

"YES, BUT . . . WHY SO MUCH OIL IN THIS DIET?
ISN'T OIL FATTENING?"

Here's an eye opener for you. Oil is a fat. And *eating too little fat is probably a major cause of overweight.* There are several reasons for this. First, many women who seem overweight are just waterlogged. A nutritious diet that includes a *modest* amount of unsaturated vegetable oils often causes seemingly miraculous weight loss because it helps the tissues release water.

Another reason that fats have an important place in your reducing diet is that they are more satisfying than any other foods. You must have about 100 calories of fat per meal (equivalent to 1 tablespoon vegetable oil, mayonnaise, or butter) or you will become so hungry that you will probably stuff yourself with 1000 calories of carbohydrates (starch and sugar) just to still the hunger pangs—a loser if there ever was one.

You'll notice that I recommend adding fats to your diet in the form of unsaturated vegetable oils. There's a special reason for this.

These oils actually help the body burn excess fat stored in the tissues. Because most of the fat in the human body is saturated, the essential fatty acids (which are found in unsaturated vegetable oils) are necessary to make these saturated body fats burn. Three tablespoons of oil daily (or 6 teaspoons) combined with your high-protein diet will help your body burn off those excess pounds.

Adelle Davis felt so strongly about this that she said, "One rule that should never be broken . . . is to obtain some food supplying a teaspoon of vegetable oil six times daily, or about every three hours." This explains why the Super-B Diet includes some oil at each midmeal, as well as at regular mealtimes.

The following foods supply the equivalent of 1 teaspoon of oil:

10 large peanuts
6 almonds or 3 pecan or 2 walnut halves
2 teaspoons sunflower seeds
3 tablespoons wheat germ
1 tablespoon lecithin
1½ teaspoons mayonnaise (made with unsaturated oil, of course)
2 teaspoons non-hydrogenated peanut butter
2 teaspoons avocado

Or you might choose to add to your food 1 teaspoon of any unsaturated vegetable oil. I prefer a mixture of peanut, safflower, and soy oil (available at health food stores) because this combination is high in vitamin E and other nutrients.

However, don't go overboard on this oil intake. Oil *is* fattening and oil-rich foods are fattening if taken in excess. Eat the suggested amounts of the above foods and avoid foods rich in saturated fats. Cold cuts, hamburger, ham and other pork products, turkey, lamb, and even roast beef can contain as much as 50 per cent saturated fats. That's why the Super-B Diet stresses fish and seafood, liver, eggs, cottage cheese, and skim milk—all low in saturated fats. However, that's not their only claim to fame.

BEAUTY-FUEL

Certain foods turn up again and again in the diets of jet-set beauties, famed nutritionists, and professional athletes. These same foods have an important place in the Super-B Diet. As you looked through the diet you probably saw many familiar food friends, but other foods I've suggested may be strange to you, or downright peculiar. Yeast? . . . Kelp? . . . Millet mush? Once again, have faith. As you will see later, these are power-packed foods that contain high concentrations of the food elements needed to turn you into the dynamic Ageless Woman. In fact, let's talk about some of these special foods —what I call beauty-fuel foods.

ADD THESE FOODS TO CREATE YOUR OWN FOUNTAIN OF YOUTH

Cottage Cheese. (An old friend if I ever saw one.) This is a favorite dieter's food, and it's easy to see why. After all, just ½ cup of this relatively inexpensive food contains 20 grams of *complete* protein— as much as a serving of meat. It's also high in calcium, an important consideration during the menopause years as we'll be finding out.

Powdered Skim Milk. Can this food *really* "beef up" your love life? Let's see.

Powdered milk is high in protein, calcium, and two of the B vitamins, riboflavin and thiamine. Laboratory research has shown that liberal amounts of these four nutrients contribute to the continued youthfulness of the sex glands in both men and women. Powdered milk was the food used in these experiments.

So why take chances? By *all* means add this high-protein food to scrambled eggs, milk drinks, sandwich fillings, meat loaf, love potions. . . .

Before you femmes fatales become too enthusiastic about powdered milk, let me add that it should always be taken with a meal that contains some oil. Otherwise, you'll be unable to absorb the valuable calcium it contains, and at the same time you will create an increased need for vitamin B_2.

Wheat Germ. High in nearly complete proteins, a source of vitamin E, it is also a treasure house of B vitamins. B vitamins, you remember, give you the energy and enthusiasm that will help beat the middle-aged blues. Sprinkle a tablespoon of wheat germ (3 protein grams) on salads, add to soups and cereals, use as a filler in meat loaf, use like nuts to top a yogurt sundae.

Yogurt. A source of complete protein, high in calcium, its unique value lies in its ability to replenish the intestinal bacteria that synthesize certain B vitamins. Put simply, yogurt creates a B-vitamin factory, right in your very own tum-tum. What's more, it is a superior source of calcium, that miracle mineral that soothes frazzled nerves. Yogurt is an exceptional calcium food because cultured milk products contain calcium that is already dissolved, making it easy to absorb.

However, yogurt has become such a fad food that people overestimate its value as a protein source. One cup of commercial yogurt contains only 11 grams of complete protein. Now that you're counting your protein grams, you can readily see that a lunch of fruit and yogurt doesn't begin to fill your protein needs. Why not mix ½ cup yogurt with ½ cup cottage cheese, add mixed fruit, and top with 1 tablespoon wheat germ? Total—18½ grams of protein. Now that's more like it.

Yeast. The taste for yeast is an acquired one. (Remember your first olive? For that matter, remember your first martini?) Well, you'll learn to like yeast too. In fact, once over your initial reluctance, you'll find that you almost *crave* yeast. That's because it's just filled with nutritional goodies that you may have a hidden need for. It's so satisfying, it's been called the perfect reducing food. It's high in complete proteins (1 tablespoon contains 7 grams), low in calories, and loaded with B vitamins and minerals. According to biochemistry textbooks, the body needs at least fifty-five nutrients daily and, except for liver, yeast supplies more of them than any other single food.

Can yeast really make you younger? Well, it will seem that way when you see how adding yeast to your diet dramatically increases your energy level, soothes jangled nerves, and creates an enthusiastic and optimistic mental outlook. Most dramatic of all, though, is the effect yeast has on skin beauty.

These typical signs of middle age—rough, wrinkled lips and tiny lines along the outline of the upper lip ("whistle marks," Adelle Davis called them)—respond to the high B-vitamin content of yeast. In my own experience, I find that during times of stress, when I need lots of B vitamins, these little mouth lines become more pronounced. But when I increase the amount of yeast in my diet to make up for the added stress, these little lines go away in a matter of days.

Yeast also seems to plump up the skin, making all "expression lines" (a gentle name for wrinkles) less pronounced. What's more, sagging facial muscles respond to an intake of yeast, becoming firmer and lifted. I've noticed this effect so many times that I call yeast the Nutritional Face Lift. Sold? Good. Now, here's how to add yeast to your diet.

YEAST FOR BEGINNERS

Mix in electric blender:	PROTEIN GRAMS
3 cups skim milk	27
1 cup plain yogurt	8
1 heaping tablespoon brewers' yeast	7
1 tablespoon honey	0
Vanilla—to taste (about 1 teaspoon)	0
1 tablespoon (heaping) powdered milk	4
2 tablespoons vegetable oil	0
	46

A dash of nutmeg on top doesn't hurt a bit.

An 8-ounce glass of "Yeast for Beginners" can be used as a be-tween-meals pickup (see the Super-B Diet). With the addition of an egg yolk, one 8-ounce glass makes a nutritious liquid lunch.

Three cautionary notes:

1. Always take yeast with some calcium-rich food. (Note the skim milk *and* yogurt in the above recipe.) Occasionally, health and beauty buffs suggest stirring yeast into water or fruit juice. This is a no-no, unless the yeast has been supplemented with calcium, an increasingly popular trend, or unless you take a calcium supplement along with your yeast.

2. Be sure to get "brewers'" or nutritional yeast, not the live yeast used for cooking or those little squares of solid yeast that were a food fad about twenty years ago.

3. Many people just starting to add yeast to their diets find that it causes gas. That's why I've added yogurt to my recipe. It makes yeast

easier to digest. The point is, build up your yeast intake gradually—or your stomach may rebel. For maximum beauty results, start with 1 teaspoon to 1 tablespoon of yeast in your recipe and gradually build up to ¼ cup.

Liver. At first glance, an unlikely candidate for Beauty Food of the Century. It would be much more romantic to believe in some exotic elixir of youth made from Queen Bee jelly or the like. A slab of liver gleaming back at you from the butcher's counter is not only unromantic but, to some women, downright revolting. And yet, if ever a woman had a faithful if ugly friend, liver is it.

First of all, liver is one of the most nutritious of all foods. An average slice of this high-protein food contains:

Calcium	8 mg.
Phosphorus	486 mg.
Iron	7.8 mg. (hamburger contains only 2.8)
Vitamin A	53,500 I.U. (hamburger contains none)
Vitamin B_1	.26 mg. (hamburger contains .08)
Vitamin B_2	3.96 mg. (hamburger contains 1.19)
Vitamin B_{12}	35 mg. (hamburger contains 2)
Nicotinic acid (another B vitamin)	14.8 mg. (hamburger contains 4.8)
Vitamin C	31 mg. (hamburger contains none)

All this may be true, but somehow, for most of us, it doesn't make that slippery slab of cold liver any more lovable. However, when you know what this food can do for you, you'll become a liver lover for sure. Liver is cherished by nutritionists and doctors as *the* blood-building food. And without healthy blood you can't have a healthy, vital body. Since liver works to build up the very essence of your entire system—your blood stream—you can expect these benefits:

Liver can make you feel ageless. That is, if you define agelessness as having the energy to play that extra round of golf, to go out for dinner and dancing after a full day, to hold down a full-time job and still have vitality and enthusiasm left over for your home and family. Liver builds stamina and the ability to withstand stress. Without these qualities, you're too pooped to play, you'd rather mope than cope. A serving of calf's liver three times a week can change all that.

Liver can make you look ageless. Listen, my friend, if you have "tired blood," all the make-up in the world won't create that priceless basis for beauty—glowing health. But liver, the classic blood-building food, can be called the supreme beauty secret.

Healthy red blood which brings a bounty of beauty to every cell in the body can be called your beauty stream. It gives skin and lips a youthful, rosy color, pinks the tips of earlobes, and adds sparkle to the eye. Does this sound like the description of a dynamic, sexy woman? You bet it does! Skin, hair, muscles, sex glands, brain cells— all are nourished and rejuvenated by your beauty stream. What happens if that stream lacks essential nutrients? The result is that condition called anemia—and there's a good chance that you've got it. One expert estimates that up to 90 per cent of America's women and girls suffer from some form of anemia. Listen to these agemaking characteristics of anemia (as described by nutritionist Catharyn Elwood) and see if that slab of liver doesn't begin to look a little more appealing:

". . . dry lusterless hair that greys prematurely; skin that says goodbye to youth and folds into wrinkles early; fingernails that dry out, flatten and break easily; an inflamed sore tongue and mouth. Even slight anemia continued over a long period sees a change in facial expression; a gay face gradually becomes haggard and drawn."

And we're all familiar with the pasty white skin tone that usually accompanies this condition.

Incidentally, if you think that some patent medicine for "iron-poor anemia" can do as much for you as a serving of liver, look again at the treasure chest of life-giving, beauty-giving nutrients that liver contains. Do you *really* think one tablespoon of "Rejuvo" can match all that?

And, while you're checking that table of nutrients, don't overlook the bonus of vitamin A that you get in a serving of liver. Vitamin A, you'll recall, is the skin vitamin, the vitamin that can give you the complexion that most schoolgirls wish they had—and don't. (What can they expect from french fries and catsup?)

So be brave. Add liver to your diet for two weeks and look in your mirror. There's your proof. Here's how to do it. . . .

GLADYS LINDBERG'S STEAMED LIVER

Heat in a skillet equal parts butter and oil.

Cut 2 big onions and sauté until they are just clear.

Take onions out. Pop in the liver. (Always cook a pound at a time.)

Cook it over low flame for a minute or two until the liver just loses its red color. Now turn it over and put the onions back on top. Pour on 3 or 4 tablespoons vinegar. Put a lid on the skillet quickly and cook 5 minutes. Turn the heat off and let the liver stand another 5 minutes. There'll be no liver taste or smell, and the dish is delightful.

Chop any liver that's left over, mix with seasoning and mayonnaise, serve later on rye crackers with grated egg on top.

DR. WHITLOCK'S LIVER STICKS

1 pound liver, ½ inch thick
½ cup dry bread, cracker crumbs, or cereal
¼ cup powdered milk
½ teaspoon salt

Cut liver in ½-inch-wide strips. Mix crumbs with milk and salt Roll liver in crumb mixture. Fry in fat until lightly browned. (Too much heat toughens liver.) This is a great "finger food." Dip the liver sticks into catsup and eat them as a snack.

Or, if the idea of eating fresh liver is just too much for you at first, try powdered liver, available at drug and health food stores. Two heaping tablespoons equal 6-ounce serving of regular liver. Here's how I take it.

LIVER COCKTAIL
(For the Brave—and the Beautiful)

Put in blender:
    4 sprigs parsley
    1 tablespoon vinegar or lemon juice
    ½ cup V-8 or tomato juice
    ½ teaspoon kelp powder or granulated kelp
Blend. Then add:
    1 heaping tablespoon liver powder (start with 1 teaspoon and
        work up.)
Add additional ½ cup V-8 or tomato juice
Blend

This combination of ingredients masks the liver flavor and, believe

me, it's really a delightful pickup. I can see that you don't believe
me. Be brave. Try it anyway. Countless students have told me that
they have more energy, feel more cheerful, and have better skin tone
and color after a regular regimen of Liver Cocktails. So drink up.

Millet. An important addition to the Super-B Diet for various
reasons. First, it is one of the oldest and most nutritious foods
known to man. Some experts declare that in an emergency situation
millet could be used as the sole source of nourishment. In fact, amid
growing rumors of impending food shortages, many farsighted and
knowledgeable people are buying bulk millet and storing it—just in
case. While I'm certainly not suggesting a millet diet, it is an excellent addition to the Super-B menus.

Millet, unlike refined cereals, is rich in high-grade protein as well
as vitamins, minerals, and that interesting substance, lecithin. (More
about it in a minute.) Millet is also an alkaline food—an important
factor in the American diet, which tends to be too acid.

But more than this, millet, like other grain and seed foods (unless
they have been nutritionally castrated by the food refiners), may
have some extra element, a mysterious *something* that is essential to
health and longevity. As Lelord Kordel says in his book *Eat and
Grow Younger,* "Modern diets ignore the axiom that seeds hold the
germ of life. Too often overlooked is the fact that nature has placed
in seed foods the concentrated essence of all nutrition in order to
provide nourishment for the sprouting plant." It's certainly true that
the diets of all those age-defying, Shangri-la type villagers, whether in
the Himalayas or the Andes, are high in unrefined grains, especially
millet.

You can add millet to your diet in a variety of ways. It's delicious
as a hot cereal in the morning. Or the cooked cereal can be packed
in a loaf pan and refrigerated. Then the sliced cereal loaf can be
fried or steamed as an additional protein food at any meal. It can be
used with meats instead of a starchy staple because it adds the contrasting bland taste we are usually seeking as an accompaniment to
meat. And 1 serving contains 10 grams of (incomplete) protein. And
millet is an excellent meat extender, good news in this era of spiral-
ing prices. Add millet meal to your meat loaf instead of the fattening, nutritionally empty cracker crumbs you may have been using.

Finally, millet is an excellent meat substitute. If you wish to cut
down on the meat in your diet, try this dish:

MILLET CAKES

1 cup *cooked* hulled millet (available at health food stores)
1 tablespoon powdered milk
2 eggs
1 or 2 tablespoons finely chopped onions
½ teaspoon poultry seasoning

Mix all ingredients in a bowl. If possible, allow to sit for an hour or two, to blend flavors.

Then drop by tablespoon onto lightly greased skillet. Flatten cakes with pancake turner. Allow one side to brown thoroughly before *carefully* turning cakes. (No flapjack dramatics. These cakes will crumble.) Serve with a tomato-cheese sauce or leftover chicken gravy with mushrooms added.

NEW EVIDENCE THAT YOU CAN "EAT AND GROW YOUNGER"

Here is some additional evidence that the fountain of youth is indeed in your kitchen and that certain everyday, prosaic foods contain substances that can stimulate the cells to continued vigor and youthfulness.

New York physician Dr. Benjamin S. Frank, whose research is the basis for so many exciting new diet findings, believes that the body ages because its repair processes are no longer efficient. While old age may manifest itself in a variety of degenerative conditions, each with its own symptoms, this degeneration stems from a single cause: the deterioration of individual cells and the body's inability to replace those cells.

Dr. Frank says, "If aging is the deterioration of our cells, then let's make them healthy again by providing those substances that nourish and repair them most directly."

The substances that Dr. Frank (and countless other researchers in this field) are dealing with are DNA (deoxyribonucleic acid), "the body's master chemical blueprint for building new cells," and RNA (ribonucleic acid), "the 'messenger' chemical that carries out DNA's work. . . . Whenever new cells are required, our DNA sends out RNA molecules to form them."

While the body does produce its own nucleic acids, as we age our bodies produce too little and of too low a quality to stimulate the trillions of body cells to replenish and repair themselves efficiently. The cumulative result? You're falling apart, my dear, that's what.

Dr. Frank feels that these nucleic acids are essential nutrients and can have a remarkably retarding effect on the aging process.

By treating his aged patients with *extracts* of these nucleic acids, Dr. Frank reported these results. After a week, 80 to 90 per cent said they felt better and had more energy. They looked better, too. Their skin quality was firmer, healthier-looking. After a month or two these additional changes in the skin were noted: deep lines and wrinkles (forehead wrinkles, smile lines from nose to mouth and, finally, wrinkles around the eyes) became shallower and less pronounced. In other words, his patients looked younger and said they *felt* younger.

Although these patients were treated with extracts, which are more potent in their action than foods, Dr. Frank believes that these essential nucleic acids can be produced in age-defying quantities by adding RNA-rich foods to your diet.

I must point out that the nucleic acid theories are quite new and have not yet stood the test of time. But look at the following list of the foods that Dr. Frank recommends as being high in nucleic acid. They are all so good for us that they belong in our diets anyway— and many are already in the Super-B Diet. So why not?

1. Fish—especially the small sardines that come from Portugal. Also lobsters, clams, crabs, and oysters. All are rich in nucleic acids. Fish is so rich in them that Dr. Frank recommends it in your diet seven times a week.

2. Peas, lentils, lima beans, or soybeans—not more than twice a week. (These legumes are fattening, y'know.)

3. Liver. (Aha! What have I been telling you? It *is* the super-food.)

4. Beets. They contain an amino acid that helps build up nucleic acid. Beets are beneficial in any form—beet juice included—and should be in the diet at least three times a week according to Dr. Frank. He also states that the amino acids in beets contribute to more efficient functioning of the brain. (An extremely useful tip. I need all the help I can get. How about you?)

5. Spinach, cauliflower, mushrooms, celery, radishes, onions, scallions, asparagus. He suggests one or two of these each day.

6. Nuts—preferably unsalted. Remember what we found out

about seeds, that they may contain some essential *something* necessary to health and the maintenance of youthful characteristics? Well, nuts are seeds.

Although the foods that Dr. Frank recommends to fight off age are entirely prosaic, two other foods that have been getting a lot of publicity in recent months are not so familiar. Are they really the Magic Diet Foods that you've been led to believe? Let's see.

HELP! HELP! WHY KELP?

Just what is in this common seaweed plant that makes it such a popular new addition to reducing diets? And does it really accelerate the loss of those excess pounds? On the surface, it may appear that the Seaweed Diet is just another of the many food fads that hits this country like an epidemic every two or three years. Yet there is a sound nutritional basis for the recent enthusiasm over kelp.

Kelp is rich in iodine, the mineral that helps the thyroid gland to function efficiently and produce the correct amount of the hormone called thyroxin. This hormone controls the speed of your life processes (or metabolism). As nutritionist Catharyn Elwood explains it, thyroxin is like a "little chemical messenger controlling the speed of your life processes. It behaves much like the accelerator in your car; when you 'step on the gas' the motor races. Just so, when your thyroid speeds up and pours out a great amount of thyroxin, your body activities are accelerated."

The woman whose thyroid is overactive is usually a candidate for the broomstick brigade. You may envy her extremely thin figure, but it's a bad bargain when you realize that this is accompanied by extreme irritability, nervousness, and seemingly neurotic excitability. The witchy hyperthyroid type drives herself and everyone around her to nervous distraction.

On the other hand, the woman whose thyroid is underactive and producing too little thyroxin feels phlegmatic and totally without energy and enthusiasm. In a word, she feels *old*. And she looks old, too. Her figure may become matronly and dumpy. Unwanted pounds seem to hang around, no matter how drastic her diet regime.

Naturally, these extreme conditions must be treated by your physician, and if either of these descriptions seems to apply to you, get thee to thy physician, posthaste.

However, a slight slowing down of the action of the thyroid seems to be very common after forty. This slowing down can be so slight that it won't be discovered by current testing methods. Even though you may feel blah and may look bloated, your physician may well say that your thyroid is okay.

Dr. Murray Israel, a New York physician who has been given international recognition for his work with thyroid activity, feels that even the best techniques for measuring metabolism and the efficiency of the thyroid gland lack precision. He believes that the hormone output of even a healthy thyroid gland steadily declines with living, and eventually stops producing enough thyroxin to keep that tiger in your metabolic tank. Perhaps this is why so many women feel that additional pounds are inevitable after "a certain age." Not so.

This is where kelp comes in. This iodine-rich food can gently nudge sluggish thyroid glands and stimulate them to produce the amount of thyroxin your body needs. Since kelp is a food, not a drug or medicine, it can be safely added to anyone's diet—with two exceptions. If you have a record of acne, iodine may aggravate this condition. And, of course, if you are already taking thyroid supplements prescribed by your doctor, you should check with him before adding kelp to your diet.

Kelp can speed up your metabolism, which simply means that you'll be operating more efficiently, you'll have more energy, and your body will process foods more effectively, which will help with those stubborn pounds that won't go away. Instead of lounging around on your hips and thighs, excess pounds burn off. When your efficient thyroid "steps on the gas," it's full speed ahead to a better figure.

Another beauty by-product of kelp is that it beautifies the hair and nails, which is not too surprising because one of the effects of an inactive or sluggish thyroid is dry, lifeless hair and splitting nails. Kelp made a believer out of me just recently.

Even though my normal diet is high in protein and calcium, the classic nail-building elements, *nothing* seemed to stop my nails from becoming brittle and splitting off in layers. But kelp seems to have done the trick. After reading Dr. Israel's comments on "lazy" thyroids, I doubled the kelp in my diet (from one to two teaspoons per day). Suddenly—almost miraculously—my nails became strong, hard, and will now grow long enough to satisfy a Chinese emperor.

Kelp is also important to you because it contains countless trace minerals from the sea, minerals that may not be available in your daily diet. The value of these trace minerals is only now being discovered in scientific laboratories throughout the world.

Many scientists engaged in trace mineral research say that kelp contains all the elements needed for cell regeneration and repair. Others have noted that kelp helps the function of not only the thyroid but also the pancreas and the sex glands and gives good results in treating premature aging.

And what does this mean to the Ageless Woman? Eat kelp. That's what it means.

AND WHAT ABOUT LECITHIN?

It, too, is a little-known food that is part of the complex nutrition picture. Lecithin (pronounced less-i-thin) is found in every cell and organ of the body and some experts feel that it is essential to cell regeneration and may retard the aging process.

Lecithin is important in weight control because it helps to redistribute body fat. Perhaps this is because lecithin is a fat emulsifier. It is used industrially to break down molecules of fat in certain products so that they can be more readily combined with other ingredients. In the body, lecithin breaks down clumps of the fatty substance cholesterol, so that it can be utilized by the body.

Perhaps this emulsifying action is the reason lecithin seems to help in redistributing body fat. Many nutrition specialists report that lecithin is helpful in shifting body weight from areas of the body where it is unwanted to places where it is needed. I think this is an exceptionally important consideration, since so many women complain, "I lose weight all right. Just where I don't want to—in my face and bust." Exercise is, of course, an important consideration in weight distribution, but many women find that lecithin seems to speed up the process.

But the value of lecithin goes further than weight loss. It can make you look younger.

1. Lecithin contains the B vitamin, cholin, which contributes to the health and strength of muscle tissue. Adding lecithin to your diet can help delicate facial muscles stay firm and *right up there where they belong.*

2. Lecithin combats those three telltale signs of the aging skin—dryness, paper-thinness, and wrinkles. Lecithin not only helps the body process all fats and oils more efficiently (it's an emulsifier, remember), it also seems to distribute them where they have been deficient. In mature women, this means in the tissues of dry and wasted skin. However it works, lecithin does contribute amazingly to skin beauty. I know. I've seen it happen on the faces of many students and members of my family. My mother, who has been a lecithin enthusiast for years, is beginning her seventies. You'd never believe it to look at her. Her skin is firm, elastic, dewy—and not a wrinkle.

An excellent source of lecithin is found in soybeans. Your local health food store will probably have soy-lecithin in several forms.

Soy-lecithin granules can be added to cereals, eggs, salads—almost any food. And the liquid blends well in any drink, "Yeast for Beginners," for example. For best results, you'll need to take two to four tablespoons daily. Since it is truly a delicious food, it seems a shame to take the capsules or tablets, which are more expensive than the nutlike granules or the liquid.

Incidentally, you have to be patient to see the results I've been describing, but don't be discouraged. Unlike those power-packed beauty-fuel foods, yeast and liver, you won't see results in a few days. But hang in there—in about six weeks you'll see your skin begin to plump up, dry patches will disappear, and lines and wrinkles will become less pronounced.

Skin and figure beauty are important, but lecithin can also contribute mightily to the mental well-being of mature women everywhere by destroying Madge. You know Madge. She is the unseen star of that most obnoxious TV commercial, the one that takes place in the telephone booth of Drugstore, USA. Remember how it goes?

Madge's friend, a doughy-looking frantic type, calls from the drugstore. "Hello, Madge? Can you help me? I just don't know which laxative to take. There are bulk types, candy types, oils, powders. I'm confused. *Please* help me."

Gee, what a career. To be the Laxative Lady in your community. The mind boggles.

I think all women loathe those commercials, with their portrayal of a woman over forty as one who is not only eternally constipated but also too dumb to make a simple decision without help from her omnipotent friend. Is Madge a M.A.M.? I'd just bet on it.

Well, constipation can be a problem, for both men and women. But the solution to this vexing problem should not be the harsh chemical laxatives that Madge recommends. You know, of course, that these work because they are *irritants.* In an effort to expel the irritating chemicals, the body expels everything, including essential vitamins, minerals, and nutrients.

A healthful, well-balanced diet will help you avoid this difficulty—and that healthful well-balanced diet should include lecithin. This substance has been found to be an amazing help in clearing up problems of chronic constipation. In a study at the Warner Institute of Therapeutic Research, it was found that inositol, a B vitamin found in lecithin, caused a marked increase in the contractions of the stomach and intestines. These contractions (peristalsis) are essential to digestion and the passage of food and waste products through the digestive tract. So a deficiency in inositol may well account for the sluggish bowel action that so many mature women experience.

Which means that, if all the women over forty gang up and add lecithin to their Super-B Diet, Madge will have had it.

"Don't call us, Madge—and we don't have to call you."

THE SKIN GAME

Every food in the Super-B Diet will ultimately contribute to the ageless beauty of your skin. If you make the beauty-fuel foods an important part of your daily menus, your face will soon demonstrate this basic truth—you must start on the *inside* to create skin beauty on the *outside.* Once you have been convinced of this by the reflection in your own mirror—you're free. Free from all those bottles and jars of miracle rejuvenating creams (at $7.50 to $10 a throw) that promise to make your skin young again.

Granted, we all need some creams and lotions to cleanse and lubricate our skin on the outside. But why go to the department stores? You can make your own face cream. Your kitchen can help you put *natural* yet luxurious creams on your beauty menu. The recipes I'm going to give you are inexpensive yet contain beautifiers that externally help control two problems so common to mature complexions—those ugly sisters, Dry Skin and Wrinkles.

First, though, I must stress the importance of leaving behind those commercial products with their high-blown promises and puffed-up prices.

THE GREAT HORMONE ROBBERY—
WHY YOU SHOULD MAKE YOUR OWN FACE CREAM

At a time in your life when you want to hang onto every one of your precious female hormones, your regular face creams may be removing hormones as well as vitamins from your system.

That's the opinion of many nutritionists, who explain that mineral oil, the base for most creams, can be especially detrimental to women in the menopause and premenopause years.

Adelle Davis said, "Although the effect of cold creams apparently has not been specifically studied, it is known that estrogen, the adrenal hormones, and vitamins A, D, E and K dissolve in mineral oils, from which most cold creams are made; and that *mineral oil absorbs through the skin when creams containing it are used.* [Emphasis added.] These hormones and vitamins are then lost in the feces. Mineral oil in all forms should probably be avoided, particularly during the menopause."

And what about face creams fortified with hormones? While there is much evidence that the external application of estrogen can improve the quality of the mature skin, these hormones are usually mixed in a cream or lotion that has a mineral oil base. There's an excellent chance that the benefits of these creams are canceled out by the drawbacks of mineral oil. Since hormone creams are among the most expensive, their use seems especially wasteful.

Of course, not all commercial face creams contain mineral oil. More and more, the swing is toward organic (vegetable oils) rather than inorganic (mineral oils) products. Just be aware that the cream advertised as an organic super-E wheat germ cream may in fact contain only one part of wheat germ oil to ten parts of mineral oil.

This is just one of the reasons that so many women have become intrigued with the idea of making their own face creams. When you mix it yourself, you *know* what's in it. And you save money, too. The most luxurious ingredients will add up to a cost of pennies a jar, compared to $5.00, $10, or even more for the commercial products. Which means you'll have some extra money to spend on something sensible—like make-up glasses ground to your own prescription, or a quart or two of Chanel No. Five.

Finally, you can screen out any ingredients that may cause you an allergic reaction. (For example, perfumed creams, pleasant as they are, often cause allergic reactions.) So put on your wizard's hat, grab that magic wand, and haul out that big black cauldron.

TRY THESE RECIPES FOR FEEDING YOUR SKIN (EAT YOUR HEART OUT, JULIA CHILD)

The idea of making your own face creams seems to have a basic appeal to all women . . . perhaps it harks back to the childhood bliss of messing around with mud pies. Whatever the reason, recipes for these concoctions abound in every magazine and newspaper.

One of the most popular recent fads has been the so-called cosmetic mayonnaise. I won't pass along my very own supersecret, exclusive mayonnaise recipe, because mayonnaise is mayonnaise. Just look in any cookbook and you'll find an excellent recipe.

While there's no doubt that the rich egg, oil, and vinegar mixture is excellent for your skin, cosmetic mayonnaise overlooks *the* essence of cosmetic magic—the psychological factor. Those rich, luxurious, perfumed commercial creams make you feel beautiful, pampered, and special—so you use them faithfully, mineral oil and all. But mayonnaise? Is that glamorous? I ask you! After the first enthusiastic application of cosmetic mayonnaise, most women are completely turned off by the idea of smelling like the leftovers from a salad bar. It just ain't got no mystique.

If this has been your reaction to these "salad ways," I think you'll respond, as so many of my students have, to the luxury as well as the purity of these cosmetic recipes.

Try this one on for size:

CLEOPATRA CREME

You'll need:
  1 small jar
  1 plastic ice cube tray (the kind that allows you to extract a single cube)
  1 pint of extra rich whipping cream

Pour about 1 tablespoon of the cream into the jar, using a spoon to include all the thick cream curd around the tip of the cream container.

Pour the rest of the cream into the ice cube tray and put it in the freezer.

That's it. You'll use cream, just rich, pure cream, to lubricate or cleanse your face. And you'll love it. The butterfat in that cream absorbs into your skin almost immediately, so there's no greasy aftereffect. And rich cream contains natural ingredients that are skin beautifiers.

First, there's vitamin A, often called the skin vitamin because it's so important in contributing to the skin's beauty. One half cup of whipping cream contains over a thousand units of vitamin A, one of several vitamins which are readily absorbed through the skin. (More about this in a minute.)

The lactic acid in cream helps your skin to maintain that all-important acid mantle, the acid-based film that is present on the surface of healthy skin and hair. This acid mantle is your body's way of protecting your skin from bacteria. It also seems to create that "dewy" effect that is so attractive. Soaps, of course, are alkaline, and remove this acid mantle. Many commercial creams also have an alkali base. But your Cleopatra Creme passes the acid test—it makes your skin look beautiful.

Naturally, you must keep your jar of Cleopatra Creme refrigerated. As long as it's absolutely fresh, you'll have no trouble with dairy odors. I find it completely odorless—my husband didn't know I used it until he read this copy—but if you yearn for some sweet-smelling goo to apply to your face, add a few drops of vanilla. It's better to smell like a cute cooky than a salad. Right?

If you have extremely dry skin, try this more elaborate recipe:

CREME DE LA CREME

You'll need:

1 small jar
1 bottle of wheat germ oil
1 pint of extra rich whipping cream

To make approximately 2 ounces of face cream, put 2 tablespoons of oil and 2 tablespoons of cream into the jar, cover, and shake vigorously. The oil and cream will mix together to form a thick, rich product. Keep it refrigerated along with the remaining oil. Freeze the remaining cream, as in the basic recipe. One batch should last about a week under refrigeration.

This luscious concoction is an all-purpose cream. Use it for cleansing, use it as a night cream, and apply it to dry skin on legs and elbows. It's a marvelous dry skin fighter, though it takes a bit longer to absorb than the basic cream recipe because of the addition of the oil.

If you want to give your skin a vitamin-rich meal, try this:

SUPER CREME DE LA CREME

To the above recipe, add:

2 capsules vitamin A, 25,000-unit strength
5 capsules vitamin E, 200-unit strength

Puncture each capsule with a pin and squeeze the contents into your Creme de la Creme. Shake well to mix. Keep refrigerated.

Why vitamins in your skin cream? Because vitamins can definitely be absorbed through the skin. Vitamin E gives especially dramatic results. Linda Clark tells about an informal survey she made, asking friends to apply vitamin E to their skins twice daily. At the end of four weeks she reported that these changes were observed:

1. Lines under the eyes smoothed out.
2. Tiny lines on upper lip smoothed out.
3. One woman found that crepy skin areas were tightened.
4. Another found that her formerly sallow face acquired a rosy glow.

My students have also experienced these results as well as the miraculous effect that vitamin E has on scarring. One woman found that acne scars, left over from a severe adolescent bout with this skin condition, became filled in and eventually disappeared completely.

I had a demonstration of the remarkable healing effects of vitamin E just a few weeks ago. When pouring a pan of boiling soup from the pot to a tureen, I spilled a stream of the red-hot liquid onto my forearm. As I watched, I could see the burned skin turning red, pulling together to form a gigantic blister. As I stood there numbly looking at the mess I'd made of my arm, my husband grabbed a 200-unit capsule of vitamin E, cut the end off, and squeezed the contents onto the burn. In an hour, this excruciatingly painful burn didn't hurt at all. The next morning my skin was unblemished with no sign of the angry blister that I had seen forming. Now I have heard countless doctors on TV pooh-pooh the idea that vitamin E has a spectacular effect on the skin. They'll never convince me.

A number of experiments have demonstrated that vitamin A, the "skin vitamin," can also be absorbed directly through the skin. Dr. Albert Sobel and Dr. Abraham Rosenberg, in a report to the American Chemical Society, stated that vitamin A absorbed through the skin can often be more beneficial in the treatment of skin disorders than the same vitamin taken internally.

Lack of vitamin A often results in dry skin, a familiar problem to many mature women. My students tell me that this vitamin A cream seems to do more to correct dry, flaky skin than any other preparation they've tried.

While your skin will definitely benefit from the vitamin-rich Super Creme de la Creme, remember that no skin cream can really help much if your diet is poor. The Super Creme de la Creme is meant as a supplement to the vitamin-rich Super-B Diet. Your skin cannot help but bloom after a vitamin feast on both the inside and the outside.

LEMON REFRESHER

You'll need:
½ pint of distilled water
Juice of 1 lemon
Several strips of lemon peel

Strain the lemon juice and add it to the water. Shake vigorously. Add the strips of lemon peel, which will enhance the fresh, lemony scent.

Use this delightful refresher to complete your facial cleansing. Apply it after you've cleansed with your Cleopatra Creme. You'll see that it removes every bit of make-up. The lemon juice tightens the pores and leaves the skin with an acid surface.

Keep this refrigerated, too.

YEAST 'N YOGURT FACIAL

Mix 1 teaspoon of brewers' yeast with 1 teaspoon yogurt. Apply to your superclean face (except the eye area).

Don't be alarmed if you seem to be experiencing an instant hot flash. Your face doesn't burn, mind you, but you do feel a surge of blood coming to the surface of the skin. Your face will feel warm, warmer, and then you'll feel as if you were sporting a real Lydia Pinkham blush. To those of you who may be saying, "Who needs that kind of facial? I can produce my *own* hot flashes, thank you," let me hasten to add this warm experience lasts only a few moments —just long enough to bring a surge of your healthy beauty stream to the surface of the skin, to nourish and stimulate the skin cells.

This is a great antidote for the "gray lady look" that many women have, especially those who are just starting on their Super-B Diets and haven't built up their health yet. Your skin will look renewed and alive for hours after this facial treatment—yet the blush effect subsides in about ten or fifteen minutes. This is a great treatment when you're planning a big evening and your face looks pale and drawn—perhaps showing the effects of a long and demanding day. This facial is the answer—it will give your looks a lift.

The long-range effects of this circulation stimulator are livelier skin color, finer texture, a softer and smoother skin surface. It is also effective in clearing up skin blemishes, seeming to dry up and heal those embarrassing holdovers from our "blossoming" adolescent years.

These beneficial effects are the result of improved circulation, the lactic acid base of the yogurt, and the high B vitamin content in the yeast. According to a report for the Lee Foundation for Nutritional Research, vitamin B, as well as A, D, and E, can be absorbed through the skin.

A PARTING SHOT

You must remember that this is not a "diet book," and the Super-B Diet is not a gimmick diet. It is a health diet. The Super-B Diet will help you become slim and stay slim, but it also does more—it helps you become ageless. It restores wasted tissues, fights premature aging, and builds dynamic energy.

Since the Super-B Diet is not a gimmick diet, not an over-simplification designed to capture the public fancy for a few profitable months, it may seem a little complicated—a little difficult at first. And this may be where we separate the M.A.M.s from the Ageless Women.

Because it is difficult—at first—to become the Ageless Woman.

You have to decide for yourself what sort of person you want to be as you mature. Do you want to waddle through what should be your best years as an overweight, middle-aged, self-indulgent baby who can't eat this and won't eat that, and *must* eat this and *must* eat that?

Or do you want to become an Ageless Woman? If agelessness is your choice, you will have to change your life style from self-indulgence to self-respect. In private, the Ageless Woman may scowl at something that's very good for her—that first liver cocktail, for example—and wrinkle her nose in distaste; but she'll say, "I *will* drink you, you S.O.B., if it kills me."

And she will, too. And she will learn to like what's good for her; because she knows that she is literally fighting for her life—the vital, dynamic, fun kind of life that she wants to live during all those bonus years that modern science has given her.

SIX

Thin Isn't Everything

Diet alone won't correct your figure problems. Diet will give your body the nutrients it needs, diet will help you lose fat, but if the muscles that remain are lax and flabby, then you need exercise. Your entire body—inside and out—needs a regular exercise program to keep it firm, vital, in proportion, healthy, and ageless.

Now don't go away mad. I am *not* going to give you the old instant-transformation pitch. You know the kind: "Give me your flabby, miserable, aging body for five minutes—only five minutes—a day while our exercise machine (or television program, or electric vibrator, or whatever) makes you into a woman whose figure Russian ballerinas will envy." You've read, and possibly fallen for, this sort of come-on many times. The exercises are slowly done to music, or while lying down, and the leaders or models who demonstrate them are always impossibly slender and beautiful—and smiling, just to rub it in. But I'm not going to let you cop out with any token, no-sweat exercise program. Getting and keeping in shape is a serious business; one that takes great perseverance and, unavoidably, a certain amount of exertion.

I'M A DIRTY, ROTTEN, LAZY SLOB

Ah, the guilt! The guilt that those exercise pitches have piled on the flabby American housewife. How about you? You know you should exercise, you *hate* exercise, you stop exercising, then you feel guilty. Right? But it doesn't end there, does it?

Someone is always nagging. You start a typical morning by waking up the family. You feed your husband and get him off to work, you feed the kids and send them off to school, you feed the cat and dog, you change the canary's water. And *finally* you settle down on the couch to relax with a cup of coffee, and who's on television? Jack La Lanne, that's who. Sixty-year-old Jack La Lanne—impossibly trim, unbelievably energetic, and revoltingly cheerful. "All right, ladies, now we'll do the tummies. Down on the floor—hup two, hup two . . ."

And all those guilt feelings are back. But cheer up a little. You probably have a sound reason for hating exercise.

THE SPIRIT'S WILLING, BUT THE FLESH IS WEAK

Let's say that it's a Monday morning and you are a person of depth. You have a sterling character and lots of will power. You've decided, "Monday is the day. I simply *have* to start an exercise regimen and get rid of these saddlebags."

So you don't turn on the television. You don't read the paper. Instead, you dutifully get out that collection of yellowing exercises, put a bouncy record on the hi-fi (as per instructions), and start with exercise number 1. Everything's going well and you're feeling pretty smug.

You start on exercise number 2. ("On count one, jump with feet apart, clap hands over head. On count two, jump with feet together, hands back at sides. Isn't this fun?") Well, no. It isn't. Because by this time you're beginning to feel distinctly uncomfortable—you're puffing, and you have a cramp in your big toe.

But you go on to exercises 4 and 5.

"Now, for our tummies, let's do some sit-ups . . . how about eight, just for starters?"

You're determined to stick it out, but by the fourth sit-up your back is killing you, you're gasping for breath, your heart is pounding, and you're developing a headache.

In short, by this time you're such a mass of wheezing, tortured flesh that the idea of continuing this masochism for four more weeks seems utter madness. Will you drag your sore body out of bed tomorrow morning and continue with the same relentless routine? Maybe. Some women do, and they deserve all the admiration and ego-building compliments that their beautiful figures command.

But there's a good chance that by Wednesday—Thursday at the latest—you'll be back in front of the TV for a well-deserved break. And when Jack La Lanne springs into the picture you'll glower at him, mutter, "Look at that darned old fool," turn the television to "A Brighter Day at the Edge of Night" or some such program, and settle down with the paper.

Lazy? You? Certainly not. After all, who changed the canary's water? But if a bout with strenuous exercise soon has you on the ropes—gasping for breath, worn out—it teaches you two things: first, you are totally out of shape physically, and second, you are attempting the wrong exercises at the wrong time. In fact, you are too out of shape to get back in shape—at least through attempting strenuous calisthenic exercises.

You are not alone. Even those naturally slender women whom you may envy probably need exercise. That friend of yours who can eat like a horse without gaining a pound is probably hopelessly out of condition. Being out of condition may not be too significant during a woman's twenties, and perhaps not too noticeable during her thirties, but during the forties, the ax suddenly falls.

Abruptly, she finds that she can't do the things she used to enjoy. A shopping trip gives her a headache—and sore feet. She gets out of breath on the escalator. And, insidiously, those deadly M.A.M.isms creep into her thoughts. "Face it," she says to herself, "we all slow down after a 'certain age.'"

THOSE OUT-OF-SHAPE BLAHS

The out-of-shape blahs come on so slowly that you don't notice them at first. But somehow you find that more and more you want to sit and relax in front of the TV. You're increasingly irritable, and when you're upset you have headaches. The vacations you used to look forward to have somehow become exhausting ordeals.

You often fall into that lethargic mood when you don't want to do anything, you don't get excited about anything, and you don't seem to have fun any more.

Well, what's happened to you? Are you really getting old? *No! No! No!* You are probably just out of condition. And if you are out of condition, chances are all the will power in the world won't keep you on a strenuous calisthenic exercise program. You will loathe all exertion.

But why drag around, half alive, when the answer to your problem is so easy? It's so ridiculously simple to attain conditioned fitness.

WHAT DOES IT MEAN TO ATTAIN CONDITIONED FITNESS?

It means:
Energy
Stamina
Endurance
Enthusiasm

In short, when you are in tiptop condition, you can laugh at the calendar and enjoy life.

In recent years we have learned that a person can be slim, with firm, elastic muscles, and still be so out of condition that she is actually sick. Being physically conditioned starts on the *inside*. If your heart, lungs, and blood vessels are out of condition, you will increasingly be the poop-out at the party. And those yellowing exercise plans *will not* make you physically fit by themselves. Something else is needed.

That "something else" is not just any old exercise. Those familiar exercises simply won't do it. The "daily dozen" won't do it. (Sorry, Jack.) Paddling around your swimming pool won't do it. A leisurely walk after dinner won't do it. That biweekly golf game won't do it. There's only one type of exercise that will bring you the rejuvenating benefits we've been talking about. And once you've tried it, you'll be sold for life.

AEROBICS IS THE MAGIC WORD

And it's a word you've probably heard often. But *exactly* what does it mean? Webster's definition is, "living, acting, or occurring only in the presence of oxygen." Which means, of course, that every human being is practicing aerobics. We're all aerobs. It's just that some of us are more efficient than others in processing the oxygen we breathe. Since oxygen is the key factor in turning the food you eat into energy, the body's ability to get and process oxygen dictates your energy level. A well-developed oxygen-processing system means that you burn fuel (your food) quickly and efficiently to produce energy.

According to Kenneth H. Cooper, father of the aerobics program, "The main objective of an aerobic exercise program is to increase the maximum amount of oxygen that the body can process *within a given time*. [Emphasis mine.] This is called your *aerobic capacity*. It is dependent on an ability to 1) rapidly breathe large amounts of air, 2) forcefully deliver large volumes of blood [throughout the body] and 3) effectively deliver oxygen to all parts of the body. In short, it depends upon efficient lungs, a powerful heart, and a good vascular system. Because it reflects the conditions of these vital organs, the aerobic capacity is the best index of overall fitness."

However, through inactivity, your processing plant (lungs, heart, blood vessels) can become inefficient to the point that the slightest exertion leaves you huffing and puffing for air. Your body needs more oxygen, but the processing plant can't deliver. The result is that the slightest exertion is unpleasant, produces fatigue, and is religiously avoided.

INACTIVE? ME? ARE YOU KIDDING?

At least once during every lecture I hear that Great American Cop-out. It goes something like this, "I must be in great condition because I'm certainly active. I take care of my big house without any help. I do all the shopping and errands. My youngest is still at home, which involves a certain amount of chauffeuring and running around after her. And then, of course, there's my twice-weekly golf game."

I've heard a thousand variations on this theme. Does it make sense? Well, test it yourself.

Think about it the next time you go to the supermarket. All the women around you run their households and regularly engage in all those "cop-out" exercises. Yet how many do you see walking with a springy athletic stride, a proud carriage, and a lively expression?

Look closely. Aren't most of them simply dragging around on doughy thighs, shoulders slumped, bosoms drooping? In fact, don't many of them look as if they're being held up by those shopping carts?

If you're honest with yourself, you can see *exactly* what the cop-out exercises really do for the health of the mature American woman.

The problem is that all those cop-out exercises overlook the essential factor necessary to obtain the magical benefits that come when you are conditionally fit. This essential factor is called:

THE OVERLOAD PRINCIPLE

In order to condition the entire body you must overload the oxygen-processing center *continuously over a period of time.* In other words, you should exercise until you begin to puff *and then keep exercising.* The overload principle helps your body build greater reserves of energy; because when the body is stimulated by above-normal exercise over a period of time, it responds by building an increased capacity for physical work. The heart becomes stronger and pumps more blood with each beat. The veins and arteries become larger and more elastic in order to carry additional oxygen to the working muscles. The lungs become more efficient. In short, the overload effect gives your oxygen-processing system a complete overhaul.

Now, the trouble with the types of exercise that most people indulge in is that they do not produce the "overload" effects. Let's look at that golf game. If you ride in a cart, you've blown it already. But let's assume that you walk those eighteen holes. You take a leisurely walk, then stop and wait for each of your foursome to take her turn. Sorry, it simply doesn't produce an overload effect. The closest you'll get to huffing and puffing is through frustration when you miss an eight-inch putt. Breaking clubs doesn't count either— you may develop firmer arms, but club breaking does nothing for your oxygen-processing system. In fact, the only measurable overload effect probably takes place at the nineteenth hole.

Suppose you're lucky enough to have a pool. Paddling around at a leisurely pace will do very little for you, conditionally. I have a friend who installed an elaborate pool, hoping that it would help with her perennial battle of the bulge. But as time went by, she became more depressed than ever over her figure problems. "I can't understand it," Claire complained to me. "I swim every day."

Ah, but *how* does she swim? An unhurried lap or two, and *then she rests*. The minute she begins to puff a little she stops to rest. Just when the exercise begins to do her some good she stops.

Put in its simplest terms, the key to the overload principle (and aerobic exercise) lies in forcing your body to breathe hard—to need and process oxygen *over a period of time*. Of course, this does not mean that you should go outside right this instant and try to run a four-minute mile. You must *gradually* develop your oxygen-processing ability by exposing your muscles and your oxygen-processing system to a progressively increasing amount of stress. Gradually these systems will develop greater strength and a greater capacity to process more oxygen. (And have faith. It can be done painlessly.)

PUFFING IS GOOD FOR YOU

Research indicates that the conditioning effect takes place after twelve to fifteen minutes of *steady activity*. Otherwise, the overload principle won't take effect. You must exercise until you begin to puff and then keep on exercising (and puffing) over a period of time to produce the overload effect. If you swim for a minute, then stop, your body recovers from the slight demands made on it—and you haven't accomplished any conditioning. (Golfers and bowlers, also please note.) This is why most calisthenic programs don't develop conditional fitness. You do an exercise, you begin to puff a little, then you stop. Even that leisurely after-dinner walk won't do it, if you're walking at a pace that doesn't push your body to some degree of stress and oxygen demand.

The overload principle answers, once and for all, those perplexing questions that I've heard at so many lectures. "I get plenty of exercise. Why isn't my figure in better shape? Why don't I have more stamina?" The answer is that you *don't* get enough exercise *of the right kind*.

As you gradually develop conditioned fitness, you will become healthier and will have more energy. Paradoxically, once you are in condition, exercise is not tiring—it is at once relaxing and stimulating. And as a bonus, most of your figure problems will disappear.

To become the Ageless Woman, you *must* exercise—and the sooner you start, the better off you'll be. Because exercise (of the right kind) is more than a vanity trip. It does more than simply get your figure in shape. It gets *you* in shape and helps develop those reserves of energy that will become increasingly important every year.

Caution! One thing's certain. If you're not in condition, you mustn't throw yourself into a strenuous conditioning program without working up to it. Chances are you spent at least twenty years getting out of shape, so it is only fair to invest about six months getting back into shape. Be prudent and progress sensibly. You want to *become* fit, not *have* a fit.

THE SUPERSIMPLE WAY TO BECOME PHYSICALLY FIT. (OR, GIVE ME YOUR FLABBY, MISERABLE, AGING BODY FOR FIFTEEN MINUTES A DAY—AND YOU'LL BE GORGEOUS.)

How do you get started on a conditioning program? First, HAVE A PHYSICAL CHECKUP. You know this, of course. But *do it*. It's essential for two reasons. The obvious one is that, if there's anything seriously wrong with you, I would feel terrible if you dropped dead with this book clutched in your hand. Second, when you have your doctor's assurance that you can undertake the kind of conditioning program that I'm going to describe, you won't be frightened by the natural physical results of the overload principle—a little puffing, an accelerated heartbeat, or even a stitch in your side—all these things are the results of pushing your body just a *little* further than that lazy, luxury-loving bod wants to go. Always remember, it is the huffing and puffing that are good for you.

The second step is so simple that you won't believe me. So I asked track coach Al Baeta to tell you how to develop conditioned fitness. And he should know. He has coached Olympics winners and has developed a fabulously successful physical fitness program for women.

Al, how can a woman get started on a conditioning program?

"The very safest and most beneficial program is to simply go outside and start walking. However, this doesn't mean a leisurely stroll.

It means a brisk but comfortable pace. At first, walk about ten to fifteen minutes without stopping. Then you might want to build up to twenty-five or thirty minutes—*without stopping.*"

Can any woman start with this initial ten- or fifteen-minute time period?

"Actually, I think she's going to be surprised at the demands this will make on her, unless she's been very active. In the beginning she'll no doubt have to work up to the original fifteen minutes, slowing down occasionally to bring her breathing back to near normal, then starting again. But—and here's the satisfying part—every day there will be a measurable increase in her strength and stamina."

Any tips on walking?

"Yes, Gloria, there are a few important points to make this walking time produce the greatest physical benefits. First, good body posture is essential. You can't slouch along like a sack of potatoes and expect your body to perform efficiently. This erect body posture has two benefits. It aids in good breathing, which is the basis, of course, for the whole aerobics approach. And it has an added bonus. It helps to develop erect posture even during the times when you're not exercising . . . not even thinking about your posture.

"The best way to describe this erect posture is to say you should 'walk proud.'

"Now, the next thing is breathing. Don't try to do anything fancy with your breathing. After all, you've been doing it for years. Just breathe naturally, but *through the mouth* as much as possible. This will help you take in a greater volume of air. As you begin to huff and puff a bit, encourage your body in this more vigorous breathing, which will ultimately give greater expansion to the lung cavity, which in turn will help you take in more oxygen."

Anything else?

"Well, sometimes people worry about what to do with their arms . . . they try to swing them too forcefully, or try to move them in some sort of artificial rhythm. Just let the arms swing in a natural, relaxed way. They will automatically work in the correct rhythm with the movement of your legs and hips. As you move faster, your arms will move faster, but you don't have to consciously increase their rhythm. This just happens naturally.

"Another consideration is the placement of the feet. Here again, just move naturally. Don't try to do anything unnatural. Some women, I've found, tend to step onto the ball of the foot. Maybe they're thinking of jogging or running. I don't know. But I do want to make the point that you should guard against staying on the ball of the foot. You want your heel to touch the ground as the body weight passes over the whole foot. If this sounds too involved, the best way is to step down almost flat-footed.

"I always think it isn't necessary to mention good, supportive shoes . . . until I see a student trying to do her walking in sandals or some such thing. And of course comfortable, supportive shoes are absolutely essential if you plan to jog." (This is the *one* time when I will recommend that the Ageless Woman wear *sensible* shoes.)

What about jogging?

"When you're at the level of being able to walk—briskly but comfortably—for twenty-five to thirty minutes without stopping, you may comfortably work into jogging. Say, walk briskly for twenty-five minutes, jog for five, and then walk slowly for five (your cool-off period, which is very important, by the way). Or another day you may alternate. Walk five minutes, jog five minutes—or adapt whatever pattern is *comfortable* for you. The most important thing is this. Don't set a distance. Set a time level. And then *enjoy* that time."

How often must you walk or jog to make the program effective?

"If you are starting on a walking program, it should be more frequent than the more strenuous jogging program—at least five days a week. A good plan, especially when a woman is just starting, is to walk on alternate days. But as the body develops a better state of conditional fitness, students find that they actually *want* to do more. Walking—or jogging—every day isn't at all too much for one who is conditionally fit. But remember, the body dictates a comfortable rate. And my students find that as they become fit they want to do more. You might say that expending energy *creates* energy.

"As far as the jogging program is concerned, the woman who has worked up to a good jogging workout should plan to jog four days a week at least. Most joggers run more often than this. But again, that's the amazing thing about this whole approach to conditioned fitness. If women will stick with it through the initial stages, they find that they *want* to engage in this activity. That it's rewarding for its own sake. In fact, it's fun."

YOU'LL BE SURPRISED

This may sound too simple and easy to be effective, until you actually get out there and try it.

Then I think you'll be surprised to find that this apparently easy program seems strenuous at first. In his successful conditioning classes at American River College in Sacramento, supercoach Baeta found that many of his eighteen- and nineteen-year-olds couldn't even jog five minutes at the beginning of their conditioning program. Eventually, though, they built themselves up until they could jog continuously for thirty minutes—a goal you may wish to set for yourself. This is a realistic goal for healthy, mature women, though it will probably take from six months to a year to reach it.

Whatever your goal, always remember that the overload principle, with all the physical goodies it implies, only goes to work after that first fifteen minutes of non-stop activity. Another point to remember is this: do what's reasonably comfortable—but not easy. The minute your workout becomes *too* easy you begin to lose the conditioning effect. So push yourself just a little farther each day, and keep yourself breathing just a little harder than you really want to.

Long-distance runner Dr. Joan Ullyot of San Francisco suggests this simple test to assure that you're not overdoing. It's called Bowerman's talk test. This test, created by an Oregon track coach, simply means that one shouldn't run any faster (or longer) than one can run along while talking to a friend. If you are too out of breath to talk, you are moving beyond your capacity to process oxygen. Slow down for a while, get your breathing back to normal, and then start to jog again.

If you enjoy a more structured program, one with specific goals, schedules of progress, records of achievement and the like, do get either of the aerobic bibles—*The New Aerobics* by Dr. Kenneth Cooper or *Aerobics for Women*, written with his wife, Mildred Cooper. They describe the whole field of aerobic exercise in great detail. These books will give you a run-down on aerobic programs for swimming, running in place, and bicycling, as well as for jogging and walking.

If you enjoy group activity, hundreds of YMCAs and YWCAs throughout the country have instituted aerobics programs. As Cooper says, "If you seek company, encouragement, advice, and expert supervision for your exercise, the Y is a good place to look." Because of the interest in this type of fitness program, many community colleges also offer courses similar to Al Baeta's.

Or you might get in touch with the National Jogging Association (P. O. Box 19367, Washington, D.C. 20036), and see if they know of any groups in your area.

SUIT YOURSELF

My personal preference is to set my own schedule. First, it's flexible, so you can fit it into your day—a special advantage to women with full-time jobs.

Second, you can take it with you. To show you what I mean, here is a postcard from Marj, one of my dearest friends—and a jogging *nut*.

> It's Tuesday, so it must be . . .   August 3, 197-
> BRUSSELS
> Hi! Now I'm known as l'américaine démenté. (That crazy American!) I've probably set back international relations 100 years, but, c'est la vie. I couldn't resist my usual jogging work-out—four quick turns early this morning around the Parc de Bruxelles. Incidentally, everyone on the tour exhausted—but not me. See? It works.

It does help to choose one specific walking/jogging time each day because it tends to establish a firm habit. But sometimes our schedules become unavoidably fouled up, and if you're used to exercising independently, you can easily make adjustments to any change of plans.

And if you exercise independently you have almost unlimited freedom of choice over where you do your jogging. You are not always confined to the sameness of an indoor track. The whole world is your track.

Of course in these turbulent times a woman alone must be prudent. (Central Park at midnight is not recommended.) Many women search out jogging buddies in their neighborhood—preferably some with black belts in karate. One friend recommends golf courses; she keeps to the cart paths and enjoys the serenity of the rolling greens.

Pleasant surroundings help make jogging a more enjoyable experience, but indoors or out, the Ageless Woman will find a way.

AND WHAT WILL PEOPLE SAY?

When I first started my solo walking and running program I was a bit deflated by the "Hey, Mommy, look at the funny lady" syndrome. But jogging has become such an accepted part of the American scene, today you'll hardly rate any attention at all, beyond a brief glance of admiration—and even envy. "By George, look at her go!" So if you choose to jog alone, don't be shy.

On the other hand, many women prefer the companionship and encouragement found in exercise groups. But the important thing is this: alone or in groups, *do it*. It's worth it.

EXPECT THESE EGO-BUILDING FIGURE CHANGES

It doesn't really matter whether you work alone or with a class or group. If you stick with it, you'll become absolutely sold on the aerobic approach to exercise in general and to jogging in particular because of what it will do for you. Here are some of the benefits you can expect:

1. *You'll probably change your dress size.* Some women find that they'll change as much as two dress sizes in six months. (From larger to smaller, naturally.) Or sometimes, instead of an over-all weight loss, they may change their proportions by converting fat to springy muscle and be able to wear styles that they couldn't wear before. This happened to Lenore.

She had had a desperate figure problem since high school, one that plagues many otherwise attractive women. Lenore was petite and beautifully proportioned from the waist up, but her hips and thighs were so heavy that they seemed almost deformed. Spot exercise did little to budge this entrenched fat. And starvation diets simply made her look gaunt from the waist up while that solid mound of fat stubbornly refused to budge. I suggested that she forget the spot exercise, embark on the Super-B Diet, and "get into" aerobics. She got her doctor's okay, read the Coopers' book, and carefully embarked on her program.

And when I say "carefully," I mean that literally. Her legs and thighs were so heavy that even the walking program was difficult for her at first. But she stuck to it. She'd read enough about aerobics and jogging to be convinced that eventually she'd get results. And believe me, she did.

In six months she was able to wear slacks for the first time since childhood. In a year her body had become beautifully proportioned. Not only were her hips and thighs inches slimmer, but jogging had also corrected another figure problem that had been lurking under all those layers of fat—that condition known as Saggybottom.

Lenore is thrilled with the changes in her figure—and so is her husband. But he does have one complaint. Since she's slimmed down, he complains, "I haven't seen her legs in months. She's *always* wearing slacks."

2. *You'll tighten your tummy and build up your bust.* Jogging flattens and firms the abdomen and also has a positive effect on the contours of the bustline. Swinging your arms as you jog tends to build up the pectoral muscles that support the breasts. Some women find their bustlines firming and decreasing in size, others find their bustlines increasing because of firmer muscle tissue in the supporting areas. According to Mildred Cooper, "We get a substantial number of letters from women who say they've noticed an increase or decrease in the bust size, and in almost all cases the change—in either direction—has been considered a desirable one by the writer."

This equalizing effect has been noticed by many joggers. It's as if the blueprint for a perfectly proportioned body is programed in each individual's genetic structure. A jogging program seems to activate this blueprint. One woman may build up too slender calves and slim down her thick waistline. Another woman, on exactly the same program, may reduce her calves and thighs and at the same time enlarge her bust measurement. In each case the changes are just what each one needs to equalize her proportions.

3. *You'll sleep better.* Your aerobic program releases tensions that may be keeping you awake and helps your body eliminate waste products that keep you from relaxing.

4. *And of course you'll have more energy.* The aerobic effect increases the efficiency of your circulatory system, so you'll find that your body utilizes its fuel (food and oxygen) more efficiently, thus producing more energy. When you get more ox-

ygen, it stimulates the muscle tissue and you find that you feel alive, you feel like wanting to do things, where before you just felt like sitting around "relaxing."

5. *You'll find that your complexion is improved.* The vastly improved circulation that develops during an aerobics program feeds the tissues, giving them renewed life. In addition, a conscientious jogger works up a sweat. And perspiration is one of your body's ways to eliminate waste products and toxins. Your own hard-earned perspiration is one of your skin's best cleansing agents.

"YES, BUT . . . I'M TRYING TO DIET. WON'T ALL THIS EXERCISE STIMULATE MY APPETITE?

No, it seems to do just the opposite. Aerobic exercise tends to regulate the appetite, perhaps because it improves your circulation, stimulates your metabolism, and helps you burn all the food you eat. In conjunction with the Super-B Diet, this stimulation of your entire system gets rid of that "hidden hunger" we were talking about in the last chapter. What's more, aerobic exercise will teach you something very important about your body.

FOOD ALONE DOES NOT BRING ENERGY

Energy comes as you build your strength and stamina and as you stimulate your system to operate at peak efficiency. As you develop conditioned fitness, you'll find that you don't need to turn to food in order to bolster your lagging energy. According to Columbia University's Dr. W. Henry Sebrell, Jr., medical adviser to Weight Watchers, "To get energy you must spend energy. With exercise your circulation heightens, your vitality increases, you feel good."

Another very important point to consider is this: a low-calorie diet *without* regular exercise results in weight loss all right—50 per cent is fat and *50 per cent is muscle tissue.* This is such an important consideration, I'm going to say it again. Without exercise, the ordinary low-calorie reducing diet will mean a loss of muscle tissue along with a loss of fat. I just wish that every woman who diets strenuously, then sits around pale and wan without the energy to do anything, could have this fact emblazoned on her . . . uh . . . refrigerator.

EXERCISE AND DIET MUST GO TOGETHER

A sensible diet *with* exercise means that you'll be burning 100 per cent fat, leaving your body both slender, firm, and strong.

Of course, by now I have made my position clear. I recommend the high-protein, balanced Super-B Diet *and* aerobic exercise. Always remember, this isn't an exercise book. And I have already pointed out that this is not a diet book. The goal of this book is to help you become the Ageless Woman.

So let's look beyond those firm muscles for a minute. There's increasing evidence that regular, challenging exercise is absolutely essential to the mature woman for reasons beyond the desire to have a slim, lithe, attractive figure.

THAT SKELETON IN YOUR CLOSET

It's been estimated that over five million women suffer from some form of osteoporosis, the bone-wasting disease that accounts for all those broken hips, ill-fitting dentures, and untold miseries in later years. Now I'm sure that the image of *you* as a dear little old lady, bedridden with a broken hip, is not only an unpleasant picture but one that seems impossibly distant. So let's think about today—and tomorrow. How nice it is to have all (or most) of your precious pearls firmly imbedded in a good, strong jawbone. Osteoporosis can destroy that jawbone and make those pearls a memory.

How confident you feel now when you can take a good fall over the handlebars of your ten-speed bike—and suffer nothing more than a scratched knee. But bone-softening osteoporosis could make that same fall a serious happening indeed. With osteoporosis, that fall could cripple or kill. Which means that, as osteoporosis sets in, you become timid about what you can and cannot do. You begin to curtail your activities—and you become old rather than ageless. And the more you curtail your activities the worse the osteoporosis becomes. A vicious circle.

Osteoporosis is extremely common in postmenopausal women, and since it's so difficult to diagnose, it is probably present in its early stages among a large percentage of premenopausal women. As a mature woman, it's a threat you should be well aware of—a threat to your health, your looks, and to your very life style during the years ahead of you. And a threat you can counteract if you start now.

Recent findings indicate that osteoporosis is arrested or even prevented by regular physical activity. Dr. Louis Avioli, director of endocrinology at Jewish Hospital in St. Louis, declares, "Any regular programed exercise, started early enough in life, should cut down on the rate of bone loss [osteoporosis]."

However, a recent study seems to indicate that it's never too late to reap the bone-strengthening benefits of exercise. In a program involving thirty-nine persons ranging in age from fifty-five to ninety-four, it was found that physical activity effectively slows down osteoporosis. Dr. Ali Seirig, at the University of Wisconsin, has also been conducting tests with laboratory animals, tracing the relationship to exercise and bone strength. His findings indicate that exercise does more than strengthen muscles. It strengthens bones too.

So the benefits of an aerobics program are measured not only in the present but in the future as well. In the present it can bring energy, a feeling of well-being, and a trim efficient body. And in the future, it can assure you of the over-all health that is essential to agelessness.

THINK OF THAT!

Regular exercise is not only good for your bones . . . it's good for your brain, too. The Rev. Dr. Thomas Boslooper has spent sixteen years trying to find out why so many women have emotional problems. And now he thinks he's found the answer—a lack of physical activity. After interviewing over four hundred women, including Olympic champions, opera singers, models, civic leaders, and four former Miss Americas, he found that all the happy women had two things in common. They all were physically active and they all felt feminine, regardless of their life styles. On the other hand, Dr. Boslooper found that "many with emotional problems tried to do things to make them feel weak and delicate. They neglected all physical activities in an attempt to feminize themselves."

This Princess and the Pea attitude is certainly common among Professional M.A.M.s. "Exercise? My dear, I simply loathe it. It ruins my hairdo"—there's that grouted Menopause Bob, again—"and what's more, I think it's so unfeminine to swe—uh—perspire. Don't you?"

According to Dr. Boslooper, a little honest sweat is exactly what M.A.M. needs to bring her back to the land of the living. He feels that the more aggressive and competitive the sport the better. "Women who don't get the positive experience of these drives become devious and bitchy." (The Reverend calls 'em as he sees 'em.) He adds, "I've found that what we call the obnoxious woman is a very aggressive woman who has no way to channel her drives." Boy, has he got the Professional M.A.M. pegged! The next time your favorite M.A.M. is picking on you, why don't you suggest that she go out and jog in the traffic? Or better yet, suggest karate lessons to her. It may be just what she needs to turn her into a real woman again.

Even though you'll find that your aerobics program isn't as competitive as karate, there is a certain amount of competition involved —competition of the best kind. You're competing with yourself as you strive to increase your performance each week. And as you continue with your program, you'll find a great deal of satisfaction in the measurable progress your body makes against the inroads of inertia, fatigue, and age.

"OKAY, OKAY. I'M SOLD. BUT WHILE AEROBIC EXERCISE IS DOING ALL THESE WONDERFUL THINGS TO MY SYSTEM, WILL IT REALLY SOLVE *ALL* MY FIGURE PROBLEMS?"

Darned near. It's especially effective for equalizing your measurements from the waist down. However, some spot exercises may be advisable from the waist up. There are some specific areas that get very little activity in any conventional exercise program. As you might expect, these areas are the "agemakers." Instant giveaways that tell the world that the pictures in your high school yearbook are beginning to fade. *But* these areas can be firmed up and rejuvenated with spot exercise—the point is, will you really do them? I think the right approach will help you stick with it.

A WEIGHTY ARGUMENT FOR RESISTIVE EXERCISE

Exercises performed with weights (or against other resistance) pay dividends by making the muscles work harder and therefore bringing results with fewer repetitions. So the first plus factor is that it takes less time to get results.

Second, and perhaps even more important, if you exercise with weights, you are forced into a measured amount of effort. There's no cheating, because the muscles *have* to work to move those weights around. And you're going to see results *soon*. Ah! Encouragement—the essential ingredient in keeping you motivated.

Finally, spot exercises against resistance are the only way to correct those "agemaking" tattletale areas that plague the mature woman. Such giveaway areas (the backs of the arms, for example) are virtually impossible to correct with the usual exercises, because the sly little muscle groups involved tend to lounge around during an exercise session, going along for a free ride while the larger muscles do all the work. As a result, those little rascals are the first to turn flabby. But you'll find that selected resistive exercise will firm these free-loading muscle groups and keep them from sagging by renewing their muscle tone. Resistive exercises will work wonders to improve lazy muscles in your bustline, your waistline, your upper back, your arms, your midriff, and your legs.

Remember now, your aerobic program comes first. Because it builds both your health *and* your figure, one of its greatest appeals is that it frees you from long and involved and boring calisthenic rituals. So get started on aerobics first. Once you feel the rewards of the extra energy that aerobics brings, it will be easy to start on these resistive exercises. And when you do start, pick out only those exercises that will solve your particular problem. Don't do them all if you don't need to.

WHAT EQUIPMENT WILL YOU NEED?

First, a set of three-pound ankle weights can be used for almost all the exercises, both above and below the waist. You can also buy a set of three-pound dumbbells if you like, but they aren't necessary. The ankle weights will work equally well for your arm exercises. I know that many articles and books will give you directions on how to make your own weights ("Simply fill two bleach bottles full of sand . . .") but don't waste your time. Chances are these makeshift weights will eventually fall apart and dump sand in your ear at some inopportune moment. A no-class operation, to say the least.

Excellent ankle weights are available at most department stores for a reasonable price—so go first class all the way. You deserve it.

The second item of equipment is something you've often read about in the back of the tacky movie magazines that we all shamefacedly read at the beauty salon. (I won't tell if you don't.) You've seen the ads, "Magic Bust Developer Increased My Bosom Four Inches." These ads always feature a smug-looking model whose almost horrifying proportions make Raquel Welch look positively boyish. You'll probably be as surprised as I was to find that these bust developers really do work. Although they may never replace the padded bra or make silicone obsolete, they *do* improve the contours of the bustline. Not only that, but they firm and shape the arms and back as well—as I'll be explaining in a moment.

With a total disregard for exotic brand names, my students promptly dubbed this gizmo the "Squeezy." What is it, exactly? The type of bust developer that I'm recommending consists of two contoured plastic hard plates with a strong spring in between. Using the palms of your hands, you simply press the two plates together against the resistance of the spring in a programed series of positions that come with your Squeezy—in a plain wrapper, too.

Finally, you'll need a broomstick, which you'll be using with the ankle weights to create a weighted bar bell. You might be able to borrow one from a Professional M.A.M. of your acquaintance, but that's risky. It would almost certainly have the broom part attached and probably a black cat, too. So perhaps it would be best to buy one. They are sold at hardware stores by the length. Get one that's one to one and a half inches in diameter and six inches longer than the span of your arms.

HOW TO GET STARTED

Look over the following list of agemakers and determine which ones apply to you. Next, read the description of the correcting exercise (The Solution) and go through it slowly—in front of a mirror if possible. Pay special attention to The Clincher—the decisive detail that will assure you of doing each exercise *correctly* and therefore *effectively*.

After you have become thoroughly familiar with each exercise and are sure you can do them *correctly* and *effectively*, you have two benefits coming. First, they will correct your tattletale trouble spots. And, second, they give you a perfectly good reason to watch that Esther Williams Film Festival—"I am not frittering away my time with television, I am *exercising*."

If you do these exercises correctly, a workout every other day should bring increased muscle tone in four or five weeks.

An important question that is always asked about resistive exercise is this: "How many times should I do each one?" Perform each exercise until you are tired and want to stop. *Then* do the exercise two or three more times than you *really want to*. (There's that overload concept again.) As your muscles become stronger you'll add a few more repetitions—always pushing yourself just a bit past the point when you want to stop. However, with each exercise I have suggested a beginning number of repetitions just to get you started.

Now, since you will be pushing those lazy muscle groups into action (when all they really want to do is relax and watch TV), you'd better wake them up gradually with a little warm-up movement. This doesn't have to be anything more elaborate than swinging your arms in several big circles—first to the front, and then in reverse direction. Next, hold onto the back of a chair and swing your legs back and forth (one at a time, of course). Or if your schedule permits you to do these resistive exercises *after* your aerobic workout, you won't need a warm-up. Believe me, your whole body will be wide awake.

Okay? Then let's take a close look at those lazy little agemakers and see what we can do about them.

THE AGEMAKERS—YOUR BUSTLINE

The Problem—As a woman matures, her breasts tend to sag or shrink, or they enlarge because of fat deposits. All of these conditions can be improved by the proper resistive exercises. Remember, the trouble is not caused by the breasts (which are glands), but by the lack of tone in the muscles that surround and support the breasts.

The Solution—Although jogging will tend to normalize the size of your bustline, exercising against resistance can actually lift the bust and dramatize your contours. If your bosom is small, resistive exercise will give you a very sexy decolletage by firming the muscles of the neck and chest as well as the supportive muscles of the breast. If your bosom is large, this type of exercise will strengthen the supporting muscles and keep you from having a matronly sag. The really full-bosomed woman often finds that the Super-B Diet, plus aerobic conditioning and resistive exercise, can ease her burdens enormously by reducing the excess fat stored in this area and by firming the muscles that support the bosom. Of course, as you've heard many times, the actual size of the breast—the gland—will not be changed. But the muscles and skin around the gland can be changed for the better.

To accomplish this change for the better, use the Squeezy according to the directions that come with it. But in the beginning don't

attempt to do each Squeezy exercise the suggested number of times
—much too difficult for beginners. I'd suggest about eight repetitions
per exercise, to start.

The Clincher—The speed at which you perform the exercises will
affect the results. If you wish to reduce fat in the bosom area, exercise rapidly. If you wish to increase the volume of the surrounding
muscles, and thereby increase the apparent size of your bust, do the
exercises slowly. For toning and maintenance, exercise at a moderate
speed. Incidentally, these tempos will affect all muscle groups in the
same way, so apply this formula to all the exercises—fast to decrease,
slow to increase, and medium tempo to tone, firm, and maintain.

THE AGEMAKERS—YOUR WAISTLINE

The Problem—Jogging will indeed firm and reduce your waistline,
but since it's going to take several months of aerobic walking to work
up to jogging condition, a few exercises with weights will speed up
this process. If you have any extra girth at all, do take the time to do
this simple exercise. That thick-in-the-middle look is so matronly and
can spoil an otherwise ageless figure.

The Solution—Stand with feet apart, one weight in each hand.
Swing your right hand over your head and bend to the left. The left
hand (with its weight) will move down beside the left leg toward
the knee. You'll find that the weights tend to pull your body in this
sideways motion. Hold this position and bounce to the left side four
or five times. Repeat the movement, this time bending to the right.
Repeat twice on each side and build from there.

The Clincher—Always bend directly to the *side*. Do not allow
your body to bend forward. You should feel the muscles at the sides
of your waist working, firming, making your waist trimmer.

THE AGEMAKERS—YOUR MIDRIFF

The Problem—If you can pinch more than a half inch of skin just
under your bra strap, or if your tummy button peaks out from under
a roll of flab, you'd better get cracking. You have a flabby midriff,
and I guarantee that, unless you *do* something, it's not going to get
better. It's going to get worse.

The Solution—You'll need your broomstick for this exercise.
Stand with feet apart, broomstick resting on your shoulders. Slide
the ankle weights over the ends of the broomstick and, with your

arms extended, hold the weights in place. Now, swing your upper body all the way around to the left, letting the weights increase the momentum of the swing. Next, swing the upper body around to the right. Start with six swings and build from there.

The Clincher—While your upper body is swinging to the right and left, the hips should be facing straight ahead. This creates a twisting motion in the midriff area and this is what does the trick. Also, if you'll keep your eyes on the weight that swings to the rear, you'll feel a nice stretch in the neck and chin area.

THE AGEMAKERS—YOUR UPPER BACK

The Problem—That bra bulge is a pet peeve of mine. It's sad to see so many stunning women with their beautiful figures spoiled by this great slab of flesh ballooning out over their bra straps. I remember one graphic example. During the highly publicized TV appearance of one of Hollywood's legendary glamor queens, the public was at first enchanted to see that the years hadn't changed her a bit. The perfect face was there, the exquisite figure was there. But then she turned around and a veritable Gladstone bag of soft flesh was there too, sagging over the top of her low-cut gown and spoiling the illusion.

My criticism of this condition would be unkind if bra bulge were unavoidable. But it isn't.

The Solution—Use your broomstick and weights in the same way as in the previous exercise. Bring the broomstick in back of your upper back, keep your elbows close to your sides. Now, straighten your arms and raise the weighted broomstick high above your head. Then lower the broomstick, bringing it back to a position behind your shoulders, again pulling your elbows close to your body. Start with four repetitions. Do the exercise at medium tempo.

The Clincher—Lower the broomstick without moving your head forward. As you lower the bar and tuck the elbows close to the body, consciously tighten the muscles that pull the shoulderblades together —*pull*.

THE AGEMAKERS—YOUR ARMS

The Problem—Look around you. You'll see that agemaking arms come in several unattractive shapes.

That swag of flab that swings from armpit to elbow is problem A.

That soufflé of fat that rises between the bra strap and the armpit is problem B. And finally, at the other extreme, that thin and wasted arm with its look of scrawniness and angularity is problem C.

Solution to Problem A—Hold one weight in each hand. Raise your arms straight up over your head. From the overhead position, bend at the elbows and lower the weights, bringing them down to the backs of your shoulders. All movement will be in the upper arms. Your lower arms remain vertical, elbows pointing to the ceiling. Raise and lower weights four times to start.

The Clincher—Keep the upper arms in line with the ears, elbows close to the head. Don't allow the arms to swing forward. Your hands should be turned so that, when your arms are raised, the knuckles are pointing toward the front, fingers toward the back. This position will give you the maximum workout in that muscle along the back of the upper arm. Can you feel it?

Solution to Problem B—As you use your Squeezy bust developer, you'll be amazed to see how many muscle groups are activated. Not only the muscles in the chest area, but also those muscles between your bra strap and armpit, both front and back, get a good workout with the bust exercises. However, if you have a real problem in this area, a little dry-land swimming will bring visible results in a hurry.

Stand straight, hands at sides, holding one weight in each hand. Now, you're going to do the backstroke. Raise your right arm up so that the elbow is pointing toward the ceiling, your hand next to your right cheek. Next, stretch your elbow back as far as it will go. At the same time slide your hand along your right cheek, then swing it back and down to complete a backward circle. Got that? It's just the basic backstroke position, but with a real s-t-r-e-t-c-h in the backward movement. Alternate four strokes to each side to start.

The Clincher—Keep your shoulders relaxed and facing forward. Avoid the tendency to tense and hunch the shoulders. Arm movements should be from front to back. Avoid any sideways movement. Try to keep the initial arm movement close to the ear. These backstrokes are controlled *movements*. Don't circle the arms wildly, allowing their momentum to carry them around.

Solution to Problem C—Scrawny, angular arms can make the slender mature woman look positively aged. But don't despair. You, too, can do a little dry-land swimming, to round and firm your arms.

Stand with feet apart, knees slightly bent, one weight in each hand. Bend forward from the waist. Now, using the classic overhand stroke, reach forward with the right hand, at the same time bringing the left elbow back and up. Start with six strokes for each arm and build from there.

The Clincher—Exaggerate all movements. Really r-e-a-c-h with your forward stroke, and as you bring your hand down and back, raise your elbow up with an exaggerated movement. Try to imagine that you are pulling yourself through the water, feeling the pull from the tips of your fingers to the waist. Even without water, swimming will beautify your arms in no time. So come on. Last one in's a rotten egg.

THE AGEMAKERS—YOUR LEGS

The Problem—At the risk of repeating myself, I want to say again how delighted you'll be at the dramatic changes in your leg contours that will be apparent after a few weeks on your aerobic walking/jogging program. However, there is one problem area that resists even this excellent exercise. The inner thighs will remain out of condition for a long time, in spite of your best aerobic efforts. Almost every woman this side of ballerina Margot Fonteyn is familiar with this problem—a fatty, dimpled bulge that envelops the inner thigh from crotch to kneecap. Because it's such a common problem, and a difficult one to solve, I'm going to give you two solutions. Try both of them for results.

Solution Number One—This is where we use the ankle weights on the ankles. With weights on, lie down on your left side, your left arm outstretched, your head resting on your arm. Use your right arm to support yourself in this reclining position. Bend your right leg so that the knee is pointing toward the ceiling, your right foot planted firmly on the floor. Keeping your left leg straight, s-l-o-w-l-y raise it up toward the ceiling. Try to raise the leg about a foot and a half off the floor (about as high as your bent right knee). Do these leg raises about four times on each side to start.

The Clincher—When raising your leg toward the ceiling, keep your foot parallel to the floor. In other words, don't point your toe. You'll feel that this increases the pull on the inner thigh.

Solution Number Two—Still on the floor, roll over on your back, arms stretched out at the sides, legs up, knees straight and feet pointing up toward the ceiling. Now, you'll simply do a scissors kick, swinging your legs open as far as they will go, then swinging them together, and allowing them to cross. Alternate; right foot swings in front, then left foot swings in front. Do six scissor kicks to start.

The Clincher—Again, keep the feet straight, trying to point the heels rather than the toes toward the ceiling. Try to swing your legs open as far as they will go. You'll feel a strong p-u-l-l on that inner thigh muscle. Good. That means, "It's working, it's working."

Remember now, these exercises are not to be considered a calisthenics program. Choose only those resistive exercises that are needed to correct your individual agemakers. The whole idea behind this total program is to free you from boring calisthenic routines. And that's why your aerobics program must come first—it's your health *and* beauty routine.

And is there any magic formula that will encourage you to stay with the aerobic program? Let's see.

WHY YOU'LL STICK WITH AEROBICS
EVEN IF YOU'VE NEVER STAYED WITH AN
EXERCISE PROGRAM BEFORE

Remember, in our discussion on diet, we found that successful dieting was much more a question of satisfying hidden hunger than of developing iron will power. In other words—dieting is essentially physical rather than mental. Conversely, the secret behind a successful conditioning program is essentially mental. And the reason for your lack of success in this area can all be attributed to the wrong attitudes.

Just what are the winning attitudes? Once again, I went to coach Al Baeta for the answer. I always go back to Al Baeta because the students in his conditioning program are overwhelming proof that he's onto something that works. When large groups of formerly out-of-condition, mature women stay with a strenuous exercise program month in and month out, never missing their workouts, you know he's found the answer to that old will-power problem. True, the fact that he's a sun-tanned, handsome charmer may have *some* bearing, but remember, these students become so inspired by Baeta's enthusiasm, and so motivated by his unique psychological approach, that they *stay* sold, long after their classes are over.

What's his secret? Let the coach explain it.

"You know, *everyone* is superenthused when they start any sort of conditioning program. After all, everyone wants to look better, everyone wants to feel better, and everyone wants to live longer. So naturally, when a person gets involved in any sort of exercise program, their mind-set is on the goal—'I want to look marvelous, lose inches, feel great,' and so forth. And they begin to program their minds so that the *only* consideration is the goal.

"Very soon the time spent in exercise becomes drudgery because the mind is completely concentrated on the goal—an abstract ideal that's in the unreal future—instead of enjoying the activity at the very moment they're engaging in it. I believe more people turn off to exercise for this one reason alone. *They are totally involved in the goal and not excited about doing the thing for itself alone.* The secret is to program yourself to consciously enjoy the time expended. Work on your attitudes (and find an activity you like) so that the time you're involved in it is worth while in itself—not just a means to an end."

GETTING THERE IS HALF THE FUN

This is one of the reasons for the tremendous popularity of jogging. It not only brings phenomenal results in the form of conditioning and reproportioning, but—most important of all—it's fun. And as a special bonus, it seems to create a unique mental lift.

In the Coopers' book, *Aerobics for Women*, Mildred Cooper says there is an "area of aerobic fitness I don't know how to label—whether to call it spiritual or psychological or emotional." She goes on to explain that almost everyone who gets into a regular aerobics program comments on this indefinable plus factor. For example, one enthusiast wrote Mrs. Cooper, "There are things about this conditioning program you didn't mention in your book. I mean, intangibles like the new attitude I bring to my children and to the relationship with my husband."

Anne-Marie Bennstrom, founder and director of The Sanctuary, the Beverly Hills health and beauty spa that is a favorite with film people, is an enthusiastic jogger. She also comments on the extra bonus of being physically fit. "It is quite wonderful to watch some-one who is out of shape gradually become turned on to an inner self and get into shape. As we feel physical and spiritual improvements, we find that there is more of life to get in touch with."

What is this plus factor? How can you *consciously* increase its benefits?

CREATIVE EXERCISE ADDS
A FOURTH DIMENSION TO YOUR LIFE

Does the rhythmic breathing that is the result of your regular walking/jogging program have an expanding effect on the consciousness? Before you smile at this idea as being fantastic, let me point out that mystics of all religions have used rhythm, chants, and the resultant rhythmic breathing as an accompaniment to exalted or inspired mental states. In the scientific realm, studies indicate that there may be a relationship between regular rhythmic breathing and the alpha state wherein the mind is operating at peak efficiency and inspirational receptivity.

Whatever the reasons, if you stay with your aerobics program for even a few weeks, you will begin to experience this plus factor. One of its characteristics is a heightened awareness—awareness of the moment.

Children have this awareness. Their time sense is geared to the present. We lose it as we get older.

We talked about this "awareness of the moment" in class one day, and Annette described it perfectly: "I took my three-year-old grandson to the beach recently, and I watched him as he built sand castles, chased a gull, played tag with the waves. He had a ball. And all because he was totally engrossed in the present. On the other hand, I thought about getting a parking place at the market (our next stop after the beach), I glanced at the water, watched him play, thought ahead to an appointment I had the next day, and remembered a TV show I'd seen the night before. In other words, I really wasn't at the beach at all, except for a few fleeting moments when I gave it my attention. I was thinking about yesterday, planning for tomorrow. When we left, my grandson was exhilarated, while I didn't feel any different at all, except that the day I had looked forward to had somehow fallen flat."

Of course, adults cannot live as children do. We all have responsibilities and ambitions that force us to weigh the past and to plan ahead. We cannot live *entirely* in the present.

Still, the only reality lies in the *now*. The past, after all, is gone; the future hasn't yet arrived. That's why we are totally alive only in those moments when our attention is entirely focused on the present. And that's why these moments are so special.

Can you think of a time when you were living totally in the

present moment? I'll bet you can, because these times are so vital, they seem "bigger than life" and stand out in our memories for years and years.

Now, the intriguing thing about aerobics in general, and jogging in particular, is that it seems to increase our ability to be aware, to live in the present moment.

And you can consciously *increase* this awareness by practicing one of the following exercises when you are on your walking/jogging program. The object is to make yourself vividly and intensely aware of the world around you.

1. *Colors*

Look around you. Can you spot three distinct shades of green in the yards and gardens of your neighborhood? If you live and exercise in the city, you're facing a real challenge—but look anyway. You'll be surprised to spot a window box or a tiny curbside tree that you've never noticed before.

Look at the sky. Is it blue? Gray? Cloudy?

Each day that you are out, choose one color—red, pink, yellow—and see how many examples of this color you'll spot as you jog along.

2. *Birds*

How many birds do you see as you are on your daily outing? What color are they? How large? It's just one jump from this kind of casual observation to becoming a full-fledged bird watcher, a fun and rewarding pastime.

Now *listen* to those birds. Can you pick out distinct bird songs?

3. *Sounds*

In addition to bird songs, what other sounds are you aware of? If you jog early in the morning, one of the most satisfying things is that you'll be consciously aware of the *lack* of sound. (But if you hear whistles, you'll know your jogging is working on your figure as well as your mind.)

After you have completed one of the awareness exercises, you can go a step further. Take advantage of the heightened receptivity of your mental state to accomplish any of the following:

1. *Deal with negative feelings.*

As you walk or jog along, consciously unload those negative

feelings. Create positive feelings by thinking, as you exhale, "I exhale anger and frustration," and then, on the ingoing breath, "I inhale serenity and fulfillment." Do this mental exercise at least ten times, trying to actually visualize the dark, confused, negative thoughts being expelled from your body and a shining, golden, vibrant awareness being absorbed into your body and mind.

2. *Develop confidence, optimism, agelessness.*

You can use your jogging time to develop success attitudes. Your mind, like a computer, can actually be programed to produce success or failure. In their book, *Success Through A Positive Mental Attitude*, Napoleon Hill and W. Clement Stone explain it this way: ". . . conscious auto-suggestion is the agency of control through which an individual may voluntarily feed his subconscious mind on thoughts of a creative nature, or, by neglect, permit thoughts of a destructive nature to find their way into the rich garden of his mind."

So, as you exercise, weed out your thoughts of insecurity, fear, and age; instead build positive, winning thoughts by repeating constructive "affirmations." They needn't be stodgy and serious. One of my students made up this "affirmation" to make her feel equal to any challenge:

"Tramp, tramp, tramp. Nothin' stops the Champ!"

Soon you will develop your own "affirmations" to fit your needs and circumstances. Do your thing. We are only beginning to learn how powerfully those positive attitudes can influence our destiny.

3. *Plan creatively.*

After your awareness exercises, you can use your time to plan your day or to map out any project. Once again, you'll find that the combination of rhythmic breathing, fresh air, and aerobic activity seems to make your mind work more creatively and efficiently.

By turning your walking/jogging session into a *creative* experience, you'll find that the time passes quickly and rewardingly. When you consciously think beyond considerations of measurements and figure perfection, and far beyond some future physical goal, you'll find that you look forward to your exercise period. It's no longer drudgery. Instead it becomes your special time to renew yourself, to get reacquainted with yourself—and just to have fun.

ANOTHER LOOK AT CALISTHENICS

Once again I would like to emphasize the fact that aerobic exercises are the key to health and fitness. They are the key to energy, vitality, enthusiasm, and ultimate agelessness. Fitness starts on the inside, and being thin is not enough. But aerobic exercises bring another surprise bonus.

Remember those eight sit-ups that turned you into a gasping blob of tortured flesh? Try them again after you have attained conditioned fitness through your walking/jogging program. You will be astonished at how easy those eight measly sit-ups have become. And what will this do for morale that has been suffering from middle-aged malaise? What do you think?

ILLUSION vs. REALITY

Knowledgeable choices in fashion, make-up, and hair styling can create an *illusion* of agelessness, and that's great as far as it goes. But the illusion is not enough. Diet (of the right kind) and exercise (of the right kind) are essential to make agelessness a physical *reality*.

An ever increasing body of scientific data proves that building a level of conditioned fitness is one of the essential ingredients in combating premature age. The old adage, "What we don't use, we lose," is especially true of the vitality of the human body. Diet and heredity also play their part, but recent medical research indicates that inactivity and premature aging go hand in hand.

So, if you want to be, quite literally, ageless—don't just sit there. Determine *now* to make rejuvenating exercise an essential part of your life. And the sooner you start, the better off you'll be. In fact, you may find that your next birthday has to be dismissed due to insufficient evidence.

SEVEN

It's Your Move

There's one thing that will date you quicker than knowing the names of all three Andrews sisters—"moving old." You can have the best figure in the world, the most fashionable clothes and make-up, but if you "move old," you will still look matronly. The final touch that determines whether or not you create a winning image depends on the message you send through your body language. Do you move agelessly—or old?

It's vitally important for you to understand this subtle beauty dimension, because your posture, your walk, your hand gestures, the way you sit—all telegraph obvious messages to those around you. Unfortunately, many mature women are sending messages that belong in the dead-letter office. The way a woman walks can say, "My body's old and tired and sexless." The way she sits can say, "I'm a passive spectator. I don't participate in life any more. I watch the action from the sidelines." Her hand gestures can whisper, "My point of view has become narrowed with age, and I'm engrossed in fussy trifles."

And these messages, in turn, create a predictable response.

WHY ACT YOUR AGE?

Suppose you are forty, or maybe you even admit to being fifty. Why blab about it with every move you make? With knowledge and a little effort, you can use body awareness and ageless movement to help you become the Ageless Woman, whose age is non-specific— and unimportant.

Body awareness and ageless movements can be learned quickly and easily; and the dividends you receive on both a visual and an emotional level are terrific. By learning to use the silent body language you can project agelessness rather than age, confidence instead of uncertainty, joy and optimism instead of depression and pessimism, serenity rather than agitation, and femininity rather than the neuter pallor of middle age.

And strangely, as you learn to act the role of the Ageless Woman and to project a vital positive image, some mysterious alchemy takes place. Suddenly you are no longer playing a role. Suddenly the role *is* you—you *become* an Ageless Woman. Great actresses know all the secrets of body language and use them. That's why so many of them remain ageless indefinitely.

Now what about *you?* You have taken your first giant step forward if you are now aware of the importance of body language. A depressing number of women don't even know about it.

When I refer to "movement" or "body language" in this chapter, I *am not* talking about the old "book on the head" school that teaches artificial movements having no relationship to real life. You want to move like an Ageless Woman, not like a model with thumbtacks in her girdle.

Every woman can learn the simple, natural movements that will enhance her ageless beauty and she should concentrate on those movements that project her image in positive ways. No woman in the world would go to a party, or a business conference, or a job interview, carrying a sign saying, "I'm nervous," "I'm unsure of myself," or "I'm getting old." Yet by movements and gestures many women are silently "shouting" exactly those messages.

Using positive body movements to project a confident, dynamic, feminine image can mean more than a simple ego trip. The image you project can mean the difference between success or failure. Your image might help your husband get that promotion; it could influence a decision to hire you or not to hire you. And if you think I am exaggerating, you just haven't been listening to the personnel men and executives who actually do the hiring these days.

The startling impact of positive body movements as compared to negative movements was recently demonstrated to me by two women, both applying for a job that was very important to them.

At the time, I didn't know them at all. I was talking to a busy executive about a self-improvement course for the women in his sales force. During our discussion he occasionally called my attention to the two women waiting in his outer office and used their contrasting appearance and mannerisms to help make his points. Within minutes it was obvious which woman he would hire.

A few weeks later, by coincidence, I met both women and I was able to piece together the entire story, which clearly illustrates the points I am trying to make. I learned that both women were equally qualified for the job and equally capable. I also learned that both women were equally nervous, but one had learned how to hide her lack of confidence and to consciously project a positive image. The other one—but let me describe the scene as it actually happened.

The first woman to enter the office was Meg Carter. She wanted and needed this job. She was forty-six, just divorced from a neurotic she should have left years before. And now, after twenty-six years as a full-time mother and homemaker, she suddenly was financially and emotionally compelled to go back to work.

Tall, slender, and red-haired, she was smartly dressed in a green suit. It was a gloomy day, but as Meg moved across the room with an air of buoyant good spirits and energy, I noticed that the receptionist brightened up in response to her friendly smile. Meg took an application form and sat down gracefully.

The door opened again and Alice came in. Her pretty face and brunette coloring were complimented by her red dress, but somehow as she walked across the room she gave the impression of being tired. Alice clutched the application form and plumped into a chair.

Both women finished the application at the same time.

Meg sat gracefully, one hand on the arm of her chair, the other casually holding a very good brown purse in her lap. She was really nervous about the interview—the job sounded just right for her. To let off tension, she took a deep breath, then exhaled slowly.

Her mind raced ahead to the possibilities the job could bring, and then back to those unhappy months after the divorce. But as she felt tension mounting, she forced herself to breathe deeply and slowly and to consciously keep her hands quiet and in a relaxed position. Still breathing deeply and slowly, she concentrated on relaxing the tight muscles of her neck, shoulders, and arms.

As the muscles relaxed, her mind became calm, and she congratulated herself for taking those drama courses as therapy during the first panicky weeks after she left Jeff. She smiled slightly as she remembered her drama teacher—an ageless pro—saying, "Darlings, everyone gets stage fright—just be sure it doesn't get *you*. Fight back with calmness. Use your mind to make your muscles relax. And once your body is relaxed, you can have the relaxed but alert mind."

So Meg sat and waited, radiating calm self-assurance.

Meanwhile, Alice sat tensely, her purse clutched in both hands and held in front of her like a shield. She too was anxious about the outcome of this interview. At forty-five, with her sons married and living out of the state, the empty nest syndrome had descended on her with a vengeance. She felt depressed and useless. When she suddenly realized that "Let's Make a Deal" and "Gilligan's Island" had become the high points of her day, she had to face the fact that she was slowly going crackers.

Fortunately for Alice, she consulted a wise doctor. Instead of prescribing tranquilizers, he prescribed work. And as Alice thought about it and talked it over with her husband, she became increasingly excited.

She grimly dieted to lose twenty matronly pounds, she purchased a new, stylish wardrobe, but she quickly learned (as many women are learning these days) that she was not considered a good employment risk—that employers hesitate to hire someone who is returning to the work force after twenty-five years as a housewife.

She sighed deeply and moved restlessly. She smoothed and re-smoothed her hair; then she began drumming her fingers on her purse. Her pretty face was twisted with anxiety, and her large, truly beautiful eyes seemed to look calculating and a bit suspicious as they moved around the room in response to her nervous thoughts.

At this moment the executive again drew my full attention to the contrast between the two women. Alice had found a handkerchief which she used to pat her mouth and then to wipe the perspiration from her hands. When we looked at Meg, she was sitting serenely poised, smiling slightly at some thought.

"Both those women may be equally capable," the executive said. "But which would you rather have contacting your clients? What I want you to do is teach more of my people to act and look like that redhead."

I don't have to tell you who got the job.

Alice lost out because from the moment she opened the door she began telegraphing negative, losing messages. Here's how it happens.

MEANINGLESS MOVEMENT IS OLD

Patting your hair, picking at imaginary lint, brushing your skirt to smooth invisible wrinkles, smoothing and straightening your gloves (gloves? an automatic giveaway), fussing with your coat when you put it on to adjust it "just so"—all these fidgety, nervous, meaningless gestures are sure signs of a spinsterish fussiness.

Actresses use these aimless, meaningless gestures as a clear indication of age. Young Cicely Tyson, for example, used gestures superbly in her socko performance as the hundred-year-old slave, Miss Jane Pittman. If you saw this riveting performance, you'll remember that her hands were never still—patting the arm of the chair, smoothing her apron, tapping, patting, fidgeting, fussing. Busy hands are old hands.

MORE AGEMAKING GESTURES

Not only are old hands busy, fussy hands, but the hands of the older woman tend to *clutch* at things. She clutches her handbag, she clutches the arm of her escort, she even clutches the arm of the chair.

Gloria Swanson used clutching hands effectively in the movie classic, *Sunset Boulevard.* Her beautiful hands became clawlike, clutching at the sweeping skirts of the gowns she wore, clutching at the script she was writing, clutching her cigarette, and, in the climactic love scene, clutching at a young William Holden. Her hands became like talons, expressing all the insecurity and jealous possessiveness of a frightened old woman.

The Ageless Woman holds things casually (even William Holden). Her hands are relaxed. When she uses hand gestures, her fingers are relaxed, flexible, and fairly close together.

Carrying too many things with you—*things that must be kept track of*—is OLD. Picture the older woman, gathering together innumerable little parcels, bits of paper, appointment books, tiny purses that must be put inside of small purses that in turn are put inside of larger purses and so on. All of this activity is inclined to make her look flustered, a bit harried—and old. Don't carry all your worldly goods with you, even on a four-week tour. Instead, pare down, simplify. Traveling light is for those who look young—and those who *think* young.

BEWARE THE "SUPERLADY" WORDS AND GESTURES

The exaggerated, crooked little finger of the "nicey-nice" lady is another age tip-off. As a matter of fact, all the "superlady" gestures or postures tend to be agemakers—the relic of another era. The lace handkerchief, for example. There's certainly nothing wrong with using a lovely lace handkerchief to blow your nose, if that pleases you. But using a handkerchief to daintily pat your forehead or your mouth gives the distinct impression of an old lady with the vapors. Fanning yourself with a lace handkerchief is even worse. It instantly puts you in that deadly line of rocking chairs on the front porch of a summer hotel.

If it's hot and you're perspiring, why not use a good, honest, modern Kleenex and wipe your brow with a no-nonsense gesture? We've come years beyond the idea that "a lady doesn't perspire, she glows." As a matter of fact, I think we've really gone beyond the idea of ladies. Period. Now, when you're through with that Kleenex, throw it away, if possible, or stow it in your purse. Do *not* put it in your sleeve, in your neckline (ye gods!), or even in your pocket where it could ruin the line of your clothes.

YOU CAN LEARN TO WALK AGELESSLY

The matron's walk is one of the most emphatic aging statements in the vocabulary of body language.

How does the matron walk? Let's sit down a minute in this shopping mall and watch some walkers. See those two women just coming out of the tearoom? They're perfect examples. If you'll notice, the one in the yellow pants suit places her feet flat on the ground as if they were solid slabs of cement. She doesn't roll her foot from heel to ball to toes, which permits, a smooth, springy walk. No, she just stumps along on those two slabs, placing them quite far apart as she takes each step. The impression is one of total solidity and weight, and her body language fairly shouts, "I weigh too much."

Because she places her feet so far apart, her body rolls from side to side as she walks. To complete the rather aggressive, masculine effect, she's rounded her shoulders, which means that her arms swing *across* her body as she moves. If you consciously imitate this walk in front of a mirror, you will see the effect it creates. Poor soul, she moves like Popeye on a rough sea, not like an attractive woman in a brand-new yellow pantsuit.

Now quick, before they disappear into the rest room, let's look at her friend. As she walks, she turns her toes out and she seems to be just mincing along, an effect that's accented by her arm position. And see, she has her elbows tucked in close to her body and is holding her arms close to her sides instead of letting them move freely. Notice, too, that instead of swinging her legs from the hip she's walking with the upper part of her legs almost immobile. Most of the forward movement is in the lower part of her legs, from the knees down.

Of course, she may be walking this way because this trip to the rest room is a desperate emergency. Unfortunately, emergency or no, that's the impression she and countless other matrons create as they walk.

WHAT GIVES A WOMAN SEX APPEAL?

In a recent "Man on the Street" column in a San Francisco newspaper, the question was, "What Gives a Woman Sex Appeal?" Every man questioned mentioned a woman's walk as a basic quality of sex appeal, and several of them specifically commented on the walk of older women as compared to younger women. "When they're older, and have let themselves go, they kind of waddle. You know, they sort of put their feet far apart when they walk." . . . "Girls walk differently than older types. I call it the Lib Walk. They swing along with those big purses slung over one shoulder. They swing their arms. The older ones really hang onto those purses [What did I tell you?] and hold themselves stiff, like they were about to break or something." . . . "Sex appeal? I don't know what it is, but I can spot it a mile away, just in the way a woman walks. . . ."

Let's see if we can spot it a mile away too. Look way down the mall. See the stunning woman in red? Let's analyze her walk as she moves toward us. First of all, she moves freely and without any impression of stiffness or restriction. Her arms swing easily from her shoulders as she strides along. Her walk is the perfect visual expression of the ancient law, "Youth is flexible, age is inflexible." She creates a picture of effortless motion by swinging her leg and hip with each stride, almost as if her leg started somewhere near her waist. The hip and leg move as one. All the movement is forward, instead of from side to side.

She *uses* her feet, placing the heel down first, transferring the weight to the arch, and then rolling onto the ball of the foot. No wonder she moves so smoothly—almost as if she were on wheels. Finally, as you can see, she's walking with her feet pointed straight ahead and fairly close together. It's not the artificial "walk on a line" slink of the professional model, but a naturally smooth movement which is the result of walking as if she were on a narrow path.

Interesting, isn't it? Now that she's closer to us, you can see that she's not as young as she appeared to be from a distance. Not old, mind you. But she's certainly a grown-up woman. She walks gracefully and becomes ageless. Chances are she's on an aerobics exercise program too because, strangely enough, the fast, efficient aerobics walk almost automatically becomes the most graceful walk at slower speeds.

The impact of a beautiful walk was demonstrated by Rosalind Russell when she starred in a television drama a few seasons ago. She portrayed a much younger woman and was totally convincing. In one scene especially, she projected the essence of ageless vitality by striding across a park, her arms swinging freely, a coat casually slung over her shoulders. That brilliant portrayal of the Ageless Woman becomes even more impressive when we remember that she was then severely afflicted with arthritis. To the observant viewer, her ankles, wrists, and hands were pitifully enlarged by this crippling disease. Yet her body movements were so skillful that she appeared graceful, vital, and ageless.

WHERE DO YOU STAND?

Look at the social pages of any newspaper and you'll see any number of "how a lady stands" photographs. Yes, you'll see examples ad nauseam of stiff, earnest ladies proclaiming to the world that they know *how*. There they are, all dutifully pointing one toe forward, the back foot turned out at an angle. When we all went to charm school (how many years ago has it been?) that was the universal pose—the ticket to Grace Kelly elegance. But somehow, today, the pose looks affected, stiff and, yes, matronly.

Today's attractive standing positions are based on that same old model stance, but there is no longer an inflexible conviction that that is the *only* way to stand. There are many variations on this theme, and I'm going to give you several suggested poses.

Poses? Does that idea turn you off? Does it sound affected? Unnatural? I'll have a great deal to say about the idea of "just being the real me" in a moment, but first, think about this. Graceful, thought-out, standing positions are the basis for poise and confidence. So often when we are standing we are in some situation that makes us the center of attention. We may be on the speaker's platform, in a receiving line, being photographed, or standing in the doorway of a personnel office. And when we are standing still, negative body language tends to come across loud and clear. The wise woman plans ahead by practicing graceful poses *before* she is in the spotlight.

The main point to remember in developing ageless standing positions is that the pose must create a graceful, female curve, which can be accomplished by using the principle of—

CONTRAPPOSTO

Although contrapposto may sound like something that goes well with veal scaloppine, it is simply a term meaning to put the weight of the body off center. This, in turn, creates a graceful S curve. I'm convinced that this S stands for "sexy," because it certainly gives a woman's figure an appealing and feminine aura. By contrast, a pose in which the weight is evenly distributed through the center of the body gives a woman all the winsome charm of Svetlana the Siberian steelworker.

You'll see what I mean if you'll try the pose yourself. Stand in front of your full-length mirror. Place your feet about eight inches apart, toes pointing straight ahead. Put your weight solidly on both feet and let your arms hang loosely, with the hands resting on the front of your thighs. Keep your hips facing straight ahead. "Svetlana, it's *you*. Solid, stolid—every extra pound magnified fivefold."

Now let's try a pose using contrapposto. Starting from the above pose, turn the left toe out, slightly. Now turn your hips in the same direction, so that the left hip is angled toward the back, the right hip toward the front. This little trick will make your hips appear to be smaller (oh, joy!). Now put most of your weight on your left foot. You'll see that this has the effect of thrusting the left hip *out to the side*. Be sure that you haven't thrust your fanny out toward the back—a very common (and appalling) pose that we often see when those ladies line up for their pictures on the social page.

By placing all your weight on one foot and pushing the hip out to the side, you have created that graceful S curve. Okay. You've taken care of your left foot. Now you have several possible positions for your right foot.

You can place your right foot directly to the side—about six inches. Bend your right knee in toward your left knee.

Or you can place your right foot directly to the right about fourteen inches and straighten the right knee—a nice pose for pants.

You could also place the right foot ahead of, but to the left of, the left foot. As you'll see when you try this, it differs from the "classic" model's pose because the right leg crosses the left leg.

Now *you* try some poses, always maintaining that S curve by keeping your weight on your left foot. (Naturally, these standing positions are just as effective with the weight on the right foot.) Is your left leg getting tired? That's because you've allowed your left knee to "lock." Keep both knees slightly flexed when you are standing. It looks better—and it feels better, too.

"WHAT SHALL I DO WITH MY HANDS?"

Please, for your sake, practice a few of the hand positions I'm going to suggest. Don't wait until you are standing before the conference table trying to present a report while looking like an eight-handed Indian goddess fighting off a swarm of hornets.

The main point to remember is this. You'll look more attractive if

(1) your hands are not too busy, and (2) your inactive hands present an asymmetrical picture. If both hands hang limply at your sides they create a provincial, awkward effect. Both hands clasped in front at G-string height is even worse. Instead, keep the hands from being too balanced by placing the right hand slightly in front of the right hip, your fingers resting on your right thigh. Your left hand will be slightly in back of your left hip. When your weight is on your right foot and your left foot is forward, you'll reverse the hands—left in front, right in back.

One hand up and one hand down is attractive, especially if you're holding a notebook, committee report, or even your purse. Don't grip objects with both hands unless it's necessary. (Remember Alice?)

Other suggestions are:

1. One hand (not both) on hip.
2. One hand (not both) in a pocket. (And remember, don't push that pocket forward or you'll pull your skirt, coat, or jacket t-i-g-h-t across your hips, leaving nothing to the imagination.)
3. One hand up, the thumb hooked into your belt, the other hand down at your side.

These are just a few suggestions. There are many other attractive hand positions, as you will see if you'll return to our trusty friends, the fashion magazines. Look at the models and see what they're doing with their hands. You'll notice one thing immediately. These vital, glamorous creatures are almost never photographed with their hands together. Instead, their hands are almost always apart, creating a feeling of movement and energy.

Hands held together are also a characteristic of old age. The hands of children are almost never together unless they've been told to fold their hands and sit quietly, a position that always creates an amusing picture because it's so incongruous. It makes a three-year-old look like a prim old maid. And it makes you look like the prim old maid too.

SITTING PRETTY

If walking and standing tell volumes about our age and attitudes, sitting can be even more revealing. Let's see how the simple act of sitting can express age—or agelessness.

The Older Woman approaches the chair warily, turns, and tries to place her hips at the very back of the chair seat by arching her back and leading with her bottom—an incredible view for those sitting in back of her. This position throws her off balance, so she falls *into* the chair rather than sits *on* it. Whoof. Once seated, she settles back, with her weight centered on both hips. Usually her hands are placidly clasped and rest in her lap. Or she may have her arms folded across her chest. These are totally passive poses and only need a pair of knitting needles and a footstool to complete the picture of grandmotherly apathy.

The Older Woman may cross her ankles or sit with both feet flat on the floor. In either of these poses, the legs inevitably relax, allowing the knees to separate—a grossly immodest pose that the older woman seems blissfully unaware of. (Could it be a subconscious admission that she no longer has anything to be modest about?)

The Ageless Woman, on the other hand, moves confidently because *she's thought about what she's going to do before she does it.* She approaches the chair, turns, and steps back with one foot so that the calf of her leg touches the seat of the chair. She now knows exactly where the chair is and doesn't have to look back or *reach* back with her hips to be sure she'll hit the chair seat. She simply bends her knees and sits *straight* down, placing her hips on the forward part of the chair seat. Then she slides back so that her hips are against the back of the chair. Once seated, she transfers her weight to one hip instead of sitting flat and stolid like a sack of prunes. By shifting her weight to one side, she again creates that graceful S curve that is so flattering.

If her weight is on her left hip, she can assume a comfortable, modest leg position by placing her left foot back, the right foot forward, and by swinging her knees slightly to the left. Then when her legs relax the force of gravity pulls them toward the left, and they will automatically remain together in a graceful, modest position.

Does the Ageless Woman sit with her legs crossed? Why not? It's a flattering pose, both young and feminine. The old-fashioned idea that "a lady never crosses her legs" is just that—hopelessly old-fashioned. Of course, a woman whose legs are heavy or extremely short will find that this position is neither comfortable nor very becoming. Each woman should let her mirror tell her the most attractive sitting positions. Remember, though, that crossing your legs is not good for your circulation, so if the position is habitual, you should change position often.

UP, UP, AND AWAY

Getting up out of that chair is another situation that separates the grannies from the glamor girls.

The Older Woman has a *terrible* time because she tries to get up while her hips are still solidly settled at the back of the chair. Her legs and feet scoot and scrape at the front of the chair in embarrassing futility until finally, in desperation, she puts a hand on each chair arm and *heaves* herself up by brute force. Or, worse yet, she may need help to get up, which may be great for the morale of any boy scouts lurking nearby—but what it does for the older woman's morale I leave to your imagination.

The Ageless Woman is ageless because she's smart. She knows that to get out of that chair efficiently and gracefully, she must put the weight (her hips) and the levers (her legs and feet) in effective alignment. So she moves her hips to the front of the chair seat, using one hand to push herself forward if necessary. And of course she moves forward in one graceful movement. No inchworm effect caused by scooting her body forward in little jerky movements.

Next she slides both feet back and under the chair (and therefore directly under her hips) so that the weight and levers are in alignment. Then she simply stands up.

I know, I know. It isn't always possible to place your feet directly under your hips because of the design of the chair. Deep couches and armchairs can be a severe challenge for anyone. But the theory is still the same—and still effective. Get the body and legs in as close alignment as possible and then just stand up. You'll see. It works.

THE THIGHS HAVE IT

Any woman who tries to stand up efficiently and *still* has difficulty in rising gracefully from a chair can blame her wobbly ascent on weak thighs. But of course *you* have been faithful to your aerobic walking/jogging program, so naturally this isn't one of your problems.

It's illuminating, though, to remember that when one ageless actor was asked how long he planned to continue his career he answered, "As long as my legs hold out." Any actor—any performer, for that matter—needs those springy, resilient leg muscles that must be earned through exercise. The moment the legs become weak, the steps falter, the movements become earthbound. And suddenly you aren't ageless anymore. You're allowing yourself to grow old—and you show it. So remember, the thighs have it. Let's hear it for aerobics!

FORWARD MOVEMENT IS AGELESS

The Ageless Woman does not settle back in her chair, resigned and stolid, meekly waiting for The End. She knows that forward movement is a not so subtle trick from the actresses' repertoire. It expresses participation, vitality, involvement. Forward movement is effective whether you're standing or sitting. If you're standing in a group and are introduced to someone, you can create this beguiling forward movement simply by shifting your weight from the back foot to the front. The subconscious impression you'll create is one of warmth and charm.

When you're sitting down, conversing with someone, you can use forward movement to indicate interest as well as ageless vitality. This gives the flattering impression that you are eager to hear every word.

Of course, when you're talking to an interesting man, you may want to give forward motion a little extra push. If you really want to have him on the ropes, use forward movement in three stages. At first, sit back. As the conversation progresses, move your head and shoulders slightly forward. Then, to indicate still more interest, lean forward from the waist. How *far* forward will depend on your décolletage, your natural endowments, and your ultimate intentions.

Naturally, you can't use forward movement all the time. ("Who *is* that woman who always seems ready to jump into my lap?") Sitting back can also be alluring rather than matronly, if it's done with style. Remember, the matron creates a neuter impression because she sits solidly, stolidly, and square on her bottom. The Ageless Woman sits so that her body line has curves by putting her weight on one hip or the other. Tucking one leg under, or sitting totally curled up in the chair (assuming that your clothes and the situation permit), is also ageless. The impression of being totally relaxed (without being dead) creates a languorous quality, like a well-fed pussy cat. This lack of tension, this aura of ease and relaxation, is also quite sexy.

"YES, BUT . . . THIS ALL SEEMS TERRIBLY
AFFECTED. I'M NOT PLAYING A ROLE, YOU KNOW.
I'M NOT TRYING TO BE ANYTHING THAT I'M NOT.
I JUST WANT TO BE THE *REAL* ME."

In every class and every lecture at just about this time, someone
comes up with a variation on this comment. And it's certainly a valid
comment—as far as it goes. Most women have an absolute phobia
about being affected—about being "something that I'm not." The
trouble with this attitude is that somehow it always seems to presup-
pose that the *"real* you" is the least attractive you. It's interesting to
note that this comment is invariably made to defend some negative
quality. "Sure I walk like a duck with two left feet—but that's the
real me."

But why should this be so? Why can't the *real* you be the very
best you? Being "totally natural" is, as I've said before, a dubious
quality. After all, the most natural persons in the world are babies—
and with all their cuddly charm, babies do many excessively unattractive things quite naturally.

But every activity beyond this baby state is learned behavior.

None of us is "natural." We are all playing roles. The distinguished British director Sir Tyrone Guthrie explained, "We are all
actors. We have to be; otherwise people in groups could not exist.
Practically no social behavior is 'natural.' It is natural to rush and
grab what we want like a baby or an animal. It is natural to growl
and scream when our desire is thwarted, be it for a bone, a rattle, or
a bishopric. Socially acceptable behavior is a highly unnatural performance, attainable only after considerable training."

So if you want to see totally natural behavior, visit a nursery
school or, better yet, go to the next month-end sale at your favorite
department store. Talk about rushing, growling, grabbing, and
screaming! And if you are lucky enough to escape from the sale in
one piece, you'll have time to reflect that all the social graces that
make us attractive and successful human beings and allow us to live
together in harmony are *learned behavior.*

Too many women use this "be natural" attitude as a cop-out. And
it is a beautiful cop-out, artistically designed to help us resist change.
And we don't want to change, do we? Because change requires effort.
But be honest. When we say, "I just want to be myself," aren't we
really saying, "I just don't want to make the effort"? After all, it's so

much easier to clump along, as we have for years, instead of consciously thinking about how to walk, how to move, and how to project a positive image. When viewed in its true light, the "be natural" attitude is not a virtue to be cherished and applauded. It is based on the purest sort of laziness and self-deception.

If you need further proof that the "be natural" attitude is a vice—the bastion of middle age and the status quo—let's tune in on our ever ready expert, the Professional M.A.M. Can't you just hear her?

"But that's the way I've *always* done things. That's the *real* me. I'm certainly not going to change *now*." And being a true pro, our M.A.M. doesn't leave it there. "I certainly hope *you're* not going to make a fool of yourself by trying to change at this stage of the game." Your buddy, the M.A.M., is always there to help you grow old gracefully. Well, at least to help you grow *old*—but gracefully? Never. After all, she's the one who walks like a duck. Remember?

But you know all about those negative techniques of the Professional M.A.M., don't you? So let's get back to the positives—and to facts. When you use positive body language (combined with fashion knowledge, beauty techniques, and rejuvenating health habits) you're not creating an artificial person. Instead, you are releasing the real you that was somehow trapped and overcome by the dreary attitudes of the middle-aged matron.

So don't give me that tired old routine, "That's not me." The *real you* is a fascinating, fabulous, Ageless Woman. Use positive body language—and all the other tools described in this book—to help you step out of the shadows and into the spotlight.

Okay. Let's not waste any more time with the drab negativism of "That's not me." Let's get back to a positive discussion of developing positive body language.

THE POWER OF STILLNESS—A TIP FROM A STAR

One of the most powerful tools in the Ageless Woman's repertoire is stillness. Along with fussy, unnecessary movements and too active hands we must mention the too active face as an agemaker. Picture the busy, busy face of the older woman, eyebrows undulating, every tooth flashing in a 32-carat smile, eyes wide in astonishment or submerged in a sea of smile lines. The too active face is an agemaker—every time.

The busy face and fluttering hands not only indicate age rather

than animated vitality, they also exhaust your audience. Think about
it. After all these flutters and facial gyrations in response to so simple
a question as "How are you?"—well, what in the world will you do
for an encore? Probably you'll make your face work even harder, because all these exaggerated, superfluous gestures and expressions soon
become entirely meaningless. The too active face is like the boy who
cried wolf. And since the message no longer comes through, even
more strenuous gestures and expressions must be added, which in
their turn become meaningless and then—good grief, where will it
ever end?

Instead of exhausting yourself and your audience with meaningless
motion, develop the quality of stillness, one of the most powerful of
all acting techniques. Once you have mastered stillness, you can use
gesture and facial expression *meaningfully*. How? By not overdoing
them. By using a few large, serene hand gestures instead of innumerable choppy, fidgety, nervous ones. By using your *eyes* instead of your
whole face to express interest and response and to create magnetism
by *projecting* your personality. We'll be learning exactly *how* to do
all these useful things in a moment, but remember, they all have
stillness as a basis.

Actress Angela Lansbury is an Ageless Woman who enchanted audiences here and in London as the high-spirited Auntie Mame and
the poignant Mama Rose in *Gypsy*. A three-time Oscar nominee, she
knows all the tricks designed to captivate an audience. She has said,
". . . the most important asset for a player is 'the quality of stillness.'
In other words, think, and let your thoughts convey emotions, but
do a minimum facially. Even at this late date, I have to remind
myself and be reminded of this necessity. John Frankenheimer,
directing me in *The Manchurian Candidate*, yelled at me one day,
'Angela, stop doing so much. Let your thoughts come over and the
acting will take care of itself.' This is also true in the theater, except
that in playing large to reach the second balcony you have to em-
bellish the basics. But it's all founded on simplicity. Nothing is worse
than a busy, busy actress or actor. They manage to convey little and
it shows they're not thinking."

TENSION: THE ENEMY OF BEAUTY

An important step in correcting this tendency to be too active is to
realize the underlying reason for this meaningless busyness. Those

clasping, clutching, fluttering hands; those fussy, darting movements; that hyperactive face—they all shout *tension*.

But you can release that tension as quickly as you would trip a switch. The secret lies in learning the techniques of breath control. Breath control is one of the first lessons in any acting class, and for good reason. Controlled breathing develops body awareness and releases tension.

Not only does controlled breathing help to control tension, it can help you to *actually create* a state of mind. We know that our emotions and attitudes are easily read in the way we breathe. It is common knowledge that the breath is short and gasping when we are under the strain of hurry, anger, fear, or uncertainty. But the reverse is also true. If we allow ourselves to practice short, gasping, shallow breathing, we can perpetuate and even exaggerate our inner tensions. But on the other hand, by consciously forcing ourselves to practice calm, deep, even breathing while under stress, we not only project an attitude of peace and serenity, we can actually create more positive mental states. By breathing peacefully and tranquilly, we tend to relax ourselves, to reduce fear and tension, and to achieve inner calmness.

Of course, this is nothing new. Actors have always known that calm, even, deep breathing not only expresses serenity and poise, it actually creates these mental states. Actors also use breathing techniques to indicate age. The older woman tends to punctuate her movements and conversation with sighs, grunts, groans, and wheezes. Her breathing is shallow and uneven, revealing more about her than she would ever tell her very best friend.

Any Ageless Woman has learned the "language" of breath—or she would never have become ageless. Meg used controlled breathing to overcome stage fright as she waited for her job interview—and remember, she learned these breathing techniques in an acting class. They are simple, and are no doubt as old as the theater itself.

BREATH IS LIFE

We can live for a long time without food, for days without water, but we can't do without breath for more than a few minutes. Yet few people breathe effectively in spite of the fact that they've been doing it all their lives.

Effective breathing is variously called *deep breathing* or *diaphrag-*

matic breathing—both good terms, since effective breathing involves full use of the deepest cavities of the lungs and is accomplished by controlling the diaphragm. Unfortunately, there is often a great deal of mysterious mumbo-jumbo surrounding this idea of diaphragmatic breathing—and there's no reason for it. It's an easy technique to learn. Let's just take it a step at a time.

1. Sit on a straight chair, body erect but relaxed. Put your hands on the lower part of your ribs, thumbs in back, fingers to the front.

2. Yawn. That's right. A real, sleepy-time yawn expands the diaphragm and fills the lungs completely. In fact, this is why we yawn when we are tired, and also why we yawn when we are in a room that's airless and warm. We are trying to get as much oxygen as possible, to wake us up and to *revitalize our bodies with life-giving oxygen.*

Yawn again. Feel how the lower part of your ribs expanded, pushing your hands out? That's deep breathing.

3. Yawning activates an involuntary diaphragmatic breath, but here's how to do it deliberately. With hands still on your rib cage, exhale. Come on. Let it all out. Now, inhaling *slowly* through the nose, consciously send a steady stream of air to the lowest part of your lungs. Imagine that you are blowing up a balloon with this calm breath, and as the balloon fills, your diaphragm pushes out, your ribs expand. Continue to inhale as much air as is comfortable, filling the middle and finally the upper part of the lungs. Hold it a moment, then exhale naturally through your *relaxed* lips.

You have just completed a diaphragmatic breath that would do credit to Caruso. Now, here's how to turn this deep breath into a tension turn-off.

1. Inhale as directed.

2. As you slowly exhale, consciously relax your lips, your brow, all your facial muscles, then your shoulders, arms, hands and fingers. Next, relax the torso, thighs, calves, feet—and don't forget your toes. Think of expelling tension as you expel breath.

3. After every bit of breath has been expelled, try to sit for a moment without breathing. Consciously *enjoy* the total feeling of relaxation and freedom that has permeated your whole body.

But as soon as you feel the least bit uncomfortable, inhale again. This isn't an endurance contest but a chance to enjoy complete relaxation and freedom from tension for a few moments.

Practice this deep breathing a few times every day. Don't overdo it. Just practice enough so that you perfect the technique. Gradually, you'll find that you will be breathing more deeply, even when you are not thinking about it.

Get in the habit of checking your body for unconscious tension spots several times during the day. You may be surprised to discover that, unconsciously, you have your teeth clenched, hands tense, calves contracted, and even your toes curled. Like slow leaks, these energy grabbers dissipate your life force in unproductive, debilitating, and *aging* tension. And they are often the cause of many mysterious cases of "nerves."

Here is another breathing exercise that not only relaxes the body but has an immediate calming effect on the mind. Much cheaper and safer than tranquilizers, it's especially useful when you have to wait—in a dentist's office, for example. This is another technique Meg used to retain her composure in the personnel office.

1. Try to sit as straight as possible, wherever you are, so that the lungs aren't pinched by a slouched position.

2. Start to breathe deeply, inhaling through the nose as directed. Of course, by this time you know how to expand the diaphragm, so it isn't necessary to sit with your hands at your ribcage.

3. As you inhale, mentally count to six. And do it slowly.

4. Retain the breath for a count of three.

5. Exhale slowly *through the nostrils*, to a slow count of six.

6. Count three beats between breaths.

Repeat a number of times, but once again, don't overdo. The increased oxygen you're getting from this deep breathing may make you a little lightheaded. It's natural, so don't let it frighten you. Just breathe normally for a while and the lightheaded feeling will pass.

The soothing effect of this one breathing exercise will convince you of the dynamic power of breath. Why does it work? Nobody really knows. It just works—ask any actor. But everyone who mentions it is *obligated* to try to explain it, so here goes. The most obvious, down-to-earth, and least satisfactory explanation is that it forces you to turn your mind from anxious thoughts to a simple, logical sequence of numbers. In addition, by taking deep, regular breaths (instead of those tense, shallow, oxygen-poor breaths), you're giving your body plenty of oxygen, which means that you are at your best—thinking more clearly and generally functioning at the top efficiency. The yogis, on the other hand, have a theory that involves placing yourself in tune with the harmonious rhythm that pervades the universe. But whatever the reasons, *it works*. As actress Margery Wilson says, ". . . breath is life—and our control of our breathing represents, to a great extent, our control of our own lives."

So far, then, we've learned how thoughtless body language—movement, gesture, even breathing—can tell more about us than we really care to have known. Our age, attitudes, and state of mind can all be revealed in bodily movements. But if we perfect positive, ageless, body movements we can *choose* the message we're sending.

Once you have mastered the physical means of communicating positive personality qualities—movements, gestures, breath control—you are ready to move on to a different and perhaps even more powerful method of communication. Once more, we can learn from the world of the theater. Throughout many centuries, actors and actresses have perfected the art of *personality projection*. Let's see how you can do it too.

PROJECT YOUR PERSONALITY—
THE SECRET OF THE GOLDEN CHORD

One of the most effective practitioners of the art of projection is Marlene Dietrich, who has mesmerized audiences for forty years through the force of her personality. Once, during an interview at the height of her career, the question of projection came up. At the time, Dietrich was expressing amusement about another glamorous star who was becoming notorious for bewailing her lack of privacy—"My fans won't leave me alone. I'm simply mobbed wherever I go. . . ."

According to the divine Marlene, attracting people is all a matter of projection, and the complaining star was actually attracting or even *demanding* all that attention through her calculated use of personality projection. And to prove this point, so the story goes, Dietrich said to the journalist, "Let's go out onto Fifth Avenue. You watch me as I walk up the street, without projection. I shall just 'turn off' my personality. Then, *Liebchen*, see what happens when I come back—when I really turn on the magnetism. . . ."

Wrapping her sable-lined trench coat around that fabulous figure, she walked up the street, pausing to look into Van Cleef and Arpels, then Bergdorf's windows. The crowd swirled by without one person giving the elegant figure a second look. Opposite the Plaza she turned and started back—this time *projecting*. Almost immediately a smiling young man stopped her, talked for a minute, and the inevitable autograph ritual took place. As she walked along another and then another passer-by stopped her. She wasn't mobbed exactly (after all, we're talking about New Yorkers). But on the trip back she had consciously projected her vibrant personality—and people responded. *That* is what projection is all about.

Another expert at the art of projection is actress Julie Harris. In explaining the power of projection, actor-director Cyril Ritchard tells this story about her. "Although Julie Harris is known among directors as one of the steadiest, clearest-burning performers on Broadway, she once left a small dinner party without being missed by any of the guests for a full hour. Yet . . . when she appeared in *I Am a Camera*, the audience not only watched her leave the set, but at one point, waited for the off-stage slam of a hall door before they could turn their attention to the actors on stage."

That, too, is projection.

Now you may not have any desire to draw a crowd as you walk down the street in your sable-lined trench coat, but it's nice to think that you can learn the art of attracting people, interesting them, fascinating them through the conscious use of personality projection. And it's nice to think that when you leave a party the other guests will darned well know that some of the sparkle has gone out of the evening.

Just what is projection? It is a way of dynamically expressing your personality in terms of emotion, energy, or life force. It is a means of communicating that goes beyond mere words. Warmth, interest, friendship, even love can be expressed through projection.

Projection comes from your "heart center." This is the sensitive spot in the center of your chest that mystics say is the consciousness center from which we experience emotion, love, compassion. You've felt a surge of energy and magnetism in this spot when an emotional experience has "touched your heart." Other well-known phrases express this metaphysical feeling—"My heart goes out to you," "My heart sings," "My heart leapt with joy." All these feelings come from the heart center.

Now, in order to consciously project your personality and to "broadcast" your feelings of warmth, interest, love, compassion, or whatever *positive* emotion you choose, you must project these emotions through this heart center. Think of projecting these emotions as if that center were a microphone and you were broadcasting your positive emotions like a golden chord of music. Or you might try to visualize these positive emotions in the form of light. Think of projecting a golden light from your heart center—imagine that it envelops the person, group, or audience that you wish to reach.

DOES IT WORK?

Absolutely. And even the most casual effort along this line will bring results. Several months ago we were discussing this idea of projection at a cocktail party. One woman, a high school teacher, was especially skeptical. "Mumbo-jumbo" was one of her expressions as I recall. Yet a week later she called me rather sheepishly for more information. "It works. It really works," she said. "As you remember, I was very critical of this whole idea. Somehow, I'm always suspicious of anything that seems mystical. But I teach one class every day that absolutely gets me down, so I thought, 'What do I have to lose?' I'll try projection and see what happens.

"The class I'm talking about is full of students who are totally bored with school. They're not bad kids. Just so—blasé. Anyway, each day I tried to project to this class, I consciously worked to project my feelings of enthusiasm for my subject and my concern and affection for the students. And you know, their response has been amazing. Suddenly, I wasn't talking 'at' them any more. We were *communicating*. Projection worked where mere words had always failed, and I was able to reach them for the first time."

She went on to tell me that she decided to try this same technique on her teen-age son—the one who never seemed inclined to talk to her in more than one or two mumbled words. Again, she found that projection worked wonders, where words had failed. She put it this way: "I've tried to talk less and project more. It seems that people 'listen' more to the feelings you're projecting than to the words you're saying."

How does projection work? There are several theories, ranging from the mundane "It's just a matter of concentration—of giving people your full attention," to much more subtle explanations involving metaphysical laws and cosmic energy. Countless great performers and actors have tied the concept of projection to the power of Universal Mind. In this form projection becomes conscious magnetism. One who masters this technique projects an almost magical warmth, magnetism, and charm. Certainly no one will ever doubt that this elusive quality exists one moment after they have come in contact with the person who possesses it.

In its simplest form, projection consists of consciously directing your own positive emotions toward others. But in its most powerful form, projection can create an aura of cosmic magnetism around the person who practices it.

If you want to develop conscious magnetism, the ultimate form of personality projection, start by simply acknowledging that there is a benevolent cosmic consciousness pervading the universe. Now, allow yourself to become a channel for this positive cosmic force. How? Caruso called it "stepping aside." Direct your ego to step aside and consciously encourage this benevolent power to flow through you and project out through your heart center. (Self-engrossed youth can seldom do this—it's one of the triumphs of maturity.) Actress Margery Wilson says, ". . . you feel its power tingling through your mind and body. Something of its largeness and grandeur becomes your own. . . ."

As you consciously acknowledge the presence of this benevolent force, the warmth, the love, the positive power of the universe flow through you to all within your sphere. And, as long as you keep your own ego in the background, people will be drawn toward the magnetic force within you, as winter-weary souls are drawn toward the life-saving warmth of a fire.

Does the concept of Universal Mind (or cosmic consciousness, as it is sometimes called) seem a bit too mystical for you? Then you'll be interested in the comments of Russian astronomer V. A. Firsoff, whose findings have led him to believe that "Mind is a universal entity or interaction *of the same order as electricity or gravitation.*" (Emphasis added.) The magazine *Psychology Today* concludes a lengthy discussion of this Universal Mind concept by stating, "The idea of the universe being permeated by Mind, or as an embodiment of Mind, is taken with increasing seriousness by physicists who propose mind stuff particles with different characteristics. . . ."

But if this idea is still a bit much for you, you might follow Thomas Edison's sound advice. He was asked by a gushing dowager to "please explain electricity to me." His answer—"Madame, electricity *is*. Use it." Well, conscious magnetism *is*. So use it.

HOW TO HOLD YOUR AUDIENCE

In addition to projection, there is another quality we can learn from the stage, a technique that will enable you to hold the interest of your audience. Whether it be your husband who is suddenly made to see you in a new light, the grown-up child who thinks, "You know, Mother's really with it," that personnel director who holds the key to an important job, or the fascinating stranger you meet some enchanted evening, you can captivate your audience of one or many by perfecting this time-proven actor's tool.

To *hold* an audience, says Cyril Ritchard, "first of all you have to exert the most tremendous concentration. You've got to keep your mind on the point every minute for as long as you want your audience. The moment you go away mentally, the audience—whether it is at a dinner party or in the theatre—will know it at once."

Total concentration on the audience, whether you're speaking the lines or listening to them, is embodied in the eyes. Eye contact maintains that electric current of concentration. But the instant your mind wanders, your eyes also wander—a dead giveaway that your thoughts are somewhere else. Your audience will sense instantly that you are no longer completely engrossed in the moment—and you've lost them. At least for a little while. Certainly this uneven current of interest will never mesmerize or fascinate anyone. This kind of fragmented attention may get by at the grocery checkout counter. It will never do as a response to conversation from the man you love.

Naturally, by eye contact, I don't mean fixing your audience with a glassy, unblinking stare. Effective eye contact establishes the concentrated interest that captivates your audience. Once eye contact has been established, the eyes can glance away, as if you were thinking about what's being said—and you'd better. You can't just *pretend* to keep your mind on the subject, or your audience will sense your lack of interest. You must continue to concentrate.

For an expert lesson in the technique of eye contact, watch outstanding television actors. You'll note how they hold the eyes of the person they're talking to, then glance away, then use their eyes for emphasis by looking straight at the other actor when they have to make an important point.

But just concentrating on your audience is not enough by itself—you must also acquire the ability to forget yourself. The minute you look winningly at your audience with the thought, "I'm going to concentrate on you so you'll think I'm terrific"—well, you've blown it. We have all encountered a bore who has read one book about charm and patronizingly sets out to fascinate us as a sop to her own ego. No, this approach will never do. As one actress says, "You have to respect your audience. The moment you exploit their attention as an ego trip, you've lost them."

It's fairly easy to hold your audience when you're playing the lead—keeping everyone spellbound with an account of your escape from Amazon headhunters, or some such tidbit. But what about holding your audience when you're playing a supporting role? On the surface, being a good listener is a passive activity, simply accomplished by keeping your eyes open and your mouth shut. But the all-time great fascinators have turned "being a good listener" into a fine art, one that is active, creative, and challenging.

HOW TO BE A CREATIVE LISTENER

The essence of creative listening was spelled out for me one evening in San Francisco. My husband and I were waiting for a table at one of the fine old restaurants and, along with others in the after-theater crowd, we were standing in the bar. The beautiful women San Francisco is famous for were well represented—elegant, sleek creatures with haughty faces and cool eyes. I remember one especially. She's a well-known model in the city, and on this particular evening she looked exquisite, her dark hair swirled high on her head, jewels sparkling on her deceptively simple black suit.

When my husband said, "Now there's the most beautiful woman I've seen in ages—ouch!—after you, of course," I naturally thought he was talking about the model. But instead he pointed out a woman sitting toward the back of the room. I glanced in her direction in a manner that I hoped was casual—but let's face it, I probably was wearing the ultimate "beady-eyed" stare. Whenever my husband says, "Now, there's a beautiful woman," you can be sure I want to get the *total* picture.

I could see immediately why he thought her attractive. Although she was sitting in a dark corner, her manner practically lit up the spot. She was totally engrossed in her escort, leaning forward and listening to his quiet conversation. But it was her facial expression that made such an impact. Even at a distance, the magnetism of her personality was shining out through her face. In comparison, most of the other women in the room looked like so many department store mannequins. Perfect—but contrived and lifeless.

And what did our friend in the corner look like? It's hard to remember physical details—tanned, I think, and with light brown, tousled hair. Sort of a European air, for some indefinable reason. And she wasn't a girl. She was a mature woman who had created an aura of fascination and beauty around herself. And as I "casually" cased the situation with my very best X-ray vision, I became aware of the fact that she was creating her aura by using three basic tools:

1. *Concentration.* She was totally engrossed in her companion. Remember, this is the secret for holding—in fact mesmerizing—your audience.

2. *Eye contact.* Unlike most of the women, she was not constantly glancing around the room. By contrast, they were eternally darting glances around the crowd, as if afraid they might miss someone more important than their escort. Our fascinating lady obviously knew the power of eye contact. She often looked directly into her escort's eyes, and I was reminded of director Michael Klinger's description of the most effective movie love scenes: ". . . they say it all with the eyes."

3. *Facial expression.* Finally, her facial expression kept her face alive with ageless beauty and magnetism. It reflected her interest and response to what her escort was saying.

Our San Francisco beauty was using the techniques of concentration and eye contact (which we have already discussed) to demonstrate her interest in her escort. Then she was reinforcing that impression of interest through facial expression—a subtle communication tool that, sadly, many women seem to have forgotten how to use. We see overactive faces or deadpan, sphinx-without-a-secret expressions, but the woman who can effectively use facial expressions to reveal her true personality seems to be increasingly rare.

FACIAL EXPRESSIONS THAT MAKE YOU AGELESS

There are certain facial mannerisms that shout age, some that murmur—*ageless.* And I'm going to give you a detailed description of both. But the most important thing to remember about facial expressions is that they are tattletales, relentlessly mirroring every thought, unfailingly revealing habitual attitudes. Your thoughts and attitudes are as plain as the nose on your face. It's easy to prove this. Just think about your friends and acquaintances. You probably know someone like Antoinette, a student of mine who has one of the most beautiful faces I've ever seen. It's a perfect oval, surrounded by a mass of dark hair, and set off by a dramatic widow's peak. She has large dark eyes and a beautifully shaped mouth. And she habitually looks as if she's just eaten something incredibly sour or swallowed a bitter pill. And Antoinette *is* a pill, suspicious, critical, always complaining, always sure she's not getting everything she deserves. So that beautiful face reflects her attitudes and is constantly twisted into a sour, suspicious expression that completely overshadows its physical perfection.

And then there's Sunny. You know how she got that nickname. Her happy, open, *accepting* nature is reflected in a dazzling facial expression. Literally, her face glows with joy, and love—and fun. And, in spite of an outsize nose and an undistinguished chin, everyone thinks that Sunny is gorgeous. And so she is.

Positive thoughts create magnetism and literally make your face luminous and bewitching. The Beautiful Bride syndrome is constant proof of this phenomenon. Negative thoughts not only create unpleasant, unattractive facial expressions, but they are repulsive in the literal sense of the word. They repel people—push them away instead of attracting them. Every negative thought is reflected in your expression and influences the way people feel about you. So before we can talk about effective use of facial expressions, we must take a cold, hard look at mental attitudes.

Certain attitudes seem to be typical of age, and so they can make even a youthful face appear old, tired, resigned. Let's see which attitudes are agemakers—and which are ageless.

AGEMAKING ATTITUDES

"So prove it"
"I'm resigned to my fate"
"Nothing good ever happens to me"
"That's just my luck"
"You can't trust people any more"
"It's my role in life to judge and criticize everyone and everything"

AGELESS ATTITUDES

"I believe you"
"Life is full of pleasant surprises"
"Everything's coming up roses"
"I'm lucky"
"People are wonderful"
"Live and let live"

Of course, attitudes are of paramount importance in winning the age game, and we'll be discussing the power of your mental attitudes in great detail in a future chapter. But for now, have fun with this list by proving to yourself how greatly the right attitudes can improve your looks—and what a mess the wrong attitudes can make of even the prettiest face. Pretend you're an actress preparing for a role. Look in a mirror and watch what happens to your face when you saturate your mind with each mental outlook.

Let's take "I'm resigned to my fate." Completely saturate your mind with that attitude. Try to *live* it. What happens to your face? Your brow furrows, the eyebrows drop down at the ends in a self-pitying droop, the lower lip may protrude a bit, and the mouth corners tense. And I'll bet anything you gave a deep, sorrowful sigh, which should just remind you again how powerfully your breathing reveals mental outlook. What a poor, sad, self-pitying creature you've become!

Now try "Life is full of pleasant surprises." Once again, live it. If you can successfully put yourself in this frame of mind, you'll see that unconsciously your brow becomes serene and relaxed, your eyebrows remain in a normal position—but your eyes are very open, subtly asking, "What wonderful thing is about to happen?" Your lips (and are they ever tattletales in the age game) will be relaxed, perhaps slightly parted—and if you're interested in how your breath reflects this mental state, see how a *slow* intake of breath seems to emphasize this expectant mood? And what a contrast to that negative expression! See how your face has suddenly become vital, interesting, appealing?

Just as you have been battling agemaking styles, make-up, and movements, you must also overcome agemaking attitudes. You must learn to emphasize positive attitudes and make them part of your personality, because those positive attitudes are the source of that inner beauty that radiates from some people.

And help is on the way in Chapter Twelve.

But having the right attitudes isn't enough by itself. Because it's easy to allow agemaking mannerisms to overshadow the effect of those positive attitudes. And many women do just that. They contradict the message they are trying to convey by using agemaking mannerisms. Think about the following list and see if you can spot any of these habits on the faces of the women you know. (Of course, *you* don't do any of these agemaking little tricks, do you?)

AGEMAKING FACIAL EXPRESSIONS
YOUR EYES

AGELESS FACIAL EXPRESSIONS

You'll looked older if your eyes:
Have a fixed expression, an unblinking stare (lack of tone in the muscles around the eyes makes them lazy, you don't blink as much as you used to)

You'll look ageless if your eyes:
Have a soft, luminous expression (created by consciously blinking, which relaxes the eyes, bathes them in "natural" eyedrops, the tears)

Are narrowed due to eye trouble or attitude and tend to peer rather than glance

Are wide open, reflecting open-minded attitudes as well as conscious control of eye muscles

AGEMAKING FACIAL EXPRESSIONS
YOUR LIPS AND MOUTH

AGELESS FACIAL EXPRESSIONS

You'll look older if your lips are:
Compressed, making you look vaguely dissatisfied or disapproving
Pursed, creating a very critical, spinsterish effect

You'll look ageless if your lips are:
Relaxed, perhaps slightly parted

You'll look older if your mouth corners are:
Tense, drawing the mouth into a straight line

You'll look ageless if your mouth corners are:
Relaxed or turned up slightly

You'll look older if your mouth is twisted out of shape because you're nervously chewing at the mouth corners

If you have to chew on something, how about a raw carrot?

AGEMAKING FACIAL EXPRESSIONS
YOUR FOREHEAD

AGELESS FACIAL EXPRESSIONS

You'll look older if you:
Constantly scrunch your eyebrows together, producing deep, vertical frown lines
Habitually lift your eyebrows in an exaggerated manner, eventually producing corrugated wrinkles in the brow

You'll look ageless if you:
Consciously relax your forehead, keeping it smooth and serene except for those selected times when you need to specifically express extreme displeasure, or astonishment, or perplexity

The best way to correct these tense and unattractive mannerisms is to become aware of what you've been doing. Then consciously relax all your facial muscles; and (again consciously) replace these misleading mannerisms with relaxed, meaningful expressions. Expressions that *accurately* reflect the positive, optimistic, forward-looking thoughts that typify the Ageless Woman you are now becoming.

And right now I can hear the "be natural" set as they chorus, "That's not honest! That's not natural! That's not *me!*"

But let's think about facial expressions for a moment. What are they really for? To communicate. They are meant to tell someone what sort of person you are and what you are thinking.

But supposing that you have developed facial mannerisms that send the wrong message? What if you are, completely against your wishes, projecting the erroneous image of, say, a tense, unhappy, critical, or perhaps completely unresponsive person. Is that honest? Or natural? Is that what you want?

Of course not! I am not suggesting that you use facial expressions dishonestly—to appear to be someone you're not. I am suggesting that you use facial expressions as *tools* to help others know the real you.

An easy way to study your facial mannerisms is to put a mirror by your telephone. Then study your facial expressions as you talk to your best friends. Are your expressions warm, friendly, responsive? Are they communicating the real you?

The old mirror-by-the-telephone trick will also let you spot the tendency to allow your expressions to become exaggerated and overactive.

Exaggerated facial expressions can involve all the features, and these overblown gyrations can "cry wolf" and prevent you from communicating your feelings and emotions effectively. However, you can learn to tone down your expressions so that they *enhance* rather than overpower the emotion you wish to express by using a technique used by many theatrical coaches. Take your eyebrows, for example. Have you been clenching them in a hammy, overemphatic expression, no matter how trivial the situation? Correct this all-the-stops-pulled reaction by thinking of this expression as having four degrees of intensity. Now, instead of completely clenching your brows, *think* a quarter frown. Now a half frown, three quarters, and finally a full "where have you been till three in the morning" scowl. As you consciously think about these levels of muscular tension, you'll find that when you program yourself for the first level of expression it will take a definite effort to squeeze your brows to the next level—you will no longer do this unconsciously.

This approach is also effective when applied to those chronic offenders, the up-and-down eyebrows. Think of your eyebrows as registering four levels of surprise:

first level: Oh, really?

second level: Paid cash?

third level: Left Harry?

fourth level: With the *Bishop?*

Now try these four levels as you watch yourself in the mirror. See how effective your expressions can be when you don't use one over-powering, top-intensity expression for every emotion?

Another way to learn control of the overactive face is to think of turning the volume down. In other words, fine-tune your facial expressions, just as you control the volume on your TV. When you feel your facial expression "blaring," consciously subdue it, fine-tune it so that it truly expresses your feelings. Countless directors have pointed out that this subtlety will make you a more impressive and convincing person. An additional bonus for the mature woman is that her face won't develop the wrinkles and grooves so apparent in the overactive face.

Good heavens! The threat of a wrinkled, groovy face should make every woman determined to tone down her facial expressions.

But suppose those exaggerated facial expressions have already formed wrinkles? And even though your thoughts are so filled with sweetness and light that you are in danger of levitating at any moment, your face still looks like it belongs six feet underground! And suppose you have that delicate bone structure that means your face has fallen like a stale joke? In short, suppose that your face is simply going to pot! Is there *anything* you can do to make your face match your ageless body and your ever youthful spirit? You'd better believe it!

EIGHT

The Lowdown on the Big Lift

Almost every woman over forty has done it. You've probably done it too. It's usually when you're putting on your make-up, combing your hair, or dressing for an important occasion. You look at yourself in the mirror, place your fingers at the sides of your face, and pull up. Suddenly you look younger, happier, more rested. Wouldn't it be thrilling to give your face (as well as your morale) that permanent lift you've just been imagining? Plastic surgery can do it. But do you dare?

Why not? Everyone else is doing it. In fact, the new patients themselves are the biggest news in plastic surgery today. The face lift, once the exclusive prerogative of the jet set or of members of the theatrical world, is now becoming commonplace among middle-income families. As a result, the number of men and women having plastic surgery has increased phenomenally, and surgeons are now complaining that they have more patients than they can handle.

Not only are these new patients from a different income bracket, but their attitude is totally different. In the past, people tended to be secretive about plastic surgery. Not any more. The new advocates are extremely vocal.

"LET ME TELL YOU ABOUT MY OPERATION"

This new attitude toward plastic surgery has become increasingly evident among my students. In the last few years they have been willing, even eager, to share the "lowdown on the Big Lift." For example, last summer one of my students, Pat Eccles, announced during her final class session that she had decided on a face lift. Everyone was so excited about her big adventure that she promised to come back after the operation and tell us all about it.

When Pat and I discussed it after class, we decided to wait for about two months after her surgery so that her "new look" would be completely established, and then to hold a small, informal get-together so the students and their friends could ask questions.

A week before the session I called to remind Pat of the date. "Not only will I be there," she said, "but I'm bringing a friend, if that's all right with you. We were in the hospital together and had similar operations, although we had different surgeons. I thought it might be interesting to hear her story too."

Well, somewhat to my surprise, our "small, informal get-together" turned into a mob scene. We had standing room only.

Those of us who had known Pat before her lift could hardly wait. The biggest question in our minds was, "How will she look? How *different* will she look?"

How did she look before? I imagine that during high school Pat had been everyone's idea of the "All-American Girl." She had a slightly round face with good cheekbones and a nicely anonymous nose. Add deep-set blue eyes and a generous smile, and you'll have a pretty accurate portrait. In her teens, Pat had been a wholesome picture of health and energy. And as Pat matured she remained healthy, happy, and full of energy; but unfortunately, sagging facial skin and muscles (especially in the eye area) eventually combined to give her a melancholy, tired appearance.

When Pat walked into the room with her friend, my first impression was that she looked marvelously rested. She didn't look dramatically different, but she had been transformed into a healthier- and happier-looking version of herself. It was as if a gentle hand had softened the marks of tension, the traces of fatigue.

For the first time I was aware that she had big, blue, highly expressive eyes. The area under her eyes was absolutely without a wrinkle, and her cheeks looked high and firm. The surgeon had done a magnificent job, and I remembered something I read in Simona Morini's book, *Body Sculpture:* "Nothing drastic should happen to a face after a good lift . . . there should never be a new face, just a face imbued with new life." And that was what had happened to Pat.

As I said, our seminar was very informal, so when everyone had settled down (and the standees were on cushions on the floor) Pat stood up and in the charming and relaxed way that had made her such a favorite in class jumped right into the subject.

"I guess that the first thing everyone wants to know is why. Why did I decide to have a face lift? Frankly, I even surprised myself a bit, when I definitely decided to do it. It's not as if I were on the stage, or even a career woman. I don't even work—that's a laugh! Actually, I work twelve hours a day taking care of my husband and my three teen-age children and our cats and our house and I'm on committees—but you know what I mean. I'm really a fairly average housewife and mother. So why did I have my face lifted?

"Well, I was just tired of looking in the mirror and feeling depressed. I have a small-boned face, and the years really began to show. Even when I felt great, I always looked tired. My eyes were especially bad. They drooped and made me look unhappy. I got tired of having the kids ask, 'Is everything okay, Mom?'

"So when Phil—that's my husband—wanted to give me a new car for my birthday, I asked him to let me spend the money on a face lift instead. So I'm still driving the old Plymouth, but I don't care. The car may be getting a little creaky, but I feel great. Maybe it's just the power of suggestion, but now when I look into the mirror I feel an extra spurt of energy. As I told Phil, it's the best birthday gift *ever*. Every time I look in the mirror, it's like getting another present."

Someone asked Pat what her husband thought about the operation.

Pat laughed. "Well, it was really funny. My husband's sense of humor makes every family event unpredictable. At first he went into the 'You don't need a face lift, I love you just the way you are' routine—a typical reaction according to my surgeon. But then he saw I was really serious and right in the middle of a sentence he looked at me kind of squinch-eyed, grinned, and said, 'Okay, Pruneface, will you trust my check or do you insist on cash?' As I recall, I said, 'I'll take a check, Banana-nose.' And I guess that completes the lowdown on my big lift."

Pat's friend introduced herself as Donna Laconni. She appeared to be about thirty-six or thirty-seven years old, with dark eyes and hair and an ivory complexion that was flattered by the coral tweed suit she was wearing. Her manner was brisk and practical as she talked about her operation. "I guess the main reason I went ahead with my face lift was financial. As I was telling Pat when we were in the hospital, I had to go back to work after my husband passed away—he was ill for a long time, and those medical bills just ate up any financial backlog that we had. I know now that I'll have to keep working as long as I can totter around on two feet. Someday I may be the oldest secretary in the world, but I know I can't *look* it. I know that my office skills are top-notch, but I also know that to hold one of the really good jobs I have to look the part.

"So I consider this operation job insurance. And that's what I told the bank when I applied for a loan to have this done. You may be surprised, as I was, that it was simple to get a loan for plastic surgery if you have a good credit record. I thought the bank would be difficult because a face lift might be considered a frivolous luxury. But the loan officer agreed that the operation was job insurance for me. He pointed out that the face lift might not be absolutely *essential*, but they loan money for vacations, and they aren't essential either. 'Lift now, pay later,' he said—which is pretty good for a banker, I guess.

"Anyway, I got the money, had my operation, and it was the best thing I ever did. It did so much for my morale at a time when I really needed a lift—if you'll excuse the pun.

"None of you knew me before so to help you see what the 'lift' can do I brought my before and after pictures."

She was right. It was the best thing she could have done to take a new lease on life. Her "before" pictures showed a woman of forty-five anyway, with a haggard face, pronounced eye bags, and a "turkey wattle" of loose flesh under her chin. The delicate bone structure had given her facial contours very little support, and time, worry, and grief had broken them down totally.

So Donna was the perfect candidate for a highly successful face lift. As one surgeon explains it, "So much depends on the general level of health, the elasticity of the skin, the bone structure. Patients who have loose skin under the chin line, or pronounced eye bags, seem to show the most dramatic results."

Pat and Donna were two extremes that demonstrate what you can expect from a face lift. Pat's bone structure and pronounced cheekbones had prevented her facial contours from completely sagging, so the changes brought about by her face lift were subtle. But Donna's change was dramatic—she looked like her younger sister.

Once the ice was broken, the questions from the group seemed to tumble over each other.

"You look so different, Donna, what did people say when you came back to work?"

"Of course, my friends were all for it—especially *after* the operation. I did have a couple of negative reactions from relatives—you know, 'I like you just the way you are.' But they know what I've been through, and now that it's been such a big success they're all thrilled for me. In fact, my sister-in-law is going to have it done too.

"At work, it was a little different. I took my month's vacation and was able to return without any obvious signs—you know, bruises or bandages. And I found that people aren't as interested in us as we think they are. Oh, the first day, lots of the gals dropped by my office to chat about the 'new me.' I mean, everyone's interested in the subject of plastic surgery today. But people are basically interested in their own affairs, and in a few days I wasn't the office celebrity any more. I certainly wouldn't let other people's opinions keep me from taking this step." (Good girl!)

"Did you experience much pain?"

Pat answered, "Really, I didn't have any pain at all—which is just what my doctor had said. Rather, he said it would be 'practically painless.' There was a little discomfort, of course. Some sensation that something had been done, but not what I'd call *pain*. I wasn't totally happy when the stitches were taken out. That's never any fun, is it? But as for real, hurtful *pain*, no, I didn't experience any. Wasn't that your feeling, Donna?"

"Basically, yes. But I did have a real emotional upset after I got home from the hospital. Even though the doctor had warned me, I looked so battered and bruised for the first few days that it was sort of scary. At first I wanted to cry every time I caught a glimpse of myself. But I suspect my depression was partly a reaction to the anesthetic, because it never did hurt. Then, as I was healing, the incisions itched terribly under all those bandages—it almost drove me crazy. But that passed in a couple of days. Certainly there was no sensation that was unpleasant enough to keep me from doing it all over again if I had to."

"Will you have to do it again? Or will this operation last from now on?"

Donna said, "My surgeon says I will probably have to come back in about two years and have a little 'tuck' to correct relaxed muscles, and then the lift should last about ten years. But everybody's different. For instance Pat, with her bone structure, won't need the 'tuck.' Then, naturally, your face ages a bit as the years go by, but if I take care of myself I will always look one face lift younger than my actual age. And when that ten-year period is up (or even before) I intend to go back for another lift. Why not? If you've done it once, then it's no big deal."

"Why ten years?"

"Actually," Donna said, "there's no ten-year guarantee that comes with your face lift; but if you follow doctor's orders, your lift should last about ten years—of course, everyone's different."

"Did the doctors give you any specific rules?"

"They sure did," Pat said. "And they said these rules will help anybody's facial beauty.

"Too much sun, for instance, is an absolute no-no for anyone who's had a lift. My surgeon showed me a chart that illustrates what happens to your skin when it is sun-tanned, and what happens to your skin as it ages. The chart shows identical changes in the skin. That convinced me to get my tan out of a bottle from now on.

"He was also a fanatic about 'clean living.' Says he can spot a gin drinker from across a room, just by the condition of her skin. So I'm drinking table wines now, if anything. He even feels that smoking causes wrinkles—something to do with the effect of nicotine on the circulation." (At this point, several cigarettes were stubbed out.)

"I think that the best advice for keeping your face lift successful is what we learned right here in our classes. The beauty-fuel foods that we've learned about in class, and the aerobic exercise, these were both endorsed enthusiastically by my surgeon. Of course, keeping your weight at the same level helps the skin to remain elastic too."

More and more questions were asked as the evening progressed. Pat and Donna answered whenever they could from their personal experience. I jotted down several of the more technical questions and promised to try to find the answers. Here are the answers to some of those questions.

WHAT'S THE BEST AGE FOR HAVING A FACE LIFT?

This is one of the leading questions, since cosmetic surgery creates a unique medical situation. That is, it's the only form of surgery based on the patient's own diagnosis. It's the one operation where *you* tell the doctor you need it—not vice versa.

How will you decide? Apart from the psychological and financial considerations, the best answer is, "The sooner the better." That seems to be the underlying attitude of leading surgeons.

In fact, many plastic surgeons feel that candidates for a face lift come to them too late. Although every surgeon could undoubtedly point with pride to older patients who have had successful lifts, any time between forty and fifty-five will give the most positive results. (And the closer to forty, the better.) Important as age is, many surgeons consider over-all physical condition to be another prime consideration. The woman who is healthy and who hasn't overindulged in food or drink will have the best results. At least one surgeon urges his patients to go into training a few months before surgery, on a regimen that makes alcohol, coffee, and even tea no-no's. He also prescribes a high-protein diet with lots of vitamin-A-rich foods.

Are you ever too young to seek plastic surgery as an antidote to those little aging lines, those tiny intimations of drooping contours? One of the latest trends in plastic surgery says no. This trend, the poroislatic approach, suggests that the patient put herself in the hands of a plastic surgeon at the first signs of aging—even in her mid-thirties. Jet-set beauty expert Luciana Avedon is probably the most famous exponent of this approach and describes her visits to the plastic surgeon with engaging frankness in her books.

Poroislatic plastic surgery is based on a program of minor corrections. At the first sign of a drooping eyelid or pouchy jaw, the patient undergoes corrective surgery. This approach has several advantages.

1. It is less traumatic to the tissues than a complete face lift.
2. It virtually prevents the face from ever looking old.

3. Its results are so subtle that there's never any need to explain how you've managed to beat the clock.

One obvious disadvantage is financial—we're talking about many operations instead of one (or possibly two) which the typical patient would undergo. It may also cause emotional problems. For most of us, the decision to have one bout with the plastic surgeon is difficult enough to make. Programing ourselves for a series of operations over the years is perhaps too much for the puritan background that haunts most of us whether we like it or not.

The poroislatic approach may not be for you, but it is definitely the wave of the future. As one surgeon said, "Young people today will probably live their middle years in an atmosphere that treats a visit to the plastic surgeon as casually as a visit to the dentist."

WILL THE SCARS SHOW?

That depends on what you have done. In the standard face lift, the hair is parted just beyond the hairline at the temple and the incision is made. It continues, within the hairline, down toward the ear, swings in front of the ear, encircles it, and curves back toward the hairline. This scar can be completely hidden by a judiciously chosen hair style.

If the operation includes an eye lift, the scars are hidden in the natural folds above the eyelid and just below the lower lash. If an eyebrow lift is needed, the suture line is concealed just within the upper hairline of the brow.

If a double chin is the problem, an incision is made just under the chin line.

WHAT'S IN A NAME?

This discussion of incisions brought out a fact that seemed new to most of the women at our seminar. That is, that the so-called face lift is actually composed of a series of operations. Depending on the condition of the patient, these operations might include:

THE RHYTIDECTOMY (standard face lift)
The surgeon separates the facial skin and part of the neck skin from the underlying muscle and tissue by means of the in-the-hairline incision described above. He then pulls the skin up to-

ward the temples and back toward the ears, cuts off the excess, and closes the incision.

BLEPHAROPLASTY (eyelid correction)

This basically simple technique consists of removing the excess skin from the crepy upper eyelid by cutting off the necessary ellipse of skin at the incision, which is made in the crease of the upper eyelid. The same technique is repeated in the lower eyelid if necessary, the incision being made just under the eyelashes to re-create the smooth and firm contours of youth. In addition to excess skin, the surgeon may need to remove excess fat from the upper and lower lids. The result is "by-by, bags."

SUPERORBITAL RHYTIDOPLASTY (eyebrow lift)

Sometimes that tired and melancholy eye expression is due to a drooping eyebrow instead of aging eyelids. Sometimes both conditions contribute to the aging appearance of the eyes. So the surgeon may make an incision right above the brow and remove an ellipse of skin to raise the brow and correct the drooping appearance of the eyelid.

SUBMANDIBULAR LIPECTOMY (chin correction)

If the patient has an usually fat double chin, the surgeon may make a horizontal incision in one of the creases under the chin and trim away the excess fat. If, however, the double chin is accompanied by wads of loose skin, giving a "turkey wattle" effect, he may also make an additional horizontal incision low on the neck, connecting the underchin and neck incisions by a small vertical cut. Or he may make a single vertical incision. This operation often leaves noticeable scars on the neck, but personally, I think an unobtrusive scar on a firm smooth neck is much better than an untouched accordion-pleated neckline and a wobbly chin any day. When this operation is considered necessary, it is usually done in conjunction with the standard face lift for best results. A chin correction had been part of Donna's operation, and the results were spectacular. The small scar under her chin line was almost invisible.

HOW MUCH WILL IT COST?

"There is no such thing in plastic surgery as a standard fee," Patrick McGrady says in his book, *The Youth Doctors.* When you realize that your face lift may include one or any combination of the operations just described, it's easy to see why surgeons are wary about quoting prices to the general public. However, it's possible to get a general estimate of the cost, and most women are surprised to find that the dream of a face lift is well within their financial means. It may require a shift in values—remember Pat's decision to have her new face rather than a new car—or it may mean a loan and time payments. But the Big Lift is certainly possible for almost everyone.

You will have to shop around. The cost of a lift will vary according to where you are, what you have done, and who does it. But to give you some specific ideas of cost, I can quote the figures given in three separate sources. In 1968, McGrady said that a face lift in Hollywood or New York could cost between $1,000 and $5,000, depending on what had to be done. In August 1973, *Vogue* reported that the cost of a lift on both upper and lower eyelids was averaging $1,000, and that a total face lift would cost between $1,500 and $2,500. In 1974 the San Francisco *Chronicle* reported that a total face lift in that city, including the hospital fees, was costing about $3,000.

However, this brings us to one of the most hotly debated issues among plastic surgeons today: the practice of office (outpatient) surgery, which eliminates hospital bills and hospital red tape. As recently as ten years ago this approach was considered the exclusive realm of the quacks and fakes and was denied the sanction of the professional community. No more. In the burgeoning Southern California area it is estimated that up to 30 per cent of local plastic surgeons are turning to this efficient and relatively pleasant approach. Respectable surgeons in Florida, Northern California, and the Southwest are also practicing office surgery. Dr. John Williams, of Century City in Southern California, is generally credited with raising the outpatient-style operation to its present level of respectability. Dr. Alan M. Steen, of Torrance, California, is another proponent. He feels that this approach is one reason more and more people are taking advantage of the miracles that plastic surgery can provide. "The reason it can be afforded by the middle class is that you don't have to use a hospital. We've done a lady truck driver who ran a food truck, construction workers, salesmen."

However, while costs are naturally an important consideration, whether you choose the outpatient approach or opt for a stay of several days in the hospital, the essential thing is to choose a highly qualified surgeon who maintains professional and accepted standards.

HOW WILL YOU FIND THE
RIGHT PLASTIC SURGEON FOR YOU?

The approved approach is to call the Specialist Referral Board of your county medical society and ask them to provide you with a list of accredited plastic surgeons living in your area. *This is essential.* For heaven's sake, don't put your precious face in the bumbling hands of Madame TuTu and her Miracle Rejuvenating Cream. This seems like an unnecessary warning, until you remember that just such a woman conducted a thriving business for years in Southern California. Instead of surgery, she applied caustic lotions that induced a drastic face peel. Hundreds of hopeful women went to her for these dangerous, ineffective, and ridiculously expensive treatments before she was finally stopped.

Be certain that your surgeon is a skilled and recognized member of the profession. The most conventional approaches to plastic surgery can create all the effects you want, so don't feel that you have to go to someone on the fringe of medical respectability for the "latest, most miraculous" techniques.

Most surgeons warn against the so-called "quickie" lift and consider it to be a totally fraudulent technique. The "quickie" face lift is a minor operation, performed quickly in the surgeon's office. It involves nothing more than removing a small piece of skin within the hairline at each temple. When the incisions are closed, there is a little lift effect. And for a couple of months the operation works. The patient looks better and within that two months she may convince several friends that they too should have this inexpensive "quickie" operation. But within a short time the swelling goes down and the lift effect disappears. All the victims of the "quickie" are right back where they started from, but a few hundred dollars poorer.

However, consulting the Specialist Referral Board will keep you out of the hands of such charlatans.

You can also learn the names of reputable surgeons through the word-of-mouth recommendations of friends who have had a *real* lift. (And which you will later check with your county medical society— promise?) There's no denying that this word-of-mouth advertising is one of the main reasons for the increased popularity of plastic surgery. Chatting with a friend about the details of her operation, about her feelings before and after the Big Lift, can all help smooth the way in a situation that is bound to be a little bit scary.

But suppose you don't have a friend who's had it done? If a heart-to-heart talk will help you make up your mind, it's perfectly acceptable to ask a surgeon (at the time of the consultation) if he can put you in touch with a former patient who would share the details of her experience with you. Many plastic surgery "graduates" are so enthused that they long to spread the word. And may indeed insist on telling you more about their operation than you really wanted to know.

People who go through the lift often become messiahs. Phyllis Diller, bless her, is an example. Although most show business personalities still tend to use the secret entrances and exits that many celebrated surgeons provide, Phyllis told the world.

When she had her face and nose "redone" at the age of fifty-four, she told women everywhere, "It isn't a sin to look better." What's more, her word-of-mouth endorsement (via the TV talk shows) resulted in such a rush of business, it became an embarrassment to her surgeon, Dr. Franklin Ashley, who finally begged her to quiet down because his stuffy colleagues were becoming critical of all the publicity he was receiving.

Magazines and newspapers can also help you find a surgeon. They increasingly tend to feature stories on plastic surgery in general and face lifts in particular. The names of prominent surgeons are often mentioned. In the past, these stories almost always discussed the work of some almost mythical artist among plastic surgeons—Dr. John Converse in New York, Dr. Ivo Pitanguy of the legendary Pitanguy clinic in Rio, Dr. Robert Alan Franklyn of Los Angeles. However, because of the increased acceptance of plastic surgery in recent years, many skilled and competent plastic surgeons can now be found throughout the United States. Chances are that during the time you are deciding on a face lift your newspaper or television station will have discussed the work of several prominent local surgeons. Once you have the names, it is a simple matter to check them out through your county medical society.

Finally, you can ask your family doctor to refer you to a surgeon— if you can trust your doctor in these cases. Remember, many of them were raised by Professional M.A.M.s "Now, Margaret, what's this foolishness about a plastic surgeon? For a woman of your age, you're in marvelous condition. . . ." As if any woman wants to be "a woman of your age." If he takes this attitude—belt him with your purse!

Now let's assume that you have the names of three surgeons—one name given to you by your best friend's cousin, one suggested by that family doctor who is still nursing a black eye, and a third who was recommended by the referral board when you called to check on the first two.

Ideally, you'll make appointments for preliminary consultations with at least two surgeons—and don't be surprised at the request to pay in advance for the consultation. Probably you will also be asked to pay the total fee in advance when you ultimately decide to go ahead.

The preliminary consultation is probably your most challenging moment in this entire experience, because at this point you are trying to decide on the *right* surgeon for you. The referral board has, of course, assured you that the surgeons are equally competent. You have talked to their enthusiastic patients. *But which is right for you?* At this point, it boils down to your personal opinion. If you and your surgeon have genuine rapport, if you both feel enthusiastic about this joint venture, if you're both in accord with the results that can be expected, your operation has the greatest chance of being a thrilling success.

It's interesting to note that Pat and Donna had both consulted Dr. X. Pat was impressed with his no-nonsense attitude and his unemotional description of exactly what surgical techniques would be involved. Although he was the first surgeon she consulted, she decided then and there to have him do the work. Donna, on the other hand, said, "I didn't like him at all. He seemed so abrupt, and was insistent that I hear all the creepy details about what he intended to do. But then I went to Dr. Y, and he was so sympathetic and seemed so interested in my reasons for needing this operation, I knew we were in accord on the results. And when he explained what he'd do, it was just in general terms, without so much mention of stitches and sutures, and cutting off exactly so many inches of skin. Ugh!"

WHAT HAPPENS NEXT?

Typically, a candidate for a face lift will see her surgeon several times before the operation. At the first session, she'll tell him just what's bothering her—"See how my eyelids droop—right here?"—

and he may suggest additional improvements that are possible. "We can get rid of this—" as he gently lifts the skin at the side of her temples, making those fallen cheeks look high and firm again. During the pre-operative sessions—usually two, sometimes three or four —the surgeon checks her skin and facial structure, watches her facial expressions, and develops a definite idea of just what he will do.

Then come the medical photographs. There are two reasons for these. The most obvious one is that they are often used as a guideline during the actual surgery. The surgeon may also use the photographs to demonstrate to the patient just what he plans to do (steady there, Donna). Another less obvious reason for the photographs is pointed out by Simona Morini. "Finally comes the ceremony of the 'before' photographs for the surgeon's record, to which the 'after' will be added once the wounds have healed. It is an unwritten law that photographs should always be taken; they are the surgeon's or the patient's best evidence, in case of a malpractice suit, of what the operation was all about."

During these pre-operative sessions the surgeon discusses the type of anesthetic used and, if there's a choice, asks the patient her preference. He clarifies the length of her hospital stay. He soothes fears about pain, and scars, and the time it will take for the bruises and swelling to disappear. A woman who has chosen her surgeon wisely will know all the answers and will feel confident and relaxed throughout the entire experience.

But still the question remains, "Do *you* dare?" For many women a "yes" answer will depend on how successfully she copes with this question.

WHAT WILL PEOPLE SAY?

If you're seriously contemplating cosmetic surgery, "What will people say?" can be your biggest psychological hurdle. Even the most self-confident among us can be intimidated by the old-fashioned attitudes toward this subject. Many people find among their family and friends tremendous reserves of moral disapproval directed against the whole idea of the face lift. Of all cosmetic surgery, to some people (especially Professional M.A.M.s) the face lift is considered the ultimate in selfish vanity. Never mind if it will bolster a floundering marriage, renew self-esteem, assure job security. No siree. To these guardians of our moral fiber, the entirely natural and healthy desire to be as attractive as possible is directly associated with sin and total moral disintegration.

All I can say is, "Hang in there, baby!" Reinforce your determination with the knowledge that this attitude is hopelessly dated, a relic of fuddy-duddyism that's thirty years behind the times. Dr. R. B. Aronsohn, in his book *The Miracle of Cosmetic Plastic Surgery*, says, "The last twenty-five years have seen not only vast improvements in techniques used by cosmetic surgeons, but a change from the stigma attached to it. If you had something done then, you were altering nature and God's handiwork. Today these attitudes are changing, at least among the well-adjusted," and Aronsohn adds, "In fact, if a person tells you today that he doesn't care if he's ugly or looks old, he's probably being irrational. . . . Many clinicians maintain that those who don't desire improvement in appearance may be the really abnormal individuals." This contemporary, open-minded attitude was reflected in a series of woman-on-the-street interviews conducted by CBS newswoman Sande Drew. To her question, "Would you have plastic surgery done?" women gave these answers:

"Yes. I'd definitely have plastic surgery done. While the rest of the world is improving, I don't want my body to fall apart." . . . "Certainly. Why? Well, any woman wants to look her best at all times." . . . "Yes, I would. Why? Well, the same reason I bleach my hair and dye it all the time, I guess. I just like to look as good as I can as long as I can. And I'd start with my face and just work all the way down." . . .

Ironically, the only negative answer was given by a pretty young girl about twenty, with a smooth, unlined face. "I don't think so. It's really not a 'natural' way. I'd rather stick with what I've got." Ah, she jests at scars who never felt a wound. Boy, will *she* ever learn!

While the attitudes of the general public are changing, what about the people in *your* life? What would they say if you had your face lifted?

If you're worried about the opinions of your acquaintances and co-workers, you're in for a shock. As Donna pointed out, most people are not as interested in us as we would like to think. They're really totally involved with their own lives, their own problems, and actually give us very little thought. What's more, our relationships with the people on the periphery of our lives can change without warning.

For instance, Lydia, an enthusiastic member of our face lift get-together, told me this story after her brilliantly successful operation.

"You know, I'd been wanting to have this done for years, but a girl in my office kept urging me not to. She had dozens of prim and very moral reasons. I'd ruin my 'natural' expression, I was being affected, it wasn't 'nice' and so forth. She was so adamant that I almost gave up on the idea of a lift just because of her comments. And I was being so silly. Without really realizing it, I was making an important life decision because of the opinion of a casual acquaintance. If my head had been on straight I would have asked myself, 'Why should I give a damn about her opinions?' I hardly *knew* her.

"I didn't really come to my senses until one day she didn't come to work. Then I realized how *little* I knew her. That supermoral little mouse had run off with her husband's tax accountant, leaving her husband and two small children.

"And she had been making me feel immoral to consider a face lift. Ha! But that's really not the point. She's out of my life now and I'll probably never see her again, and yet I'd let her influence my life. How foolish! I've really learned from this, not to care so much about what other people think—at least those people who only belong on the fringes of my life."

But what about the important people in your life? Your husband and family. In her book, *Beauty You Can Buy*, one surgeon told Harriet LaBarre, "A majority of husbands feel there isn't any necessity for the operation. They accept their wives as they are. They say, 'Oh, you don't need it; you look fine to me.'

"'Well,' the wife usually says, 'I know I don't need it for *you* . . . but I need it for *myself*.' This is a familiar exchange in my office. The husband usually agrees, not with any enthusiasm, but at least with an 'All right, go ahead.' Afterward, however, he is pleased; he begins to enjoy going out with this more attractive woman."

Still, many women can expect to have some trouble with their families over the Big Lift. But attitudes are changing rapidly, and generally these problems can be worked out. As. Dr. Franklin Ashley says, "I think most people who have any intelligence and are fairly broad-minded have come to the conclusion that people have the right to do whatever they can to improve themselves."

Of course, it's a long step from all those broad-minded, intelligent people to the Professional M.A.M. in your life. You *know* she's going to be there, ready as always with her helpful advice. What does she say about your face lift?

"If God had meant for us to look young forever, He never would have invented bags and wrinkles," she sniffs.

Next to the menopause, plastic surgery is the area in which the Professional M.A.M. seems to do her negative best in spreading doubt, anxiety, and misinformation among her relatives and friends. Often she cleverly entwines the two subjects, identifying plastic surgery with mental imbalance and other old wives' tales associated with menopause.

"My sister has really flipped, I tell you. Can you imagine? She's actually having her face lifted. I'm sure it's just part of the 'change.' She takes after Mother's side of the family, you know, and they always have a bad time of it." She taps her forehead significantly.

Or she'll dredge up a horrendous story or two about Cousin Letty ("she was the wild one, you know") and how her face was absolutely ruined by some charlatan at a remote clinic in Switzerland after that ski instructor ran out on her.

Never one to be deterred by facts, she may even take the approach that plastic surgery is a dangerous, "newfangled" fad. Not true. In fact, forms of cosmetic surgery were performed by the ancient Hindus—and without the benefits of anesthetic. If that doesn't prove that the desire for beauty is basic, I don't know what does. But the modern face lift was perfected by a charming Frenchwoman (wouldn't you *know*), Madame le Docteur Suzanne Noël in the early 1900s. The techniques that she pioneered remain basically the same today, although naturally many refinements are being added all the time.

As usual, facts are your best defense against that Professional M.A.M. in your life—facts and knowledge that *dominance* is the name of her game. It's not disapproval of the face lift that's her main concern. Nor is it a desire for your welfare (though she may sincerely think so). No. It's dominance of *you* that's the issue here. In making your decision, remember that it's *your* face and *your* emotional needs that are of prime concern. You'll be strengthened in your decision by the awareness that you can't please everyone. In fact, this realization is one of the great bonuses of the mature years. You really can't please everyone. And if you have to choose someone to not please, doesn't the Professional M.A.M. make a lovely choice?

After all, at this stage of your life, the most important person to please is—*yourself*. That's the ultimate answer to "What will people say?"

"YES, BUT . . . I'M STILL NOT QUITE READY
TO TAKE THE BIG STEP UP TO COSMETIC SURGERY.
IS THERE AN ALTERNATIVE TO
THE SURGICAL FACE LIFT?"

Nothing will be more effective than a surgical face lift in rolling back the years. But there are some medical procedures that are recommended to correct specific conditions.

The plastic surgeon may use face planing, the face peel, or silicone injections in conjunction with the face lift.

What can they do for you? Face planing or a face peel can give you a younger-looking, less wrinkled skin, after the scars have healed. Though I have to add here that improving your health habits (the Super-B Diet, aerobic exercise) can produce almost the same rejuvenating effect. It takes longer—but it lasts.

You must use caution and be aware of the fact that these treatments are also the realm of the quack, the charlatan, and the dangerous amateur. Proceed with caution. I cannot stress too often that no one should be allowed to treat your face except reputable medical experts—experts that have been cleared by you through the referral board of your local medical society. Remember, if some charlatan makes a mistake on your face he can say, "Oops," and skip town. You, on the other hand, have to wear your face—you can't run from it.

What about silicone treatments? Silicone can be used to plump up the face, to fill in wrinkles, and to improve contours in the cheek or chin area. This is a technique that is still being debated in medical circles. But in specific cases some plastic surgeons may use silicone injections to fill in the smile lines at the sides of the mouth or to erase the deep frown lines between the eyebrows, because neither of these two areas is significantly affected by the surgical face lift. But the widespread use of silicone is still in the very experimental stage, and unless it is used as part of a surgical face lift you should certainly proceed with caution.

However, one highly successful New York dermatologist, Dr. Michael Kalman, has been using silicone injections for five years on some of the most famous and beautiful faces in jet-set and show-biz circles. It may be that his work is setting the pace for the future. He points out that silicone is non-allergenic, does not cause cancer, does not change with time, and can be used to fill in wrinkles and expression lines or for facial contouring on the cheekbones and the chin.

How does it work? "The whole process is very simple and only costs a little more than an average office visit," says Dr. Kalman. "What we do first is have the patient sit in an upright position, because that is the way most people see her or him—we get more and more men all the time.

"Then we mark off those areas which are to be injected with an orange sterile solution. . . . Then we have the patient lie down and inject him with a ¼-cc. syringe with a 30-gauge needle—which is the finest needle made. We start injecting the silicone, a fifth of a drop at a time, about 5 millimeters apart. We never use more than ½ or 1½ cc. per session or per face.

"After the injections have been given, we ask the patient to press firmly over the areas to prevent bruising—just to prevent black and blue marks. There might be some pain if the patient is supersensitive. If that is the case, we deaden the area with a cold spray. After the patient washes his face, there might be a slight redness or a slight swelling if he had not applied enough pressure."

However, Dr. Kalman says he has seen many patients go right on to the TV studio and before the cameras, just minutes after a treatment. Not only is silicone injection quick, painless, and economical but, according to Kalman, it has a specific physiological benefit as well.

"In addition, silicone works advantageously by stimulating cells in the skin called fibroblasts, which produce collagen, the main structure of the dermis of the skin. The final effect is that silicone is incapsulated in the tissue while forming new tissue. There is absolutely no chance of infection providing you use the medical grade of silicone."

He concluded, "Silicone is not a youth pill and it is not a miracle, but we have seen some marvelous results with it."

WHAT TO DO TILL THE DOCTOR COMES

Still, all these methods are based on complex medical techniques. The question remains, "Is there anything *I* can do either before (or instead of) my visit to the youth doctors? Is there a non-medical approach to lifting and rejuvenating my face?" The exciting answer is, *yes!*

There *are* several things you can do—simple, inexpensive, safe techniques—which will make your face appear lifted, younger, vital. I am always surprised that these techniques are unknown to so many women. They are all easy, inexpensive, and readily available.

THE BEAUTY SECRET OF A LEGEND

In France, in the seventeenth century, a courtesan named Ninon de Lenclos became a legend in her time, not only because of her beauty and her sizzling private life, but because in her later years she retained her youthful appearance to a startling degree. It's been said that young men fell madly in love with her when she was well past seventy years old—of course that may or may not appeal to you, but it would be fun in the future to have the chance to say no.

Mystery and legend surround the means she used to retain her beauty, but one of her secrets is said to have been a series of facial exercises that kept her skin elastic and firm and lifted her facial contours in a perpetually youthful manner.

Although the actual techniques she used are lost in the mists of time, some very contemporary beauties are using modern, scientific facial exercises—and getting age-defying results.

HOW DO THEY WORK?

On exactly the same principle that body exercises work. After all, the face is composed of nerves, bones, and muscles, just as the body is. If the facial muscles are kept toned and firm, the face will retain its youthful contours. The skin will be firm because it is supported by the solid muscle underneath, and the skin will have an improved color, texture, and elasticity. Why? Because any exercise, whether it's for the face or the body, not only tones the muscles but improves the circulation which feeds the cells and helps with the disposal of wastes. This is why facial exercises, consistently practiced, bring such satisfying results, lifting facial contours and at the same time minimizing wrinkles.

Yes, facial exercises *do work*. Many plastic surgeons (Dr. Mar McGregor of San Francisco and Dr. Harold Holden of Los Angeles, for example) have pointed out the benefits of facial exercises. However, they only work if you keep at it. Unfortunately, most people do them for a week and stop. Which is why their miraculous results are not too widely known. But for the exceptional woman (and that's you, isn't it?) who will follow them consistently, the results can be spectacular. Will you look as if you've had your face lifted? No, but as a student of exercise specialist Marjorie Craig said, "You won't look as if you need it, either."

Some of the most effective facial exercises have been described by Marjorie Craig in her book, *Miss Craig's Face Saving Exercises*. She has developed a series of thirty easy-to-do exercises based on familiar facial expressions. For example, the exercise to lift a sagging jowl (or even the suspicion of one) goes something like this. Pull the left mouth corner *to the left* as far as you can. At the same time, raise your eyebrows. Keeping the mouth pulled to the side, slowly wink the left eye. Now tightly squint the left eye and wrinkle your nose. Hold for a moment and slowly release the muscle tension.

Her exercises sound utterly mad and somewhat spastic, but they work. If you follow her exercises faithfully, you'll see an immediate improvement in your facial contours. The changes will be subtle at first, but they will be there. And each day the "lift" will become a tiny bit more pronounced. At the end of a month you'll see some readily visible results. (And so will your friends.)

There are several other approaches to the subject of facial exercises, including a complicated but effective method based on the isometric principle of working a muscle against resistance. Do a little detective work at your public library. You'll be surprised at the number of books on this subject.

But whichever system you follow, the results of regular facial exercises will soon convince you of their value.

Charlene, a student of mine in the Los Angeles area, owes her career to facial exercises. She was a stunning girl, about twenty-five at the time I first met her. She knew she could become a top-notch model in the fashion-photo field if only her face were thinner. As one photographer said, "I want to see cheekbones, luv, not the round face of a milkmaid."

Instead of being discouraged by this and similar comments, Charlene searched for a solution. When she asked me about plastic surgery I suggested facial exercise instead. Charlene was determined and persistent. She worked out her own exercise schedules using several techniques. It took her almost a year, but at the end of that time she had actually changed the shape of her face. Not the bone structure, of course. But her tightened and firm facial muscles now allowed her delicate bone structure to show through. In short, she became a knockout. And that photo career did materialize. She has been a successful photographic model for fifteen years now in the highly competitive Los Angeles fashion world. And she's still doing those exercises faithfully. Need I add, she looks about thirty, and her jealous contemporaries call her Dorian Gray.

Facial exercises? *They work.* If you do.

MASKING? TAPE, RUBBER BANDS, AND BUBBLE GUM

Horizontal lines on the forehead are one of the most common forms of wrinkles. Many women appear to have corrugated foreheads instead of the smooth, serene brows that we associate with feminine beauty. What's more, plastic surgery won't remove these. Silicone treatments may—but why not get rid of them yourself?

I learned the simple way to correct forehead lines from drama coach Josephine Dillon, the first Mrs. Clark Gable. I had been studying film acting techniques with her, and this lesson, as with all lessons in her acting classes, had a dramatic flair.

I was in the middle of a scene, emoting happily for the imaginary camera, when she swept across the studio and rapped me sharply on the forehead. "That's monkey motion," she said brusquely. "Constantly raising the eyebrows and moving the forehead are monkey expressions. . . . In correctly expressing human emotions, the eyebrows are seldom moved. And look at those wrinkles on your forehead . . . the camera will make them look like canyons."

She also explained that forehead lines are never the result of age but only of faulty facial habits. Her solution? Apply three horizontal strips of masking tape to your *relaxed* forehead whenever you are at home alone. The tape will tell you when your forehead wrinkles. You'll be surprised to note how often you are raising (or trying to raise) your eyebrows. Some women do this only when they're talking. The phone rings. "Hello?" And the eyebrows shoot up toward the hairline. Others find that the active forehead is a constant accompaniment to their thoughts.

Whatever the degree of your problem, the old masking tape trick pays a double dividend. Not only will you break yourself of this unattractive facial habit eventually, but your forehead will remain smooth and unlined for several hours after the very first tape application. Great preparation for a big evening.

We experimented with this tape trick in my classes and found that it works very well for correcting other "set expressions." For example, to minimize the vertical frown line between the eyebrows, smooth out the wrinkle by pushing the eyebrows apart with thumb and forefinger. Then apply tape to the now relaxed area. Each time you feel yourself trying to frown against the tape, consciously relax those forehead muscles.

The tendency to pull the mouth to one side or bite the corner of the mouth is another wrinkle-making facial habit that can be corrected with tape. Relax your face and apply the tape from the corner of your mouth to the side of your nose, starting at the mouth and gently pulling the tape up as you apply it. You may apply tape to just one side or both sides, depending on your particular facial habit.

The rubber band trick is another of Miss Dillon's techniques. It was used in her classes to help us develop awareness and control of our facial muscles. But it is also an excellent workout for the muscles of the lower half of the face. It's a great icebreaker, too. Try this at your next bridge party, and I guarantee hysteria will reign.

You'll need a large rubber band, one quarter to one half inch wide. Slide it over your head and place it at the base of your neck *in back* and just under your nose *in front*. Now, using facial muscles only, work the rubber band from under your nose, down past your mouth, and over your chin. You'll find that you have to be very active—working the lips, raising the cheeks, jutting the lower jaw forward. It's a great general workout to tone up the facial muscles— if you don't die laughing.

A recent *Glamour* magazine suggests that good ol' bubble gum is effective in firming a double chin. In order to blow bubbles (you remember how, don't you?), you have to keep smoothing the gum with your tongue. This gives your tongue a real workout and is effective in firming the underchin line. To prove it, place your fingers under your chin line. Now, wiggle your tongue up and down. Feel the movement of that muscle? That's why this works. *Glamour* adds that, while actually blowing those bubbles, you'll be working your cheek muscles—an added benefit. (Of course you'll do all this while you're alone—probably at the same time your forehead's taped up. Aren't you gorgeous!)

One of Hollywood's most timeless and regal stars is an advocate of gum chewing. Between "takes" she chews three or four sticks of gum at a time. Working on this huge wad really gives the muscles of the face and neck a workout. This vigorous chewing works on a condition that is often overlooked in a woman's concern over wrinkles and surface imperfections. With soft foods so prevalent in the modern diet, we don't chew enough to keep our jaw muscles developed, so the face becomes smaller and thinner as the years go by. To give you an idea of how important chewing can be in maintaining ageless facial contours, place the fingers of each hand on the cheeks just in front of your earlobes, and place your thumbs under your chin. Now chew vigorously several times. Really press those back teeth together. Feel the muscle action?

Another point about chewing. Do you always chew your food on one side? Try to switch from side to side, so that both sides of your face will get equal exercise, thus keeping your face more symmetrical.

IT'S A SNAP!

However, all these techniques take time to show visible and lasting results. How would you like to have an immediate preview of how you will look after cosmetic surgery? With cheeks lifted, smile lines diminished, eyes wide and rested. In other words, how would you like to have an instant face lift?

One simple gadget can give you a "mini-lift" until you muster up enough courage (or cash) to call on that plastic surgeon. I'm talking about the trusty Hollywood headband. It will lift years from your face. (And you'd be surprised at how many famous beauties would not leave their boudoirs without one of these painless, do-it-yourself face lifters.)

The headband is just that—a band of specially treated elastic that you slide up over your face and above your hairline. The band pulls the hair up and back and gently lifts your facial contours in the process.

After you're through gazing at yourself in pleased amazement (allow about fifteen minutes for pleased amazement the first time you experience this uplifting miracle), you can arrange your hair over the headband and add a pretty scarf to cover the elastic. Or you can wear it with a wig, as many enthusiasts do. I kid you not—you'll drop ten years in the time it takes to put on one of these headbands.

Is it comfortable? Yes, when correctly applied. Pure hell if you don't get it on just right. So *practice*.

"QUICK. WHERE CAN I BUY ONE?"

There are several good headbands on the market. Many beauty salons carry them. And you can also find them under the hair dryer. You'll often find them advertised in the back of one of those tattered movie magazines—perhaps right next to and overshadowed by the spectacular ad for the Squeezy. Like the Squeezy, the headbands work, regardless of their somewhat tawdry surroundings.

THAT AGELESS FACE—CAN IT STOP A CLOCK?

It's all very well and good to say, "You can be younger than your years." But in spite of our best efforts to be slim, attractive, unlined, and ageless, we women have a biological time clock that makes it impossible to ignore the calendar. Unlike men, women must go through an obvious, physiological menopause which implacably demonstrates that time is passing by.

As this clock ticks away, we often find that the spirit may be willing to be ageless but the flesh is weak and tired. We'd like to put a spring in our step but we're just too exhausted. We choose clothes with an eye to temperature control rather than fashion. ("Can I fling off the jacket in case of a 'hot flash'?") And what's the point of having a young, glamorous face if the expression is twisted by anxiety or depression?

Can we really be Ageless Women when menopause comes along? Is it possible? Or are we just kidding ourselves? Let's see.

NINE

The Pause That Distresses

There's no doubt about it. Menopause couldn't come at a worse time. It descends upon us at the advent of middle age, when we already have enough problems, thank you. Our children are growing up, becoming involved in their own problems and glandular discoveries, and blundering into all sorts of troubles. Many of our loved ones are nearing the end of their lives, and this sometimes forces us to face other difficult decisions. Do we place that loved one in a rest home? Or do we turn our own house into a convalescent home, creating even greater tensions?

And believe me, the tensions are there. Because just as the children are growing up, moving away, and leaving us with the empty nest syndrome, our marriages are also undergoing a period of strain and all our personal relationships are in need of re-evaluation. Then, just when we need him most, that Rock of Gibraltar husband begins to have problems of his own.

With an exquisite sense of poor timing, our society loads such difficulties on us just as nature slugs us with the physiological fact of menopause. And women often must wrestle with all those domestic crises while plagued with chronic sleeplessness, periodic hot flashes, leg cramps, headaches, and heart palpitations.

And who can blame a woman if, as a perfectly sensible reaction to all these disturbances, she suffers from anxiety and tends to burst into tears at inopportune moments?

For relief she may turn to the women's magazines. And how do they help? They tell her she must become *involved*. She must support political causes, join N.O.W., immerse herself in community affairs, recycle her old bedroom set, build a new wardrobe from "designer" patterns, become a "tiger" in the boudoir, and finally, provide gourmet meals for a family of five. And if she can't succeed in all these roles simultaneously, she's failed as a woman. Just the verdict she needs at this time!

The problems of menopause may be far in your future. But since menopause can occur any time between the ages of forty and fifty-five, you may already be involved, or it may be just around the corner. In either case, you most certainly have heard enough old wives' tales to make you look forward to the "change" with uncertainty and dread: "Well, the change does that to some women. My Aunt Patty just went all to pieces. They finally had to put her in a sanitarium. . . ."

WHAT DOES THE MENOPAUSE REALLY HOLD IN STORE FOR YOU?

According to those old wives' tales, the symptoms range from losing your mind to losing your libido. Most physicians are only slightly more encouraging. "Some women go through the menopause with almost no difficulty," they say. And it's true. Some women do; but there are others who suffer from mild to severe depression, insomnia, chronic fatigue, headache, heart palpitations, aches and pains, leg cramps, vaginal irritations, dizziness, anxiety, and other unpleasant and diverse symptoms. And why do some women have an easy time and some women a difficult time? Sadly, too many members of the medical profession answer this question resignedly, "Nobody really knows." You are expected to give up, endure stoically, and grow old gracefully.

DO YOU HAVE TO SETTLE FOR THIS?

Do you have to wait passively, watching the calendar, dreading the approach of the "change," and wondering if you will be one of the lucky ones—one who breezes through? Or if you are already involved in menopause, do you have to endure—to stoically endure what should be some of the happiest years of your life?

No. No. And again *no!* You can decide right now to be one of the lucky ones. You can decide right now to sail through the menopause with a minimum of difficulty, both physical and psychological. You can decide to be one of those remarkable women who copes with her *real* problems with clear-eyed, clearheaded logic, and who leaves the *imaginary* problems to the soap opera queens. In short, you can be an absolute *doll* as you quietly experience an uneventful menopause.

By now you probably think I'm about to give you a pep talk on meeting these crises with will power, patience, and fortitude. Not on your Lydia Pinkham, I'm not. Because the most maddening, most humiliating thing about this whole process is the patronizing attitude of too many people, including doctors, that your menopausal difficulties are "the product of an overactive imagination."

That is simply not true. Many women do have a terrible time during menopause and it sure as hell is not their imagination. Many a woman experiences severe physical problems, and they can be serious enough to eventually cause mental problems if she doesn't receive help.

MENOPAUSE: THE DOUBLE WHAMMY

The menopause experience is complicated by the fact that it takes place on two levels—chronological and physical. As we have mentioned before in this book, a mature woman in our youth-oriented society goes through an identity crisis at this time in her life. "I'm no longer young, yet I'm certainly not old—so what am I?" The menopause causes her to ask herself a more perplexing—even traumatic—question. "Am I still a woman?" At this difficult time in her life a woman's very sexuality is threatened. *These are the chronological stresses.* And of course they can cause depression and anxiety. What else would anyone expect them to cause? And this entire book is designed to help a woman recognize, understand, and triumphantly overcome these chronological stresses.

But profound physical stresses are also brought about by the impact of the physiological changes of menopause—the second powerful blow of the double whammy. And these physiological changes can express themselves in mental difficulties. Just at the time when a woman's psyche is reeling under the impact of chronological stress, her poor psyche is clouted again by chemical changes.

What makes this double whammy so devastating is that the chronological and physical symptoms are mixed up together in the minds of the woman who is having the problems, her perplexed family, and good old Dr. Daddums, who so often fails to help her.

Recognition of the dual nature of menopausal symptoms is the first step toward solving them. And these problems can almost always be solved, as you shall see.

So at the risk of sounding repetitious, I must emphasize that this entire book is designed to help you recognize, understand, and triumphantly overcome the chronological stresses brought about by our youth-oriented society and its puritanical background. This one chapter, however, will concentrate primarily on helping you isolate and *solve* the physical, chemical, and glandular problems that can turn the menopause years into a shattering experience for many women.

"YES, BUT . . . AREN'T YOU BEHIND THE TIMES?"

At about this point in any discussion of menopause someone is certain to insist, "It's ridiculous to paint such a gloomy picture when '*everyone*' knows that supplemental hormones take care of all these menopausal problems."

But do hormones *really* solve all those mysterious and vague physical problems that are common during menopause? Let's see.

It's certainly true that when you go to your doctor complaining of any of the familiar menopausal symptoms he'll probably suggest hormone therapy. And this may help. If so, count your blessings. You are one of the lucky ones. But there is a fifty-fifty chance that these hormone treatments will cause more problems than they solve. Many women find that some common menopausal symptom may be cleared up after supplemental estrogen, but several other vague and apparently undiagnosable symptoms often take their place. And at this point there is an excellent chance that good old Dr. Daddums will say patronizingly, "You'll learn to live with these small discomforts. Remember, in about ten years they'll go away." (But don't kill him yet. Help is on its way.)

The fact is that some women can't tolerate hormone therapy, for one reason or another. And if she can't tolerate them, no other treatments are offered beyond the inevitable tranquilizers, sedatives, and that maddening advice, "Now, Margaret, you just have to expect these little things at your age."

As the physical symptoms increase and the glandular stresses multiply, the woman in menopause may very well develop problems with anxiety, depression, and faulty memory. And the kindly, fatherly old Dr. Daddums will prescribe still more tranquilizers, pat her shoulder more frequently, and refer her to a psychiatrist. And by this time she may need one. She is probably being plagued by recurrent dreams in which she messily murders Dr. Daddums with a double-bitted ax and loves every minute of it.

The tragedy is, she may then undergo years of futile psychiatric treatment when in reality her mental problems are not a reflection of the chronological stresses we've discussed but rather a mental reaction to physical stress. Psychiatry can no more help her physical problems than it can cure a broken leg. *These very real physical problems can only be corrected by physical means.*

LET'S TAKE A LONG HARD LOOK AT ESTROGEN THERAPY

As you know, many of the common symptoms I've been describing have been attributed to the reaction of the body to the waning output of estrogen by the ovaries. A school of enthusiasts has developed that considers estrogen therapy to be a veritable fountain of youth. These enthusiasts are extremely vocal. Hardly a week goes by that doesn't see a newspaper or magazine story extolling the miracles of estrogen therapy and proclaiming that it's a cure-all for any menopausal difficulties. And even some of the more conservative practitioners agree that estrogen therapy can perform miracles in situations where the patient's symptoms *are directly related to estrogen output.* Some of the conditions that estrogen therapy can help are: hot flashes, insomnia, depression, anxiety, and vaginal irritations due to hormone changes. Some physicians estimate that estrogen therapy gives marked relief to fifty per cent of their menopausal patients.

But what about the other fifty per cent? In non-medical terms,

"tough luck." No, let me be fair. Certainly, there's a desire throughout the medical profession to help these women, but as gynecologist
Sherwin A. Kaufman said during a TV interview, ". . . there are
other ways of dealing with menopausal symptoms. They are not at
all as effective as estrogen but at least they are helpful—not in hormonal ways—there are some sedatives and tranquilizers that will help
and for such women [who are unable to take estrogen] this becomes
a method of choice." This opinion summarized the point of view of
the panel of experts. In other words, it's estrogen or tranquilizers.
Take your choice.

Then, too, there are the women whose past medical history makes
the use of estrogen therapy dangerous. Any woman who has a he-
reditary history of gall bladder problems should think twice about estrogen therapy. Recent studies indicate that postmenopausal women
taking estrogen are two and a half times more likely to have gall
bladder problems than those who are not taking estrogen.

The conservative *Medical Letter,* in a recent article, warns against
the routine use of estrogen to treat anxiety, depression, headaches,
crying spells, insomnia, lassitude, and other emotional complaints associated with menopause. Actually, the letter states that for some
women use of estrogen may promote or aggravate cancer and "there
is no adequate evidence that such treatment is beneficial . . . or
promotes either the feeling or appearance of youthfulness." They do
say estrogen can be helpful in overcoming the physical discomforts
of flushing and sudden perspiration common to many women during
menopause. The also say that low oral doses of estrogen or vaginal
creams containing estrogen may relieve vaginal discomforts.

If you're one of the 50 per cent who have experienced remarkable
results from hormone therapy, good for you. You and your doctor
can have a good laugh over these conservative evaluations of estrogen
therapy.

But suppose you're one of those women whose medical history
precludes the use of hormones? Or suppose your physician has
prescribed hormone therapy with disappointing results. If hormones
aren't the answer . . .

WHAT'S A WOMAN TO DO?

In the past, a woman was supposed to accept these discomforts as
her lot. On a subconscious level, perhaps it was just more applesauce
about the sins of Eve and how women must pay and pay and *pay* for

that ill-advised picnic in the garden. Whatever the reasons, it is really an eye-opener for the twentieth-century woman to read some of these medical approaches to the menopause from the recent past.

In a medical book published in 1897 (and quoted in Dr. Kaufman's book, *The Ageless Woman*), these were the suggested treatments.

"[For] the congestions of the genital organs, which are sometimes particularly distressing in causing sexual excitement . . . relief may often be obtained by the abstraction of blood from the *os uteri* either with leeches or by means of puncture with a tenaculuum or scalpel; an ounce or more of blood being removed . . . there is little additional which can be said in regard to the general treatment of those who are passing through the menopause. *Those who are not sick, but think they are, must be disillusioned with gentleness but firmness.*" (Emphasis added.)

And in 1894 an article in the *Journal of the American Medical Association* explained, ". . . excessive sexual desire at the menopause is indicative of disease," As a cure it recommended ". . . hot douches, gradually increased up to ten quarts twice daily." The article concluded with this classic example of male chauvinist piggism: "Such patients have so much lack of confidence in themselves, their physicians and their friends that they have not the will power to keep up a systematic course of treatment. Hence they go around from one physician to another."

Appalling, isn't it? If you've ever longed for "the good old days," that should be enough to cure you. No wonder Granny nipped away at the elderberry wine. It was either that or the double-bitted ax.

YOU'VE COME A LONG WAY, BABY

Whether or not estrogen therapy is for you, it has made one precious contribution to every woman's life. It has brought about a more realistic attitude toward the menopause, taking it out of the realm of whispered tales of odd behavior and mysterious maladies.

We can now look at the problems of menopause and see them for what they are—*deficiency conditions that are correctible.*

WHICH DEFICIENCY? THAT IS THE QUESTION

Most of the medical profession has concentrated on one deficiency —hormonal deficiency. But there is a new approach to the deficiency theory that is now gaining momentum. Simply stated, it's this: *most so-called menopausal symptoms can be traced to specific nutritional deficiencies. And they can be corrected as easily as you eat your lunch.*

Dr. Abram Hoffer, the Canadian psychiatrist who is often called the father of megavitamin therapy, has specialized in the nutritional approach to treating specific mental disorders. When I asked Dr. Hoffer if any studies had been made on the relationship between nutritional deficiencies and the mental disturbances that we associate with the menopause—anxiety, depression, and so on—he said, "I don't think there is such a thing as a menopausal symptom. I consider menopause a natural state that men and women go through . . . the women who are placed upon a proper diet, occasionally with supplementation, especially vitamin B$_6$ and zinc, will sail right through the menopause without difficulty."

STRESS: THE NAME OF THE GAME

Poor eating habits, of course, cause nutritional deficiencies. But nutritional deficiencies can also be caused by stress. And the menopause years are filled with stress. There is the physical stress as the body undergoes hormonal changes. There is mental stress, because during the menopause years a woman must make her most important decisions—about her growing children, her family, her career, and her marriage. Then there is chronological stress, as a woman undergoes an identity crisis and must re-evaluate her role as a woman. These stresses interact with and magnify each other.

Dr. Hans Selye, recognized as one of the world's foremost authorities on stress and its causes and effects, has this to say in his book, *The Stress of Life:* ". . . stress can be caused by anxiety, overwork, drugs (medications) and chemicals, psychological upsets, even air pollution and noise. The important point to remember is this: stress, no matter what its origin, has certain predictable effects on the body. Through a complete system of alarm reactions, *stress increases the body's needs for all nutrients.* If these needs are not met, the body will supply the emergency nutrients from the body's various storage areas."

Continued stress means continuing this "robbing Peter to pay Paul" reaction and brings about numerous conditions that nutritionists call "stress-caused" deficiencies. You'll be amazed at how often these stress-caused deficiencies resemble typical menopausal symptoms. Would you believe hot flashes, insomnia, headaches, anxiety, depression, mental confusion, bursitis, vaginal inflammation, incontinence (loss of bladder control)—all could be related to nutritional deficiencies?

According to Adelle Davis, "When menopause symptoms are severe, the condition should be looked upon as another form of stress. . . ."

She felt that stress increases the body's needs for all nutrients and that problems at menopause are caused by a diet deficient in the many nutrients required to meet the body's pyramiding needs at this time. *When all nutritional needs are met, a healthy woman is unaware of disturbances.*

Gladys Lindberg, the prominent Los Angeles nutrition consultant, also agrees with this nutritional approach to the unpleasant side effects of the menopause. She told me that in her opinion almost every physical symptom (and most psychological ones) associated with the menopause can be eliminated by correcting our diets to meet our increased requirements. "In many cases, the unpleasant conditions that we associate with menopause are merely the result of long-term nutritional deficiencies," she said. "As the stresses pyramid during menopause, those deficiencies that we've been limping along with for years suddenly become acute. Correcting these deficiencies means that you'll clear up the problem, and menopause will simply mean that a woman stops menstruating, that's all."

Prolonged periods of stress cause many destructive changes in our glandular balance. The first victims of prolonged stress will probably be the adrenal glands. As we shall see, their condition has a special relationship to the menopause.

WHERE ARE YOU, NOW THAT I NEED YOU?

Let's get back to hormones for a minute. Did you know that you have a second source of estrogen? As the hormonal output of your ovaries gradually slows down, the adrenal glands often step up their production of estrogen, and this can help the body adjust gradually to the changes taking place at menopause. The condition of the adrenals may well explain why "some women have a difficult menopause—and some don't."

If your adrenals are exhausted because of mental and physical stress and nutritional abuses, they cannot produce this buffer of estrogen that you so desperately need—*natural* estrogen, geared to your system.

The result is that your female body is not getting the female hormones it needs to function efficiently, and all manner of problems result.

How can you relieve the stress on the adrenals and keep them in shape to produce that buffer of estrogen?

HOW TO KEEP THAT SECOND TEAM IN THERE PITCHING

Well, Coach, the first move is to remember that stress, no matter what its cause, stimulates the adrenals to action. At the alarm signal (the onset of stress) the pituitary gland secretes two hormones (or messengers, as one physician calls them) that dash through the blood stream to the adrenals shouting, "To arms, to arms, the British are coming," or some such message. The adrenals, those two small glands above the kidneys, in turn send out *their* messengers (adrenal cortex hormones) to all parts of the body and many emergency preparations take place: proteins are broken down to form sugar for quick energy, blood pressure increases, minerals are drawn from bones, the blood sugar soars, and many, many other changes prepare the body for an emergency.

A woman who is under continued stress is, in effect, constantly rousing her adrenals to action. Unless steps are taken to protect these glands, they can become exhausted—too pooped by incessant emergencies to produce the supplemental estrogen that will make her menopause a smooth and uneventful one.

How do you protect your adrenals from exhaustion? It's easier to explain how *not* to treat these poor overworked glands.

THE "I GET A KICK OUT OF YOU" BLUES

The initial abuse of the adrenal glands usually starts first thing in the morning. You get up feeling droopy and not quite awake. You aren't hungry (too much dinner the night before), but you do need something to get you started—an eye opener.

Ah . . . that first cup of coffee. It tastes so good—because it makes you *feel* good. The caffeine in the coffee performs this humanitarian service by giving your adrenals (probably still pooped out from the day before) a swift kick, forcing them to send an alarm throughout your body and raise your blood sugar level. As your blood sugar goes up, life seems worth living again. Things look so bright, in fact, that you just may have a doughnut with your second cup of coffee. And since you'll forgo breakfast, it won't really be all that fattening, now will it? And all that sugar means yet another kick, and your faithful adrenals send your blood sugar level even higher. You feel so good, so full of energy, that you're not even hungry. So of course you don't eat the nutritious breakfast that your body really needs.

Then comes the inevitable letdown. At ten-thirty you begin to droop again. You feel drowsy, dopy, and have no energy at all. What you need is a coffee break. Another cup of coffee, or tea. Maybe even a cola drink. The caffeine and sugar in those drinks deliver another stiff kick to your already overworked adrenals.

This dietary pattern is just one of many ways you can keep your adrenal glands exhausted and unable to cope with the continued demands made on them. They are always too worn out to make those precious auxiliary estrogens that you need after forty.

How can you relieve the stress on your adrenals? By following these simple suggestions.

1. "Eat breakfast, you idiot!" That's Helen Gurley Brown's advice. And it's excellent. We've seen what horrible things happen to your poor adrenals when you use artificial stimulants to raise the blood sugar. But a nutritious, high-protein breakfast raises the blood sugar naturally, without a shock to these glands. What's more, that blood sugar stays right up there for hours after your first meal of the day. Which means you feel energetic, optimistic, clear headed, and able to cope.

2. Follow the Super-B diet as explained in Chapter Five. It's just what the doctor ordered for several reasons. First, a high-protein diet is essential to offset the demand of stress. In her book *Let's Get Well*, Adelle Davis said, "During a single day of severe stress, the urinary loss of nitrogen has shown that the amount of body protein destroyed equals that supplied by four quarts of milk [approximately 144 protein grams]. Yet if such a tremendous quantity of protein can be eaten during that day, the tissues are unharmed." Although your diet may not give you this much protein daily, it is certain that high levels of protein (as suggested in the Super-B Diet) are advisable during the stressful menopause and premenopause years.

And speaking of the Super-B Diet, remember those beauty-fuel foods: liver, wheat germ, and yeast? They contain certain vitamin-like substances which are called anti-stress factors. Although much remains to be discovered about these nutritional elements, what *is* known is this: they have a fantastic ability to help the body withstand the ravages of stress. Another anti-stress factor is found in the pulp of green, leafy vegetables. (See? Your mother was right—again.) So eat your spinach and broccoli and lettuce. They're good for what ails you.

There is still another reason for eating the beauty-fuel foods. They contain an element that is directly related to the condition of your adrenals—pantothenic acid, one of the B vitamins. The richest natural sources of this vitamin are liver (did you ever get the feeling that you were being stalked by a plate of liver and onions?), yeast, wheat germ, soybeans, peanuts, egg yolks, and kidneys.

In addition, the vegetable oils that were stressed in the Super-B Diet are also essential to the healthy functioning of your adrenals. The unsaturated fats present in these oils contain an element called linoleic acid. A deficiency of linoleic acid causes a degeneration of the adrenal cortex and limits the production of adrenal hormones. In laboratory experiments, rats that were lacking linoleic acid, and therefore suffering from impaired adrenal function, increased their production of adrenal hormones almost 90 per cent when oils containing linoleic acid were added to their diet. The mixture of peanut, safflower, and soy oils that I mentioned previously is an especially healthful combination that will give you the essential fatty acids you need.

3. Avoid sweets. (And I'm as sorry to hear this as you are.) The unpleasant fact remains that sweets deliver that "below the belt" kick that helps exhaust your adrenal glands. Sweet as they may taste for the moment, you must decide whether the consequences are worth it. When you find yourself compulsively drawn to that box of candy—think! *Many authorities feel that the women who have a particularly difficult menopause are those whose adrenals are exhausted.*

The Adrenal Metabolic Research Society suggests that, in order to maintain the health of the adrenal glands, "We cannot overemphasize the importance of the proper diet—specifically the strict elimination of *rapidly absorbed carbohydrates* in order to obviate the sudden rise in blood sugar with its subsequent fall." Although you may not feel that you want to avoid these foods *completely*, it's certainly a good idea to go very easy on sugars (candy, cake, all those luscious goodies) and prepared cereals (Wheatos, Flakeys, junk like that). Even those natural sweets—dates, raisins, dried fruits—should be eaten with discretion. And remember that soft drinks are high in sugar content. Which brings us to the subject of colas, tea, and coffee.

THE CASE AGAINST COFFEE

Look, I know that I seem to be taking all the fun out of your life. But don't give up. The theme of the next chapter is, "Sex is Swell," so I'm really not a total killjoy. But the case against coffee is so astonishing—and so important to your well-being—that we simply have to face up to it.

Now everyone knows that most people are sensitive to the stimulating effects of coffee. That familiar phrase. "No coffee for me, or I'll never sleep tonight," is well known to hostesses.

But limiting your caffeine intake to the hours before four o'clock still won't take the sting out of this superstimulating chemical that we all imbibe so casually. Keeping you awake is one of the least damaging things that caffeine does. As I mentioned before, caffeine drinks beat those tired adrenals and stimulate them to further action. These poor old glands then give you a momentary lift, but it's a lift that lets you down, because the result will eventually be exhausted adrenals. Consequently, the Adrenal Metabolic Research Society includes coffee in its list of foods to be strictly avoided.

But the effects of too much caffeine can be even more serious. Psychiatrist Dr. John Greden (of Walter Reed Army Medical Center in Washington, D.C.) suggests that doctors should routinely ask their patients about caffeine intake. Speaking to the American Psychiatric Association, he explained that overdoses of caffeine can bring on all the symptoms of an anxiety state. Other symptoms can be an irregular heartbeat, irritability, muscle twitching, diarrhea, drop in blood pressure, and even circulatory failures. He told about one of his patients, a young woman of twenty-seven, who was suffering from headaches, lightheadedness, and an irregular heartbeat. These symptoms developed over a three-week period.

She rejected a diagnosis of anxiety reaction caused by something in her life. Instead she did some detective work and traced the symptoms back to her purchase of a new fresh-drip coffeepot. "Because this coffee was so much better," Dr. Greden says, "she had begun consuming an average ten to twelve cups of strong black coffee per day—more than 1,000 milligrams of caffeine."

That's four times the 250 milligrams that are considered a large dose. When she reduced her coffee consumption to normal her symptoms disappeared.

Coffee is the worst caffeine villain—but that meek cup of tea, so famous for its comforting qualities, packs a wallop too. A strong cup of tea will also give your system a good jolt of the old caffeine. And cola drinks are likely to contain a strong dose. (These are especially bad because they contain both caffeine and sugar—known as the old one-two punch to your adrenal glands.)

But beverages aren't the only common source of caffeine. Aspirin compounds contain it, and Dr. Greden says, "Two over-the-counter headache tablets along with three cups of coffee and a cola drink can double the normal caffeine dose. And even drugs can't neutralize the effects of caffeine." Even so, many physicians and psychiatrists try to tame these unrecognized cases of "coffee nerves" with calm-down drugs and side trips into your psyche.

I can vouch for the insidious effects of coffee on the nerves. I seem to be one of those not so rare people who are extremely sensitive to the effects of caffeine. More than two cups of coffee make me not only nervous but also anxious and depressed. A sunny day can turn into a gloomy one with that third cup. And if I'm ever so foolish as to have four or five cups, I'm a neurotic mess. Luckily, I discovered many years ago that coffee is simply poison to my system. Even though I love it, I limit myself to a couple of cups of coffee *per week*. Peace of mind is worth the sacrifice.

So, if you're suffering from unexplained irritability, irregular heart-beat, a madly racing, palpitating heart, constant diarrhea, or anxiety attacks—take a good long look at your friendly coffeepot, especially if your doctor can find no other reason for these conditions beyond that grab-bag explanation "nerves." Perhaps you're one of many women who should consider drastically limiting *all* caffeine stimulants. In view of the case against coffee, it's worth a try.

THOSE "YOU'VE GOT TO EXPECT THIS, AT YOUR AGE" SYMPTOMS

Although your adrenal glands are often the first casualties in this battle against stress, specific nutritional deficiencies can be another result of stress. It's amazing how often these nutritional deficiencies masquerade as the classic "untreatable" and "unavoidable" menopausal symptoms.

CALCIUM

Probably the most widespread nutritional deficiency among women in their forties and fifties is a calcium deficiency. What does this mean to you? Simply this: a calcium deficiency can turn any woman into a textbook case of "The Screaming Menopause Mimis."

Take poor Mrs. C.D. (Calcium Deficiency), for example. For the last few months she's been keeping her family in an uproar because of her quick temper and irritability. And to add to their confusion (and hers), she can just as quickly and unexpectedly turn an impossibly cranky tirade into a flood of tears. If you'd been there last Monday night you might have witnessed something like this.

"I've told you a thousand times not to leave the newspapers in that chair. *I won't tell you again.*" ("Big deal," thinks her son. "Why does she get so upset over every little thing?")

"Bill, you're at least five minutes late for dinner *again.*" ("That's a nice greeting after a long day at work," Bill mutters to himself. "What in the world is the matter with her?")

But because Bill loves her and is truly concerned over this transformation in his usually carefree wife he goes into the kitchen to make amends. And when he says, "Gee, honey, I'm sorry," Mrs. C.D. suddenly bursts into tears and sobs, "Oh, Bill, I just don't know why I'm so jumpy lately."

It may be a mystery to Mrs. C.D. and her family, but really the answer is often simple. Irritability, depression, headaches, night sweats, hot flashes, and leg cramps—all these typical menopausal conditions—can be symptoms of a calcium deficiency. Calcium deficiencies are common during menopause because the hormonal output of the ovaries and the amount of calcium in the blood are directly related. Estrogen not only increases the body's ability to absorb calcium, it also causes calcium to be held longer in the body so that it can be used over and over again. But as the ovaries gradually reduce their output of estrogen, you need more calcium to prevent a calcium deficiency with all its unpleasant manifestations—especially if your exhausted adrenals can't contribute their auxiliary estrogen supply.

Many women have found that taking enough calcium to meet the body's increased needs during menopause can overcome those apparently mysterious menopausal symptoms in record time—sometimes even in one day.

In fact Mrs. C.D. can often change from an old witch to a frisky lamb by eating a balanced diet—and by substantially increasing her calcium intake. The reason for this miraculous transformation can be understood when we realize that calcium is . . .

THE NERVE MINERAL

Calcium is the element in the body that aids in the transportation of nerve impulses. If the body is undersupplied with calcium the nerves become tense and *you* become irritable. This is turn causes stress, which again clobbers our beat-up old friends, the adrenal glands. And as we've learned, when they feel put upon, they sulk and don't produce that supplemental estrogen, which thus increases the need for calcium still further, and so—it's a vicious circle.

Another stressful result of this calcium deficiency is water retention. When the body is undersupplied with calcium, salt and water are retained and contribute all those unpleasant symptoms of premenstrual tension, a condition that many menopausal women seem to experience even though they are no longer menstruating. You know the symptoms I mean—suddenly your weight balloons up five or even ten pounds, your breasts, hands, and face may swell, you get headaches, and most of all you're so nervous, irritable, and just plain bitchy that you and your family both wish you could hop on your broomstick and go someplace else for a few days—*any* place else.

But you can trade that broomstick for a pair of angel wings by correcting that calcium deficiency.

HOW MUCH IS ENOUGH?

Dr. Herta Spencer, who does extensive studies in calcium metabolism, feels that 1,200 milligrams of calcium daily (instead of the usually recommended 800 milligrams) is essential for adults. Most nutrition counselors would recommend even more. Adelle Davis suggested that every mature woman needs at least two grams of calcium daily.

The most convenient source is milk, of course. One quart of skim milk fortified with one half cup of powdered milk will do the trick.

However, it is possible to drink milk until you gurgle and still suffer from a calcium deficiency. There can be several reasons for this. For instance, if you are on a fat-free diet you will absorb little or no calcium from your food. If your diet does not contain some fat *your body cannot absorb calcium.*

Many a mature woman has turned herself into a nervous wreck by following a low-fat reducing diet. Just when her body desperately needs calcium, the low-fat diet makes it impossible to absorb it. Whenever you want to absorb calcium—regardless of the source—you must take it with some food that contains oil. You will remember that the Super-B Diet recommends adding three tablespoons of unsaturated vegetable oil to your daily menu; just make certain that you take the calcium-rich foods and the oils at the same time.

Calcium deficiency also occurs if large quantities of liver, yeast, or wheat germ are eaten. (This means *you* if you've been following the Super-B Diet.) The mature woman *needs* these foods, but she must be aware of the fact that they increase her need for calcium. All of these high-powered foods are high in phosphorus, in addition to all their other nutritional goodies. Because calcium and phosphorus are interdependent in complex ways, a phosphorus-rich diet increases the need for calcium. So read the Super-B Diet carefully and be certain that the phosphorus-rich foods I've mentioned are always eaten with calcium-rich foods. In addition, you may find it helpful to supplement your diet with calcium lactate or calcium gluconate tablets.

If this is beginning to sound a bit complicated, it might help to think of these nutritional equations like a recipe. The familiar recipe for baking a cake involves a rather complex chemical process; and if you leave out the baking powder, for example, you're not at all surprised that the cake doesn't turn out as expected. The same is true of our recipe for good health. Filling your nutritional needs involves a complex chemical process. One element reacts with another. If you leave out an essential ingredient you won't get results.

An excellent example of the interaction of various nutritional substances was demonstrated by Dr. Jenifer O. M. Jowsey in a study at the Mayo Clinic. Dr. Jowsey is an expert in osteoporosis, that insidious bone-wasting disease that has long been considered an inevitable accompaniment to the menopause. This is the condition, you'll recall, that causes jawbones to atrophy so that those gorgeous "pearls" just fall out, that's responsible for so many fractured hips among the elderly, so many aching backs among the not so elderly, and finally, it's the culprit that causes women past the menopause to lose an average of one and a half inches in height.

Initially, Dr. Jowsey and her associates treated affected bones with fluoride alone. This fluoride treatment did form new bone tissue, but the end result was always resorption of the bone. But when they added calcium and vitamin D to their fluoride treatment the new bone that was formed was properly mineralized and actually increased in density.

So you can see that correcting that calcium deficiency isn't simply a case of closing your eyes and swallowing calcium supplements. To correct that calcium deficiency, several other ingredients must also be added to your nutrition recipe.

D DOES IT

Which brings us to vitamin D. Your diet may be high in calcium but if you're not getting enough vitamin D your body can't use the calcium it so desperately needs. In her book, *Let's Eat Right to Keep Fit*, Adelle Davis said, "The hot flashes, night sweats, leg cramps, irritability, nervousness and mental depression so frequently experienced [at menopause] can usually be overcome in a single day by giving calcium and vitamin D; when the calcium intake is already adequate, vitamin D alone can relieve these symptoms."

People have become so familiar with the warning "Excess vitamin D is toxic" that there is an unwarranted fear of taking this vitamin. It's true that too much vitamin D is certainly bad for you, but how much does it take to induce a toxic reaction? The Merck Index says that the danger level comes at "prolonged daily use of 50,000 I.U. [International Units] or more. . . ." *Prevention* magazine adds, "Few —if any—would reach this level except through appalling ignorance. It is rare that a vitamin D supplement has a potency of more than 1,000 I.U. And one a day is all you should ever take except on the advice of a physician."

Certainly no one should take *massive* doses of vitamin D (or any other vitamin for that matter) without her doctor's approval. But since studies have shown that *substantially increasing the intake of vitamin D can increase the amount of calcium absorbed by the body up to tenfold*, it seems wise to ask your doctor about taking additional vitamin D along with your calcium supplements. If he has any nutritional background at all and can think beyond the entrenched "it's all nonsense" attitude about vitamins, he will be able to give you expert advice on the supplementary amounts that you can *safely* take.

Meanwhile, an excellent source of vitamin D is part of Nature's bounty. Vitamin D is the sunshine vitamin, so slather yourself with some perfume-scented vegetable oil, put on a sun hat, and get your body out into the sun. The oil's important beyond any beauty reasons, incidentally, because the body absorbs this vitamin from the sun-drenched oils on the skin.

GOOD NIGHT, SWEET DREAMS

But for many women in the menopause years "good night" just means hours of tossing and turning. Calcium can help here too. In fact, calcium is often called "Nature's sleeping pill."

Just before you go to bed, drink a cup of hot milk that you have fortified with one teaspoon of calcium-rich powdered milk. Add a dab of soy butter for that essential oil you will need. Supplement this drink with a couple of calcium tablets. For many people, this jolt of calcium works better than a sleeping pill, and it has none of the sleeping pill's unpleasant side effects. Not only will you sleep better, but you will be helping your body maintain that essential calcium supply.

As an added bonus, an article in the *British Medical Journal* tells of a study that seems to indicate that calcium taken at night, just before retiring, is especially influential in helping the body combat osteoporosis. The doctors found that, among postmenopausal women, more calcium was absorbed when the calcium supplements were taken in one dose just before retiring, rather than in extended doses throughout the day. Although this test involved only post-menopausal women, it seems reasonable that "calcium at night" could be a good schedule for any mature woman to follow.

LET'S MENTION SOME UNMENTIONABLE SUBJECTS

Let's face it, it's hard to feel ageless, confident, and beautiful when you live in constant fear of wetting your pants. Yet this is a very common problem during the menopause years.

Sometimes the cause is physical and may require surgery. But because surgical results can never be guaranteed, the operation may or may not result in greater bladder control. Sometimes the condition is simply called "muscle relaxation," and a series of muscle-strengthening exercises are prescribed. These exercises can be effective, but not on debilitated muscles that won't respond. If these treatments are the extent of your physician's advice (beyond the suggestion that you avoid giggling or sneezing) you may find that another approach to your embarrassing problem will be the answer to a prayer. *There is a nutritional approach to incontinence that often brings immediate results where other methods fail.*

Apparently deficiencies in magnesium and vitamin B_6 can cause incontinence (or lack of bladder control). I had read of the sometimes dramatic results that have been obtained by meeting the body's magnesium requirements. However, San Diego's Dr. Bernard Rimland, a psychologist who has been getting remarkable results in treating autistic children with megavitamin therapy, reinforced my findings that incontinence is a common symptom of magnesium deficiency. In a recent interview he told me, "Every time I read a letter in 'Dear Abby' that tells about someone's bedwetting problems, I'm tempted to write to her and suggest that these people supplement their diets with magnesium and vitamin B_6." To illustrate the relationship between magnesium and incontinence, he talked about one of his studies that was concerned with the effect of diet on mental problems. Magnesium was not included in the experimental diet, and pronounced incontinence within the test group was an unexpected development. He stated emphatically that magnesium would certainly be added to all such diets in the future.

Loss of bladder control is an embarrassing nuisance, but a deficiency of magnesium and vitamin B_6 can also cause serious mental and emotional problems—the kinds of problems that are familiar to a woman who is "going through a difficult change."

AM I REALLY LOSING MY MIND?

Mrs. M.D. (Magnesium Deficiency) has been having those vague menopausal problems that her doctor says she must expect at this time. Although she eats a well-balanced diet, takes supplementary hormones, and uses diuretics to combat her tendency to water retention, Mrs. M.D. still suffers from irritability, anxiety, and more recently some new problems. Let's listen as she explains it to her doctor.

"I really don't know what's the matter with me. I've been playing bridge with this same group for years now. But last week my hands shook so much that I could hardly hold the cards. I didn't think I was that nervous about the outcome, but suddenly I just got the shakes. And I kept making the most ridiculous mistakes. I couldn't seem to remember the bids. I mean, I couldn't even remember what I'd bid for a minute. It really shook me up. I felt so foolish.

"Then, when I got home, Debbie dropped her schoolbooks on the table, and I nearly jumped out of my skin. I jumped all over her too, poor kid.

"Even the TV irritates me. Steve and I used to enjoy it so much. It was a relaxing way to spend the evening together—but now it makes me so nervous I could scream! What *is* the matter with me?"

Mrs. M.D., like many women in the menopause, is displaying symptoms of still another nutritional deficiency.

MAGNESIUM AND YOUR MIND

The medical profession has long recognized that there is a relationship between magnesium and a person's mental and nervous state. In fact, hospitals have used magnesium to cure the confused mental states brought about by alcoholism and senility.

But it is only recently that a few members of the medical profession have begun to suspect that magnesium deficiency is the cause of many of the disturbing mental and nervous problems associated with a difficult menopause.

Nutritionists, though, have recognized for years that hand tremors, vertigo, numbness or cramps in the hands or feet, mental confusion, irritability, and extreme sensitivity to noise (all problems associated with menopause) can often be traced to magnesium deficiencies. Sensitivity to noise, for example, has long been accepted by women as "one of those things we must put up with." And it is just one more thing that makes a woman a bundle of nerves and a trial to her family during menopause. But laboratory animals with a severe magnesium deficiency become increasingly sensitive to noise; such animals have gone into convulsions at such slight noises as the turning on of a faucet.

Some experts estimate that up to 80 per cent of Americans suffer from a magnesium deficiency caused by the widespread use of high-nitrogen fertilizers that rob our food of magnesium. And that deficiency is magnified by the physical changes of menopause. Magnesium is lost in the excessive perspiration that accompanies "hot flashes" and "night sweats." The diuretics that are prescribed during menopause also rob the body of magnesium.

At any age, but especially in menopause, magnesium must be added to our diet. Reporting in the June 1964 issue of the *American Journal of Clinical Nutrition* on her massive, world-wide study of magnesium deficiencies, Dr. Mildred S. Seelig wrote, "Contrary to the consensus, the customary diet in the Occidental countries cannot be relied upon to provide sufficient magnesium to maintain equilibrium."

HOW MUCH MAGNESIUM?

Dr. Seelig suggests a *minimum* daily intake of 385 milligrams for a 140-pound woman. However, because of complex chemical relationships, you'll need more than this amount if your diet is rich in protein, calcium, and vitamin D, or if you do any social drinking.

Can you take too much? According to Dr. Seelig, there is little danger, since, in a normally healthy person, the excess is excreted. However, I have to add my usual word of caution. Don't go overboard on any single nutrient. Remember that cake . . . and think about what would happen to it if you added two cups of baking powder instead of a half teaspoon.

One readily available and inexpensive source of magnesium is Epsom salts (magnesium sulfate). To supplement your diet, take a very small amount—one eighth teaspoon. This will yield close to Dr. Seelig's recommended requirement and is such a small amount that it will not have a laxative effect. Although this is a convenient and inexpensive way to add magnesium to your diet, it's probably best to take magnesium with other minerals, because magnesium is closely allied to your body's ability to utilize calcium and vitamin D. I'd suggest instead that you take a multimineral tablet that contains balanced amounts of magnesium, calcium, and trace minerals. Multimineral tablets are available at any health food store.

MORE ABOUT NUTRITION AND YOUR MIND

Calcium and magnesium aren't the only nutritional deficiencies that can cause depression, irritability, apathy, and other negative mental states that often accompany menopause. For example, in experimental situations, mild deficiencies in any of the following B vitamins have produced similar symptoms in dozens of experiments on both men and women volunteers:

1. Vitamin B_1 deficiencies result in

Fatigue	Apathy
Depression	Confusion
Forgetfulness	Anxiety
Irritability	Restlessness
Quarrelsomeness	Lack of co-operation

Some of the volunteers suffered from insomia, nervousness, sensitivity to noise, and even hypochondria and paranoid tendencies.

2. Niacin deficiencies can cause these disturbing mental conditions:

Irritability	Imaginary unfairness
Suspicions	Depression

3. Pantothenic acid deficiencies caused
   Irritability
   Depression
   Quarrelsomness
   Some volunteers became hot-tempered and easily upset over trifles.

4. Biotin, another member of the B-complex family, is definitely related to mental equilibrium. A deficiency in biotin caused mental depression which sometimes developed in intensity and became panic.

These symptoms might well describe the mental state of many women who seem to change from normal, well-adjusted, functioning individuals to negative, neurotic, whining, downright weirdos during menopause. The very important point to remember is this: many times these mental conditions develop even though a woman's life situation is happy and stable. And in many instances her only problem is malnutrition. And malnutrition can be quickly corrected if you know how.

MYSTERY ON THE MENU

I have seen many examples in my work and personal life of the relationship between mental well-being and nutrition, but I think

Ruth's experience is one of the most astonishing that I've ever encountered.

I had known Ruth for years, and although she has the sensitivity and awareness that usually accompany artistic ability, she had always been extremely well adjusted and stable. In spite of the ups and downs that come into everyone's life, she always bounced back from every crisis—and with a grin on her face, too. So I was totally unprepared when her personality changed completely.

She was her familiar easygoing self when I saw her shortly after her twins went away to college. No empty nest syndrome for her. With her usual bouncy approach to things, she informed me that she was tired of sitting at home on her tuffet and had taken a job as the art director of a small advertising agency.

We got together for lunch a little later, and Ruth was still thrilled with the challenge of her new job. Her brown eyes sparkled as she said, "It's a bit hectic, but just what I need at this stage in life. I feel twenty years younger. And David is as thrilled as I am."

The only cloud on her bright horizon was a skin problem that had developed suddenly—almost overnight. "I don't know what's the matter with it," she said. "But my dermatologist seems to think it's some kind of 'bug' and so I'm taking antibiotics. I'm sure it will clear up soon."

But it didn't clear up, and that's one of the reasons we made another lunch date several months later. "Maybe you can suggest something that will help my skin," Ruth sighed. "Heaven knows I could use some good news."

When we met at the restaurant I was totally unprepared for the change in my friend. Her skin problem was noticeable and certainly a cause for concern, but I was even more surprised at her totally negative and depressed state of mind. And, as lunch progressed, it became apparent that something serious was bothering her. She fidgeted and squirmed in the comfortable banquette, seeming unable to sit still for a minute. I'm sure she wasn't listening to half of my chatter.

Suddenly, with a wild look, she said, "I've got to get out of here." And she lunged out of the booth, bumping the table as she went, and rushed into the powder room.

Naturally I rushed right after her, ignoring the curious and concerned glances of the other diners. When I opened the door there was Ruth, hunched in the farthest corner of the sofa, clutching her head in her hands. I went over to her and put my arm around her.

She started to sob and the story poured out. "I don't know what's the matter with me. *I don't know.* I just couldn't sit there any longer. I feel this way at work, too. I don't know what comes over me, but suddenly I'm just overcome with fear and I have to rush out. I know that I'll have to quit my job if this keeps up. And I really love it, except for these waves of panic that come over me with no reason. I can't even relax at home. David is worried sick about me and—oh, God, do you think I'm going crazy?"

I looked at my old friend. With her frightened eyes and hysterical sobbing—well, I wouldn't have bet she wasn't headed for a complete breakdown. I tried to soothe her as well as I could, and learned that she hadn't been to a doctor for a checkup. She was afraid he would send her to a psychiatrist. But after I drove her home I finally convinced her to call a doctor.

And this is where Ruth had a lucky break. Because good old Dr. Kannon was out of town, and this emergency call was referred to a new, young associate who agreed to see Ruth that afternoon.

When I called Ruth the next day she was still unnerved but feeling much relieved. "Well, the best news is this. Dr. Freeman, who is just marvelous by the way, asked a lot of questions about me and my home life and my habits. He thinks that it's something I ate . . . and something that I didn't eat. Listen, I'll explain when I see you. I know how interested you are in this 'food for thought' stuff. Anyway, when I asked him if I was a candidate for the looney bin, he said rather stuffily, 'We prefer to call it psychiatric therapy. But whatever term you use, I think that's the last thing you need.'"

When I finally saw Ruth two weeks later, I learned the fascinating nutritional detective story that Dr. Freeman had unraveled. Ruth had been suffering from a severe deficiency of the B vitamin biotin, which had been brought about in a number of ways. First of all, as is the case with so many weight-conscious American women, her diet had been inadequate for years. She was just starting the menopause, which, as we have seen, causes general stress throughout the system and increases the body's need for all nutrients. And finally, although her new job was fun and challenging, it also added one more stress factor at exactly the wrong time. These combined conditions had caused a general deficiency in most nutrients, but most of the problems had been caused by a deficiency in biotin, which had also caused the dermatitis. As the deficiency became more acute, she developed a general mental depression that sometimes turned into panic.

In addition to menopause and the stress caused by her new job, other factors contributed to Ruth's problems. When she started her hectic new job routine she didn't have time for breakfast. So she prepared an eggnog that she could drink "on the run." This seems like an excellent solution to the breakfast problem . . . milk and eggs, what could be better, more nutritious? Right?

Wrong.

Ruth used the *whole* egg—both yolk and white. And that was her mistake. Because *raw* egg white contains a substance, avidin, that combines with biotin in the system, prevents it from reaching the blood, and ultimately causes a deficiency in this vitamin. Ruth's Dr. Freeman, apparently one of the growing number of forward-looking young physicians who are knowledgeable about nutrition, explained that all foods containing *raw* egg white should be avoided by *everybody*.

Anyway, these eggnogs started the deficiency, and one of the first signs of this deficiency is dermatitis which, in Ruth's case, was incorrectly diagnosed as an infection. So her dermatologist dosed her with antibiotics, which further reduce the body's supply of biotin. Finally she was taking one of those tablet-a-day vitamin preparations that is out of balance in the B department and, instead of helping, actually created an increased need for biotin.

It is ironic that with the best intentions in the world—with the "nutritious breakfast," the additional vitamins, and with the "expert" advice of her dermatologist—Ruth almost wrecked her happy life. But Ruth was lucky. With a new high-powered diet (rich in yeast, which is the best source of biotin), some balanced vitamin supplements, and a little rest, Ruth was her former self in two weeks. And the frightening, disturbing symptoms have never recurred.

But I can't help wondering about other women who aren't lucky enough to find a Dr. Freeman and who go the psychiatric route instead.

Dr. Abram Hoffer, father of megavitamin therapy, says, "Many people have been kept in psychotherapy for years without improvement when they could have been treated with vitamins and nutrients. Once nutritional factors in emotional problems are fully understood, nine out of ten people now being treated by psychiatrists will be able to be cured by their family doctors."

Now isn't it nice to know that whatever is happening to those glands of yours, and in spite of the whispers about "nutty Aunt Pat" and all those other horror stories you've heard, you don't have to lose your mind?

So let's turn to another, less dramatic problem that plagues almost every woman at some time in her adult life.

NUTS TO YOU

Would you believe that eating twelve raw pecans daily can correct the water retention that plagues so many women before their menstrual periods or during menopause? It sounds fantastic, but the experiments of Dr. John Ellis of Texas indicate that the vitamin found in raw pecans can relieve the bloating, sore breasts, and mind-blowing tension that many women experience at this time.

Diuretics are often prescribed to correct these symptoms, but Dr. Ellis found that, since vitamin B_6 works in conjunction with sodium and potassium to regulate the body's fluids, vitamin B_6 acts as a natural diuretic. And deficiencies in B_6 cause water retention with all its unpleasant side effects. However, Dr. Ellis' patients who were taking B_6 not only lost waterlogged pounds, but some of them lost up to three inches in the waistline after a few short weeks.

Other symptoms which were relieved after taking B_6 for several weeks were: tingling and numbness in fingers and toes, excruciating cramps in the calves of the legs, and hand tremors—all familiar symptoms of the menopause. Another condition common during menopause, itching and inflammation of the vaginal area, has been relieved by adequate B_6.

Pecans are one of the richest sources of B_6, but since this vitamin is destroyed by heat, be sure to buy *raw*, untreated pecans if you wish to increase your B_6 intake.

Another rich source of this vitamin will be familiar to followers of the Super-B Diet—brewers' or nutritional yeast. In some cases, supplements may be more convenient. Dr. Ellis treated his patients with 50 milligrams of B_6 daily; and after three years of this dosage, none of his patients showed any negative side effects.

Vitamin B_6 is another of the nutrients that can help you to maintain that balanced, serene, and easygoing disposition that makes you

such a living doll. But if you do find yourself more irritable of late—
a bit snappish—don't just chalk it up to the "Change" and let it go
at that. A B_6 deficiency may be responsible, so it's important that
you know how adequate amounts of this vitamin can help you
maintain your emotional equilibrium.

Vitamin B_6 serves many functions in the body, some of which may
not yet be clearly understood. But one of its most important functions is that of helping the body to use magnesium. Apparently the
soothing effect of B_6 is due to the better utilization of magnesium,
which, as we've seen, has far-reaching effects on the nervous system.
(See how the ingredients of the "nutritional recipe" act together?)
Because of the interaction of these two nutrients, it's important that
they should be taken together.

From the preceding pages we have learned that the natural physiological changes of menopause can bring about a variety of nutritional deficiencies, which in turn can cause mysterious and vague
maladies having no perceptible reason or cure. Estrogen therapy is a
standard treatment for these maladies. But the tragic fact is that this
treatment can often magnify the maladies and even cause new ones.

DOES ESTROGEN THERAPY CREATE NUTRITIONAL DEFICIENCIES

Although the use of supplemental hormones to relieve the distress
of menopause has been heralded by some as the greatest gift to
women since Steve McQueen, response to hormone therapy is as
unpredictable as the plot of an underground movie. Some women
respond dramatically and have a permanent cessation of their menopause woes. Others respond for a while and then, inexplicably, the
same symptoms—or others—return. Then there are those for whom
the hormones don't give relief at all. Perhaps one answer to this mystery is the relationship between supplemental hormones and vitamins. Remember, too, that the Pill is also made up of hormones,
and even though you may be too young for the hormone therapy
used during menopause, your Pill may be causing exactly the same
deficiencies.

Dr. Dorothea Kerr relates progesterone, the hormone frequently
used in menopause therapy, to headaches and depression. Writing in
Vogue, she says, "The menopausal and post-menopausal women taking hormones, like the oral contraceptive users and pregnant women,

may have changes in vitamin and mineral needs. Research with the Pill shows massive amounts of vitamin B_6 (pyridoxine), and increased amounts of vitamin B_2 (riboflavin) may be required to restore protein and enzyme metabolism to normal." She adds, "I recommend that all my patients on oral contraceptives or a menopausal estrogen replacement program use vitamin-mineral supplementation."

Vitamin B_6 isn't the only vitamin affected by hormone therapy. There are other deficiencies which can create familiar maladies that are usually explained away as just another inevitable part of the menopause mystery—"just your imagination."

For example, deficiency in folic acid, another of the B vitamins, is common among women taking the Pill. Since, as we have mentioned, hormone therapy for menopausal problems closely resembles hormone intake for the Pill, it seems plausible that this deficiency would also occur frequently in older women who are on a regimen of supplemental hormones.

What are the results of a folic acid deficiency—and what can it mean to you in terms of over-all health, energy, and a general feeling of well-being? A deficiency in folic acid can cause a type of anemia, one that doesn't respond to either iron or vitamin B_{12} supplements. (Those of you who are taking those patent medicine tonics to cure "iron-poor anemia" should note that iron isn't the only answer to building up your beauty stream.) And some of the commonest symptoms of anemia—weakness, dizziness, depression, forgetfulness, shortness of breath, that dead-tired feeling, and a pounding heartbeat—are also some of the common and "vague" distresses of menopause. If no other physical cause can be found for these symptoms, and if you're not responding to the iron approach to your anemia problem, you might ask your doctor about the possibility that your condition is related to a deficiency in folic acid, especially if you're taking supplemental hormones or the Pill.

What foods contain folic acid? If I said liver, would you throw this book at me? It's true. That miracle food is just loaded with all the goodies you need. (And I'm just as sorry as you are that chocolate cake isn't the richest source of *everything*.) However, in spite of a good diet, supplements that include folic acid will probably be necessary if you're taking hormones.

The use of oral contraceptives can also affect the levels of certain mineral elements in the blood. According to Doctors Roslyn Alfin-Slater and Derrick B. Jelliffe in an article in the Los Angeles *Times*,

"The levels of calcium and zinc in blood are lower, and copper is higher, in women taking anovulatory drugs."

The vitamin E requirements are also affected by oral contraceptives. Doctors Alfin-Slater and Jelliffe say, "It would not be surprising if the requirement for vitamin E was increased by the continued use of oral contraceptives." Dr. Evan Shute, the Canadian gynecologist who is one of the world's authorities on vitamin E, had this to say about vitamin E and the Pill: "The great danger of the progestogen pill is that it contains estrogen, which can bring on thrombophlebitis [blood clots in the veins]. . . . Vitamin E, the natural antagonist of estrogen, can prevent and treat the condition."

MORE ABOUT E AND ESTROGEN

According to the World Conference on Vitamin E, *a woman's needs for vitamin E increase tenfold during the menopause; and if estrogen is given, the need for E increases still further.*

Because vitamin E stimulates the body's hormone activity, some nutritionally oriented physicians even prescribe E instead of supplemental estrogen, with very successful results.

Dr. Shute described his use of vitamin E for problems of the menopause in an article in *Ladies' Home Journal.* "For menopausal women, vitamin E in sufficient doses can sometimes take the place of estrogen therapy and, of course, is preferable to it. Estrogen has so many drawbacks. Not only can it bring on thrombophlebitis, but it can also cause embolism. [In an embolism, blood clots detach themselves from the vein walls and move through the blood stream to block the brain or lung.] Estrogen is so suspect here [in Canada] that letters have been appearing recently in the British medical journals recommending that it not be given after delivery, even to dry up breasts. Estrogen is a two edged sword; it can do harm as well as good. For instance, doctors use estrogen suppositories for senile vaginitis in old women and estrogen creams on the vulva to eliminate itching and burning. But estrogen often makes these conditions more distressing. I prefer to use vitamin E. It isn't effective all the time, just as estrogen isn't. But if you can't use one with good effect, you can almost always use the other."

Many nutritionally oriented physicians are following Dr. Shute's lead and prescribing E instead of estrogen with very successful results. One friend told me that her hot flashes and night sweats disappeared entirely when she started taking 500 units of vitamin E daily.

OUT, DAMNED SPOT!

Another annoying problem during the menopause years (and before) is the appearance of brown pigment spots on the backs of the hands ("granny freckles") or on the face ("liver spots"). Larger deposits may appear around the edge of the hairline or on the neck. These "age" marks are just one more piece of the deficiency puzzle.

Research indicates that this pigmentation is the result of a vitamin E deficiency. It's not surprising that these pigment spots occur during menopause, since the need for vitamin E skyrockets at this time, especially if supplemental hormones are taken.

I am convinced that there is a dramatic increase in the need for vitamin E when taking hormones for any reason. I have noticed that since the Pill became popular at least 70 per cent of my students have showed some dark pigmentation on their faces or necks. The significant point is that these spots, formerly associated with age, are now becoming common on girls in their early twenties—on women of all ages. Strangely, many of them seem to develop this dark pigmentation on the upper lip.

THE STRANGE CASE OF THE VANISHING MUSTACHE

An exceptionally beautiful girl, a student of mine who became a successful model, developed such a dark mass of pigment on her upper lip that she could no longer work. It looked like a Groucho Marx mustache. She told me that she had recently started taking the Pill and a few months later—voilà! Groucho Marx. Her doctor sympathetically warned her that the sun would increase the pigmentation but could suggest neither a cure nor a cause.

I helped her plan a superdiet that would include most of the vitamins that anyone needs. However, in the case of E, it is difficult to get *enough* from basic foods, since it is present mainly in oils and is destroyed by heat, hydrogenating, refining, and all the other things we do today to make our food "better." So she decided to take a vitamin E supplement, along with vitamin A since the two work together. In addition to taking these vitamins internally, she also applied both vitamins directly to the skin by pricking the capsules and applying the vitamin oils to her upper lip.

She used the vitamins faithfully and little by little the brown shadow faded (though it never disappeared entirely) until it could be covered by make-up. We found that sunlight did indeed tend to darken the shadow, but we learned that an ointment containing Paba (another of the B vitamins) was a superb sun screen and kept her "mustache" from darkening.

Other students found that spots on their hands, faces, and necks seemed to fade if they increased their intake of vitamins A and E, applied both vitamins directly to the spots, and protected their skin from exposure to the sun.

AGE? FIGHT BACK WITH VITAMIN E

Remember Dr. Hans Selye? He's the expert on stress whom I mentioned before. He has been producing premature old age in laboratory rats by exposing them to various stresses (noise, pollution, etc.) and at the same time feeding them a diet deficient in vitamin E. When large amounts of vitamin E are given, however, the premature aging does not take place.

In fact, there is much evidence to indicate that a vitamin E deficiency, coupled with poor nutrition, is a factor in bringing about a premature menopause. One prominent nutritionist advises her mature clients to maintain an exceptionally nutritious diet along with plentiful vitamin E supplements and says, "I do think, after observing many, many women, that those who have a delayed menopause seem to stay physiologically young. What's more, those who are in the menopause, and who do not get increased vitamin E, appear to age rapidly."

WHAT ABOUT MIDDLE-AGED SPREAD?

Can vitamin E be a factor there too? One doctor I talked to said, "The truth of the matter is that no one knows why a woman's body goes through this process of fat redistribution at middle age . . . but it's clear that many women find their thighs, hips, upper arms, and especially waists tend to grab fat and fill out, even if the woman isn't exceptionally overweight. But we can see that this isn't related to the waning estrogen output because, after all, middle-aged spread is common to men too."

But Adelle Davis said, "I suspect that the middle-aged spread of men is not so much the result of age or too many calories as of an undersupply of hormones caused by cumulative multiple deficiencies, of which vitamin E is one." She added that she has recommended 100 units of this vitamin after each meal to women whose weight was correct but whose "faces were too thin and hips too large." She said, "Though vitamin E may not have done the trick, the weight of most of these women has been redistributed, which was all they or I care about."

Because vitamin E is so closely allied with the healthy condition of the sex glands (in both men and women) it is sometimes called the sex vitamin. Well . . .

IS IT TRUE WHAT THEY SAY ABOUT THE BIG E?

More vitamin E is found in the body than any other vitamin. Apparently, every cell needs its full supply to function at top performance. There is a heavy concentration of the vitamin in the pituitary, adrenals, and sex glands, which has spawned (if you'll pardon the pun) all kinds of fantastic stories about vitamin E, the S*E*X vitamin. I am constantly surprised at the number of people who think that it is a superaphrodisiac and seek it (or shun it) according to their temperament.

So let's set the facts straight. Vitamin E is *not* an aphrodisiac. Since the libido is a mental rather than a physical quality, vitamin E won't turn you into a tiger if that isn't your sexual temperament.

But numerous studies do indicate that vitamin E is necessary for the health and vitality of the sex glands, so it is easy to see how all these juicy rumors got started. What vitamin E *does* do is maintain the youthful function of these glands. It will keep you and your glands young and vital. In other words, vitamin E helps arrange things so that when the spirit is willing the flesh will not be weak. Truly a friendly vitamin in that respect.

PLANNING A DIET FOR THE
MENOPAUSE YEARS, OR HELP! HELP! I HAVE
ALPHABET INDIGESTION

Vitamin B (in all its complexities), vitamin D, vitamin E, calcium, magnesium . . . yes, we have talked about many vitamins and minerals that are especially important to women who are approach-

ing or are in the midst of the menopause. I hope that I've convinced
you that your nutritional needs at this time of life are exceptional.
But how can you be sure you're getting all the vitamin and mineral
goodies that you need?

Well, the standard answer is, "Eat a balanced diet," but of course
that mythical balanced diet is designed for the mythical "average"
person. A woman enmeshed in the menopause doesn't have average
needs—and does she know it! As I mentioned previously, the Super-B Diet is an excellent start for the woman who wants to build
optimum health. But during the menopause years *it's only a start.*

I don't see how you can get all the vitamins and minerals you need
at this stressful time without supplements—and lots of them.

Take vitamin E for example. If you try to get all your vitamin E
from that old faithful "balanced diet," you are in big trouble. In
order to take the 400 to 600 units that Dr. Shute recommends for
mature women in good health, you will have to swallow *from one to
one and a half cups of wheat germ oil a day.* If you insist on going
this route, you can end up being the healthiest (and maybe the
sexiest) Fat Lady the circus has ever had.

You're up against the same sort of problem with the other vitamins and minerals. The beauty-fuel foods are vitamin-rich, it's
true; but in order to fill your increased needs for certain nutrients
you'd have to eat like ten lumberjacks.

No, you'll just have to consider adding supplements to your diet,
always keeping in mind that they complement your diet and are not
a substitute for nutritious, healthful food.

And how will you know which vitamins to take and in which
quantities? Naturally, your first thought is, "Why, I'll ask my doctor."

VITAMINS AND YOUR DOCTOR

And what happens when you ask kindly old Dr. Daddums about
vitamin supplementation? Unless he's one of the growing number of
forward-looking physicians who recognize nutritional therapy as the
wave of the future, you're likely to get this typically negative answer,
"Now, Margaret, what's all this nonsense about vitamins? You certainly don't need supplements. You'll get all the vitamins anyone
needs from a well-balanced diet. If you want to throw your money
away on vitamins, go ahead, but I do think we can do something

practical about this anxiety and depression you've been experiencing. It's nothing unusual at your age. Here's a prescription for a mild tranquilizer." And so you go to a pharmacy—probably in your doctor's own medical building—and pay hard cash for $12 worth of tranquilizers. What a good little patient you are! You haven't thrown away $12 on vitamins that could remove the *cause* of your nervousness. No, you've wisely invested $12 in a *drug* that will mask the symptoms and keep you dopy for what should be the best ten years of your life.

Would it be fair to say that, in general, the medical profession is prejudiced against the whole idea of vitamin supplementation?

Nobel Prize-winning physical chemist Dr. Linus Pauling thinks so. At a nutritional symposium held at Stanford University recently, he chastised the nutrition and medical establishment for "ignoring the question of optimum amounts of vitamins and minerals people should take to be in the best of health." He said, "I think they [the medical establishment] have committed themselves to an unwillingness to examine the evidence in an unbiased way. And even when the evidence is clear, they ignore it without having a sound basis for doing so."

A highly revealing example of the medical establishment's entrenched prejudice against vitamin therapy was described by Dr. Evan Shute in an interview in the *Ladies' Home Journal*. He mentioned the case of a thirteen-year-old boy whose legs were almost destroyed when he was run over by a bus. After seventeen months of standard treatment all the skin grafts had failed and "he was sent home from the hospital to die." As a last resort he was taken to the Shute Institute where he was treated with vitamin E. The vitamin was administered orally and also a vitamin E spray was used on his damaged legs. In twenty-four months, according to Dr. Shute, the boy was healed. His legs were completely restored—and this without the use of skin grafts or a stay in the hospital.

Before and after photographs illustrating this phenomenal treatment and recovery were at first accepted for display at the annual meeting of the American Medical Association. But then suddenly the photographs were arbitrarily rejected. "Why had the AMA changed its mind?" asks Dr. Shute. "If we were wrong, the best way to have destroyed us would have been to expose our results to the judgment of our peers. But long ago the AMA took a stand against vitamin E, and it *can't* be wrong. How could American medicine have made such a gigantic mistake?" He goes on to ask, "Why are doctors so skeptical of vitamin E? It is because they haven't tried it—or haven't used large enough doses or a reliable preparation. . . ."

Another opinion comes from Dr. Bernard Rimland. He feels that "There is an extraordinary amount of prejudice against the idea that a vitamin—a perfectly safe, naturally occurring chemical that we all need to sustain life—can be required by some people in large quantities." Citing a study by Dr. Leon Rosenberg of Yale University, Dr. Rimland said nearly a dozen metabolic disorders have been discovered—all since 1954—which impair the body's utilization [of vitamins or minerals] to such an extent that the person may require hundreds of times the "so-called minimum daily requirement."

And just to emphasize that a blanket of misinformation is being handed out to the general public regarding the whole vitamin question, Senator William Proxmire tells us something we all should know about that sacred "minimum daily requirement." In a recent speech before the Senate, Proxmire blasted the Recommended Daily Allowance (formerly called the Minimum Daily Requirement) as a "capricious, unscientific and illogical standard." He further charged that "the Food and Nutrition Board of the National Research Council . . . is influenced, dominated and financed in part by the food industry. It represents one of the most scandalous conflicts of interest in the federal government."

What does all this mean to you? Simply that the Recommended Daily Allowance (RDA) is not set as a standard to assure you of optimum health but is rather an arbitrary figure designed to make the devitalized foods produced by the food industry appear healthful and nutritious. Senator Proxmire adds, "It is in the narrow economic interest of the food industry to establish low official RDAs because, the lower the RDAs, the more nutritional their food products appear."

In a neat demonstration of double-think, the 1974 RDAs are lower than previous standards. In other words, if foods aren't as nutritious as they should be to meet human standards of health, let's just tell people that they don't need so many nutrients. Whew!

Well, what can you do other than picket the Food and Drug Administration with a sign saying, "Repent"? For the present at least, you can treat the recommendation of the Food and Drug Administration with grave suspicion.

WHAT YOU CAN DO

Knowledge is your best weapon. The foolproof way to assure that you'll sail through the menopause is to take an *active* rather than a passive approach to your health. Determine now that you won't settle for less than vibrant, energetic, joyous, good health. Here's how:

1. Learn about your body's changes at this time—and learn about your body's needs. I'm certainly *not* suggesting that you ignore medical help. Of course you should have periodic checkups and consult your physician in case of any unusual condition. What I am suggesting is that you take some responsibility for the care of your body. Remember that dear old Dr. Daddums is often twenty years behind the times and losing ground fast; *so search out those physicians who are interested in building health rather than just treating symptoms.*

2. Learn to recognize Dr. Daddums. Here are some clues. Dr. Daddums is the oracle—the bringer of truth and light; so he at least mildly resents any hint that you might have ideas about the care and treatment of your own body. Dr. Daddums does not believe in vitamin or mineral supplements. He progressed as far as tranquilizers and estrogen, but there he stuck fast. Dr. Daddums—the source of light and wisdom—wants you to bring that body to him in a reasonably neat and washed condition. He wants you to listen respectfully to his pronouncements, take the pills that he prescribes, pay your bills on time, and trouble him as little as possible.

It is important to recognize Dr. Daddums for what he is, but it isn't easy. For one thing, it's hard to keep your cool around the good doctor. (Years of experience have taught him how to disarm you.) Usually you are at a distinct disadvantage, having waited (naked) for half an hour, clutching a wisp of fabric that's mislabeled "a gown," and trying to keep your eyes from those grim metallic stirrups on the table. By the time Dr. Daddums makes his grand entrance you are no longer in a condition to question anything.

But let's review some of the other clues. Dr. Daddums' conversation is larded with stereotyped one-liners that are filed in his mind under M for menopause: "At your age, Margaret" . . .

"When we're upset, it's easy to imagine things" . . . "No one really knows why". . . "These are minor problems that will pass in time" . . . "Well, if vitamins amuse you, I suppose they won't do any harm. . . ."

It is astonishing how courageously doctors—mostly men—endure the problems of menopause.

A rule of thumb is this: if your doctor displays more than *one* of the clues listed here, *find another doctor*.

3. Resolve to supply your system with all the nutrients it needs to meet the increased stresses, both physical and mental, of the middle years. However, don't become enthused about a single "magic" vitamin. There "ain't no such animal." As you can see from this chapter, various nutrients must work *together* to build health.

4. While the RDAs of vitamins and minerals are much too low for your needs in the stressful mature year, for heaven's sake, be sensibile. Don't take gigantic amounts of *any* vitamin— and don't take the extra amounts you need without the knowledge to back up this approach. Which means—

5. Build your own knowledge of nutrition. It's a fascinating study—because it's all about *you*. I've just touched the surface in this chapter. Three authors who will help you gain a basic knowledge of nutrition are Adelle Davis, Carlton Fredericks, and Linda Clark. They have all written best sellers—you'll have no trouble finding their books.

Building your own knowledge of nutrition (starting right now) can be one of the most important things you will ever do.

My friend Linda is a good example. She was in the midst of a terrible menopause. As she put it, "I had all the symptoms ever described and had invented some new ones."

Her family doctor had tried all the customary treatments, but nothing helped. Then one day she picked up a book on nutrition at a church rummage sale and began to leaf through it. To her surprise, there was a section on menopause; and vitamins and minerals were suggested as a treatment for all her mysterious maladies.

Armed with her book and a list of vitamins and minerals she wanted to take, she marched down to her doctor's office. Fortunately her doctor was not a Dr. Daddums. He was not one of the doctors who insist that you either get well or die his way and no other.

He glanced through her list of supplements said, "Well, vitamins sure as hell won't hurt you, and nothing else has helped. So why not? Give me a day or two to read up on this and I'll call you."

When he called, he not only approved her list of supplements but added a few more. Within a week Linda felt like a new woman, and the intrigued doctor, who has since become an expert on nutrition, was spending all his spare time reading up on the new discoveries in the field.

Linda's case is not unusual. For every Dr. Daddums, there are other doctors who will be willing to work with you to discover your nutritional needs. But sometimes you have to point them in the right direction. You will probably have to learn for yourself enough about nutrition so that you can ask the right questions. Once you have a sound body of knowledge about nutrition, you will have the confidence needed to seek out the doctor who will at least say, "Vitamins sure as hell won't hurt you. . . ."

Is this an easy approach to the problems of menopause? No. Not exactly. You will have to give up the passive approach and really study nutrition. For some women it may seem much easier to spend the next fifteen years on those "mild tranquilizers" that doctors are so partial to. Fifteen years is just about the time it will take before the entrenched medical establishment begins to realize what vitamins can do for the woman in menopause. According to many experts, the field of vitamin therapy is the wave of the future in medicine.

And after those fifteen years that you could have spent *living* rather than existing in a drug-induced haze filled with "mysterious" maladies, you may wonder what ever happened to good old Dr. Daddums, the one who pooh-poohed your questions about vitamin supplements. Oh, he died years ago—from a heart attack that could have been prevented by sound nutrition.

TEN

Love and the Age Game: Play to Win

But when it comes to playing this most important game of all, many women find they are losers. The proof is all around you—in the divorce statistics, in the vacant faces of that overly married couple at the next table, and maybe, just maybe, in your own bedroom.

Why are mature women so often losers in the love game? There's no chronological reason for it. If life begins at forty, so does love. Or, rather, it should and for very valid reasons.

First and foremost, if you've reached forty or there about, remember that you've only reached the halfway mark in the life of modern woman. And with the long-overdue awareness of woman as a sexual being, not just a childbearing machine, those old-fashioned puritanical concepts that tied a woman's sexuality to her childbearing function have gone out the window. As Jane Ogle says in her article, "Sex Begins at Forty," "The anxieties, the tensions, the inhibitions of your twenties and thirties are behind you. So relax. Sexpress yourself to the fullest." In other words, play to win, girls!

But instead of being winners, so many women find that they are losing at the game of love. Wistfully, they see themselves gradually disqualified as players. They often see that their marriages have slipped into a faceless limbo—or become battlegrounds—or have ended in the divorce courts. And the woman alone, whether through divorce or widowhood, often faces the bleak prospect of being *permanently* alone.

Yet this doesn't have to be the case. And once again, the proof is all around you. There are some women, ageless every one, who have maintained fulfilling marriages or exciting affairs (seldom at the same time—no need to be greedy). Still others have embarked on romantic second marriages.

What's their secret? Maybe you already know it.

These women live life to the fullest because they have refused to relinquish their sex appeal. They know that without this essential quality it's impossible to play the Love Game. Rather like attempting to find a partner for tennis when you don't possess a racket.

SEX APPEAL: AT YOUR AGE?

Have you still got it? Can you get it back? Well, I have some good news and some bad news. First the bad news.

Any woman in her right mind knows that a certain type of sex appeal is the sole prerogative of the very young. That wide-eyed, round-bodied, smooth-skinned animal magnetism that almost any girl/woman under twenty possesses is a force all by itself. Trying to compete with the total fallout produced by such creatures is like trying to compete with an atomic bomb. And no wise woman even tries.

But—and this is the important point—any man worth your trouble will not be permanently engrossed by the sex-bomb phenomenon. And that's where the appeal of the Ageless Woman can be irresistible. Because, while the sex kitten is essentially concerned with *being* loved—"How to Turn Him On" as one *Cosmopolitan* article put it—the Ageless Woman creates a more profound relationship because she is interested in *loving* or, as Eric Fromm says, "radiating love."

Now don't misunderstand me, I'm not talking about that tepid dish entitled "joy through companionship, a guide to the twilight years." No, I mean s-e-x, but sex in all its myriad and delightful connotations. And here the Ageless Woman has an undeniable advantage in the sex department. Of course, I mean experience.

I recognize that today's liberated sex kittens possess technical knowledge that would put the Sultan's favorite to shame. But if technical knowledge is everything, why are psychiatrists' offices and encounter groups filled with members of the "now" generation—men, women, and miscellaneous—who plaintively complain that their personal relationships are not satisfying?

If technical knowledge is everything, why is impotence one of the most prevalent sexual problems among young men today? It is becoming increasingly apparent that technical knowledge of the sex act—who does what, with which, and to whom—does not guarantee success in the Game of Love. As Anita Loos pointed out in a recent article for *Vogue*, ". . . the ballad makers of today turn out lyrics that ask 'Is That All There Is?' That hard-bitten song, recorded by Peggy Lee, was bought by millions of young people, who apparently agreed with Peggy."

No, when I say experience, I mean a quality that goes beyond exper-tease. I'm talking about a compassionate knowledge of the human heart. A knowledge that can make love—and sex—the totally fulfilling experience it was meant to be.

Still, it isn't as simple as that. Experience, a knowledge of human nature, is a starting point, but there are many subtle qualities that the Ageless Woman has developed that give her her own arsenal of secret weapons.

I'll be discussing the qualities that create the appeal of the Ageless Woman in great detail, since they are, after all, qualities that any woman can possess. But first, an object lesson in what *not* to do. Let's look at our old friend, the M.A.M., and see how she has effectively killed off her sex appeal.

THE CASE OF THE MISSING SEX APPEAL

The Professional M.A.M. has been so efficient in neutralizing herself, it's hard to know where to start in explaining the long list of her sexual transgressions. Interestingly, many Professional M.A.M.s had plenty of S.A. at one time. Often, as young girls, these women possessed that type of animal magnetism that I described earlier. Because of their youth, and without any conscious effort or emotional involvement, they were attractive to the opposite sex. But often they never understood men, in fact never liked men, and just accepted the homage to their youth as their due. For women of this sort, men have been an ego trip, someone to take them out, buy them things, and generally make life pleasant for them. And the price for all these goodies was—well, you know. . . . "Men are all *animals*, and you just have to humor them."

But when the magnetic youthfulness is gone, these women have nothing to take its place. Since they don't understand men, in fact, don't really like men, they don't see them as people at all. They *do* reduce men to an animal state—and *how* they hate those animals when they will no longer jump through the hoop.

So the essential quality of the sexless Professional M.A.M. is this: she doesn't *like* men. And feeling this way, naturally she can't really understand them. As a result, she lives in a totally female-oriented society where Man is the enemy. It's Us and Them. Françoise Sagan was certainly speaking to the M.A.M.s of this world when she said, "Stop braying in the name of all women, 'They owe us this or that'; become more interested in men. There are women who say, 'we women,' who refer to men as 'them,' who never stop gossiping with their girl friends, about men, of course. They want a man so they can go out with him, but they don't want to know anything about him."

Charles Revson, the Revlon man who made millions because he was one of the few men in the world who understood women, described our neuter friends in this way: "The 'Groupies,' as I call them, are women who surround themselves with other women . . . who join women's groups because *men are a very little source of pleasure and satisfaction to them.*" (Emphasis added.) He goes on to say, "I feel the [sexually] attractive woman is not a joiner. Not that she doesn't have women friends. But she is not one to go through life surrounded by groups of other women. Her orientation is toward the man, because she is happiest with him."

But is M.A.M. comfortable and happy in masculine company? About as happy as a cat in a dog show. And so, as much as possible, she has removed herself from the world that men inhabit—not for her the easy and stimulating camaraderie of the sexes. Her objective is to control men for her own purposes. Because of the fact that she doesn't like men, distrusts men, she has allowed her point of view to become hopelessly narrow and stunted. No wonder she doesn't understand the man in her life. Her interests are totally female-oriented in the worst sense of the word. And all she has left is that limiting mental outlook that the women's liberation movement is railing against. And rightly so.

As a result of this limited viewpoint, not only has her physical sex appeal vanished with her youth, but her mental sex appeal—that intriguing, mysterious, feminine quality that can spark his imagination, challenge his composure, and just generally get under his skin—has never had a chance to develop.

But does M.A.M. care? "Listen, you know they're all animals—just after one thing." Of course, by now good old Harry doesn't seem too interested anyway; because, while M.A.M. has been accenting the mental differences between the sexes, she has also been minimizing the physical differences. In all the ways we've discussed in detail —clothes, make-up, hair styles, movements—her entire physical personality is neuter.

Is there a cure for the Professional M.A.M.'s lack of allure? I don't really think so. Not for the real Pro. But don't worry about the Professional M.A.M. She's pushing man away with every conscious and subconscious weapon she has—because she *wants* him out of her life. To the Professional M.A.M.s of this world, his only real purpose is as a sort of drone. Actually, whatever she may say, this Queen Bee is quite happy with things the way they are. No, instead save your sympathy for the man in the Professional M.A.M.'s life—and for our next case.

SEX APPEAL AND THE UNWILLING M.A.M.

It can happen any time—that moment when the Unwilling M.A.M. realizes that she is losing her sex appeal—in fact, her very identity as a woman. It might be the occasion of her twentieth wedding anniversary, when her husband presents her with a gift. "Well, Mother, here's the vacuum cleaner you've been wanting." She wants a vacuum cleaner like she wants a hole in the head. What she's *really* yearning for is a black lace nightgown—or some similar symbol that says, "You're still the most exciting woman I've ever known."

Or perhaps it happens at a party, the one she dressed for so carefully, the party she had looked forward to for so long. When she was seated next to that interesting stranger she realized that, in spite of her best attempts at conversation, he was (oh, God!) being *polite* and, even worse, deferential. The way one would act toward the Queen Mother.

However it happens, somewhere, sometime, the Unwilling M.A.M. realizes that she has traded her identity as an exciting, female woman for the neuter image of the middle-aged matron. And in panic and dismay she asks herself, "What happened?"

Well, what happened is this. After twenty years as a homemaker and mother, our Unwilling M.A.M. has become so locked into these roles that she has forgotten the art of being a *woman.* In our culture, at least, this can mean too many concessions to "the children," so that after twenty years she isn't the queen in her castle but rather a barely tolerated servant. And any attempts to break out of her role into a new, exciting image are greeted with catcalls. "Honestly, Motherrr—you aren't *really* going to take dancing lessons?"

These years of letting life revolve around the children take their toll in her marriage, too. If all of your children are over sixteen and your husband is still calling you "Mom," look out. It's time to update your image.

And what about those twenty years as a wife? Well, unless a woman has been paying attention, she finds that she has slipped into the female-dominated social life we were talking about earlier. Because she hasn't really thought about staying an exciting female, she has instead become a Groupie and has somehow embraced all those dreadful Professional M.A.M.s we've been discussing. All of her social activities revolve around women's clubs, the PTA, the hospital auxiliary, and so on. Naturally she and her husband have nothing to talk about.

And even those social occasions that are co-educational are usually afflicted with suburban apartheid—men on one side, having one too many and talking football or tennis, women on the other, locked into the type of conversations that grace the afternoon bridge table. The type of conversation one woman has described as "dishes, diapers, and douches." No wonder our Unwilling M.A.M. feels dull. She *is* dull. And no one knows it better than the man in her life.

And so our Unwilling M.A.M. becomes unhappy and increasingly uncertain about her role in life. She grows a little bitter—*demanding* her husband's attention instead of charming him—and often becomes neurotically possessive. And because she feels bitter and frustrated it becomes increasingly easy to slip into the spirit of those hate sessions that are the spécialité of that all-female world ruled by the Professional M.A.M. "I told Harry, 'Listen, if you think you're getting out of this house without doing that list of jobs I set out for you . . .'" "You should have seen the ghastly sweater that George bought me for my birthday. I have to return it, of course—but then I always do, his taste is so terrible . . ." "Then right in the middle of the afternoon, he got romantic—you know what I mean—and the lawn wasn't even mowed yet, so I just told him . . ."

And since her social life is governed by the approval of groups of middle-aged women who also have problems, when our Unwilling M.A.M. tries to break out of the mold she faces social ostracism. Just try crossing that Mason-Dixon line at any suburban party—and see what happens.

Well, what's the answer for our perplexed and unsexed heroine? First of all, she has to break away from that all-female peer group that has dominated her personality and limited its growth. This takes courage—and the willingness to be alone with her thoughts once in a while. Someone, somewhere, said, "Solitude is the price of greatness." Well, we're not talking about being great perhaps, but taking time to know yourself is an essential step in letting your personality grow.

My advice to the Unwilling M.A.M. is this: learn to say no! The Headdress Ball will get along without you this time around. Let someone else have the satisfaction of being chairman.

And what about "The Group" at the office? Do you really have to have lunch with that same closed corporation *every* day? Once in a while, spend that lunch hour by yourself—walking, browsing in the shops, or just getting in touch with "who you are." Perhaps you should examine all of your social contacts from time to time to see if you are continuing some that you have outgrown. There is nothing more exhausting than trying to maintain a relationship that is past its prime. It takes courage to change, but maybe it's time to say by-by to "that old gang of mine."

Of course, you aren't going to turn into a hermit. And you aren't going to abandon all of your women friends. But you'll concentrate on your women friends as individuals, not as members of a vast pressure group that forces everyone into a middle-aged mold.

And what of that suburban social life? Here's where you have to use your ingenuity. Every individual will face different problems, so I can't have exact answers for you. But here are some suggestions.

Man-woman get-togethers that have a *reason* will allow you to participate as an individual, and not merely as somebody's wife. Even the
Committee to Save the Blue-footed Booby or to Preserve the Long-
toed Stint can be a step away from the suburban crabgrass syndrome
and may allow you to relate to other people (even your husband)
in a new context.

Think about joining political committees, sports-oriented groups—
tennis, bike touring, backpacking—or cultural groups—the Arts
Council, the Opera Guild. And of course, classes and courses of all
kinds.

Mixing with the opposite sex on a purely social basis is necessary
for a healthy personality and has been endorsed by many counselors
and psychologists. "Seeing how the other half lives" is just as important for the happily married woman as it is for the woman alone.
And for the widow or divorced woman, this mixing with men is essential. In his book *Aging Successfully*, Dr. George Lawton prescribes, "If there is one thing a man or woman needs all his life it is
to remember that he *is* a man and she a woman. I can give no better
prescription to older women who want to keep their femininity
than this: at least once every day, have a conversation with a man."

It may not be easy at first to change your attitudes—not after
twenty years of self-imposed exile in the housewifery world ruled by
the Professional M.A.M.s. And if you do want to change attitudes,
you may have to develop the tools needed to express the change. So
here we have our Unwilling M.A.M. at her next dinner party, seated
beside an attractive and interesting man. Does she know how to talk
to him? Can she turn this brief encounter into a relaxed and pleasant
moment that salutes the difference between the sexes? Unfortunately, she cannot. She's forgotten how. Which also means that she's
forgotten how to fascinate the *really* important man in her life.

But the Ageless Woman remembers. She remembers how to talk
to a man—and she remembers a lot of other things that make life in
a world of men and women fun and stimulating. In fact, she's never
for one moment forgotten what it means to have sex appeal. And
the Unwilling M.A.M. can learn it all—if she chooses to.

SEX APPEAL: THE AGELESS WOMAN NEVER LOST IT

The primary quality of sex appeal has nothing to do with age. As
my friend Sheila said, "I learned my first lesson in how to be attractive to men from my beautiful older sister. I remember as a knobby-

kneed and desperately unpopular thirteen-year-old watching my sister Marjorie getting ready for still another date, and I asked, 'Gee, Marj, do you think the boys will *ever* like me?' Marj gave her soft blonde hair a final pat. 'Sure they will, punkin'. If you'll remember one thing.' She enveloped us both in a cloud of perfume. 'The reason that boys like girls is because we're different from them.'"

Sheila patted her own soft blond hair and continued. "Well, I've never forgotten her advice. And while I wouldn't consider myself an expert, I really find that as a divorced, forty-five-year-old woman I have a marvelous and varied social life. I know lots of interesting men—and they like me. What's more important, they still seem to desire me as a woman." She smiled smugly. "And I'm sure that one reason is that I always accent the physical differences between the sexes. While the twenty-year-old can get away with tailored hair styles, raucous laughter, an arrogant manner, I know that I must accent my femininity in every *subtle* physical way."

Well, what have I been telling you? Your clothes, your hair, your walk, your manner must all whisper, "I am a woman—and you'd better believe it."

Charles Revson said, when describing the woman with sex appeal, "She does everything she can to attract without becoming a slave or hysterical about the way she looks. . . . Of course a lot of it has to do with her inner view of herself, and that's what's going to be revealed in her appearance."

And what about that inner self? Does any man really love a woman because she has a beautiful mind? Beautiful, probably not. Intriguing, yes. In fact, one of the world's greatest lovers has called mind—

THE FIRST EROGENOUS ZONE

Anatole Broyard says, "In these days of sexual revolution, instruction manuals, sensitivity therapy and 'raised consciousness,' the case of the Italian writer Gabriele D'Annunzio should be instructive . . . he was certainly one of the greatest lovers in history. Compared to him, Casanova, for example, seems a mere sensualist. [D'Annuzio] . . . was a true believer who made a religion of love, a man who proved something our age seems to have forgotten: that the mind is the first and foremost of the erogenous zones."

To any man whose emotional level goes beyond two disheveled

bodies shuffling wordlessly toward an unmade bed, a woman's mind, personality—in fact, whatever it is that makes her uniquely herself— is indeed the first erogenous zone. Not the last, mind you, but definitely the first. As columnist Charles McCabe says, "I've been attracted to unbrainy women in my time, mostly because of their physical beauty, and I can tell you it's been a torture. You just can't be *interested* in a woman's face and form for that length of time. The lady must be a person, above all else, to be permanently interesting."

If you're still skeptical of the idea that a man can be attracted by your mind, remember that this whole concept involves an element of mystery. It involves that indefinable female quality that affects men like catnip.

Of course we're not talking about the type of mental approach that says, in effect, Look how bright and intellectual I am. This type of mental show-off isn't popular with anyone. (Nobody loves a smart-ass.) Nor do I mean the compulsive woman, always involved with multitudinous activities, who grabs an arm and says earnestly, "Oh, Mr. Calder, let me tell you *everything* about the latest project of the League . . ." Good Lord, no!

I mean the kind of brains that create for you a full and exciting inner life. A man is intrigued and challenged by a woman who is an interesting person in her own right, whose personality has enough depth to provide that essential ingredient for any successful relationship between men and women: the masculine need for meaningful conquest.

The woman who relies on the appeal of physical conquest alone finds, to her chagrin, that this appeal is very short-lived indeed. The conquest of Bunny Booby entitles a man to a few slaps on the back and sly winks from his male contemporaries, but Bunny Booby is soon forgotten. She does not wear well—and thank God for *that*. The real man needs a worth-while challenge and that must come from the mind.

The implication of this intriguing inner life is the secret allure of the world's most fascinating women. Garbo, Marlene Dietrich, and Jacqueline Onassis all have this quality of depth and mystery. And every Ageless Woman can and must develop this same quality of depth.

As one man who wanted a divorce told his wife, "You never stimulated or challenged my ideas, so I never felt you were a person." Easy for him to say. He hasn't been chained for fifteen years to a houseful of small children and an endless cycle of repetitive jobs. So what's a woman to do? How can she develop her self-identity?

"YOU WILL MEET A MYSTERIOUS STRANGER"

For starters, she must recognize the inevitability of her need to get in touch with her own personality. She must restore her own identity. As her children grow up the entire focus of her life *must* change. If it doesn't, she will either become a neurotic, meddling mother-in-law to her grown children or a sort of emotional vampire to her husband, trying to fill the void in her life by an unnatural and negative attention on him. So it's essential that she change the focus of her life from one of selfless concern for her family to a selfish concern for herself and her own development.

For many women, this change in emphasis will occur almost unnoticed. As the children are launched, a woman who has had both a career and a family will sigh with relief and achieve even greater fulfillment in her chosen career once she can give it her total attention.

But for many other women this other "change of life" will find them unprepared and lost. They have been so accustomed to fulfilling the needs of others, they can't even recognize their own needs—the paths to their personal fulfillment.

This can be a long odyssey, and the enormity of the choices available can be a little frightening. For women who are in this position, I recommend two very simple, comfortable steps. If you remember that childhood game, these aren't "giant" steps, meant to launch you pell-mell into the unknown. These are comfortable "baby" steps that enable you to feel that your feet are planted on solid ground.

So, to begin, a woman can ruthlessly set aside *at least* one afternoon or evening each week for herself alone. A time when she can do anything she likes. But she must constantly guard against feeling *guilty* about spending this time for herself alone. She must also guard against any mawkish inner voices that assure her, "I'm doing this for the children." Because it is absolutely essential that she start to develop a healthy attitude about her right to a life of her own.

Next, it will help her to make a list of all the things she likes and all the things she hates. Her finished list would have the things she likes most at the top and the things she hates most at the bottom.

Making up the list will not be easy. It will call for a great deal of introspection, because the object is to list what *she* really likes and dislikes—not what the Professional M.A.M.s have convinced her that she ought to like and dislike.

When the list is completed to her satisfaction, her work is not over. Suppose cooking is high on her list. Good grief! She already spends two or three hours each day planning and cooking meals. The last thing in the world she needs for a stimulating diversion—for self-expression—is a gourmet course in Cordon Bleau techniques.

No, she should choose subjects from near the top of her list that will bring stimulating *contrast* to her life. Then she should attend classes, read books, consult experts, and above all join men-and-women groups that share her interests. She should choose interests that take her *out* of that house—not only physically but mentally. Her new interests must encourage creative, stimulating thought processes. And creative thought becomes habit-forming. Once the mind wakes up and stretches a bit, it becomes greedy for new experiences.

As the reawakened Unwilling M.A.M. revels in new thoughts, new experiences, new emotions, and new relationships, she not only becomes more interesting to herself, *she becomes more interesting to everyone*. She will begin to reawaken some sex appeal without even trying. (But she will try a little, of course.)

WHAT ELSE IS SEXY?

Health is sexy. As I've said many times throughout this book, the Ageless Woman pursues vibrant good health with a passion. She knows that diet, exercise, and a positive mental attitude are essential ingredients to her allure. Health is positive, dynamic, creative. Bubbling good health is LIFE. And *that's* ageless.

But what of the woman who isn't blessed with good health? If she's the Ageless Woman, she keeps her health problems to herself. Her answer to "How are you?" is always something positive—"Fine" . . . "Just great" . . . "Never felt better"—unless there is a specific reason for her to explain why she feels miserable and ill. *There is nothing that will age you more than "enjoying" poor health.* Detailed descriptions of hysterectomies, sinus infections, and ingrown toenails are the exclusive province of the Professional M.A.M.

VANITY IS SEXY

A good healthy dose of self-esteem is terribly attractive to men. Once again, this creates an aura of conquest. The man senses that you are a person of value in your own eyes and therefore in the eyes of others. He's challenged and intrigued. Can he hold your interest?

Physical vanity is also sexy. Men love to tease women about their primping and fussing over perfume and make-up and such. But they're secretly flattered at all this trouble just to please *them*. Of course the woman who wanders around in a gray flannel bathrobe when her husband is home, then dresses to the nines for her club meetings gets failing grades in this department. She's made it pretty clear that she doesn't give a damn how she looks for him. And he has every right to be irritated by her misplaced vanity.

WHEN SHE WAS GOOD, SHE WAS VERY, VERY GOOD

And when she was bad she was—adorable. There's nothing less appealing to a man than Goody Two-shoes. And nothing more beguiling than a certain wickedness. Now I don't mean a depraved wantonness or a mule skinner's vocabulary, but rather a glorious and amused acceptance of the human condition—warts and all. The woman who can be mischievous, playful, a bit devilish will always be attractive and appealing to men. After all, as V*ogue* says, a bit of devilish playfulness means "laughter, and laughter is one of the basic ingredients of love. A man senses that, with such a woman, romance would be glorious fun."

HAPPINESS IS SEXY

The joyful, fun-loving, positive, enthusiastic woman will always attract men like a magnet. It's only in books that men like "problem" women. In real life, the woman who is a constant worry, who is unhappy and depressed, simply drives a man to distraction (or to his secretary). Men don't have the temperament for these long-term sacrifices. They become irritated and bored with the problem woman. Then, naturally, they feel guilty because they can't cope. And when they feel guilty they feel uncomfortable. And what does every man do in the face of discomfort? He leaves. Sometimes physically—always mentally.

The Ageless Woman is attractive because she isn't neurotic. She loves life and enjoys life to the fullest. And she knows that sex is only one of the sensual pleasures. She enjoys them all—good food; comfortable, even cozy surroundings; soothing and stimulating music; perfumes, potpourri, scented candles, or the pungent smell of a crackling fire in the grate; all these contribute to her zest for living. And to her appeal. After all, around her, everything is so pleasant, so comfortable. Why, he never wants to leave.

A DASH OF IMPERFECTION

While the problem woman is something a man can't cope with, the vulnerable woman will capture his heart. A woman should never give the impression that she is so capable, so self-sufficient, that she doesn't need him at all. Men are enchanted by minor, even amusing frailties.

A high school friend of mine has become the dean of one of our large universities. She flies across country to speak at educational conferences, briskly manages all of the complex administrative duties that are essential to her position—and goes into a complete flap when it comes to balancing her checkbook. She simply can't do it without her husband's help. She's also terrified of moths—and he has to "save" her from one of these winged "monsters" every so often.

An affectation? Not really. I believe that she, and many other women I could describe, are simply saving their emotional energy (and their relationships). They're highly capable about most things. And about a few unimportant things that "bug" them, they've decided to let the men in their lives be strong, stalwart, masculine, and indispensable. Which keeps everybody happy.

This quality of vulnerability, of needing a man, is something that the mature woman should study very carefully. Because it's the quality that she loses most easily. Years of dealing with home and family, of making decisions, of coping, can turn the woman of forty-plus into a brusque, cold-eyed, and somewhat frightening figure. Certainly not a figure a man would want to snuggle.

The cure is simply a readjustment of values. Is efficiency *everything*? Or are a few foibles, a few minor weaknesses, too stiff a price to pay to capture the heart of that man in your life?

The woman who has a career outside the home must be especially aware of the need to live a double life, at times. She may be totally decisive and in control on the job (and she'd better be), but the same take-charge attitudes will slowly and surely erode her relationship with the man in her life. A conscious awareness of substituting the "*I* think *you* must do thus and so" attitude to a "What do *you* think *we* should do?" approach will subtly bind the ego wounds he may have been sustaining. Do I hear screams of anguish from the women's liberation front? Sorry, ladies, but the Ageless Woman knows that in the battle of the sexes you can win the battle and lose the war. As Kirk Douglas points out, "Many women are currently paying the price for their so-called liberation: loneliness. Many a woman is liberating herself right out of her man's bed."

THE LAST WORD ON SEX APPEAL

I guess that the most fascinating woman I've ever known is—well, let's call her Madame de Z. Born and raised in Brooklyn, she earned an art scholarship that took her to Paris. There she met and married a young diplomat and under his tutelage became an outstanding hostess and sophisticated woman of the world, meeting people from international society, cultural leaders, and the conservative aristocracy of Europe. Quite a career for a little girl from Brooklyn, as she candidly admits. She often said, "I became more European than Europeans." When her husband died, she returned to the United States and turned her talents toward dress designing, which is how I happened to meet her.

Marina de Z. has a marvelous sense of humor, and the fairy-tale aspects of her career were a constant source of amusement to her. While I was working as her model and assistant, she would regale me with intriguing and intimate stories from *le beau monde.*

Now, if anyone knows the finer points of attracting men, it's Marina—combining as she does the engaging honesty and humor of the American woman with the seductive wisdom of the European woman. And most important of all, she's a fascinator who does it all with the force of her personal magnetism. A beauty she's not. So I wrote and asked for her secret. And here's her advice.

My dearest G:

Well, I am indeed flattered that you consider me to be an expert on the fine art of attracting men. I must admit that I have always liked men and felt enormously grateful that *le Bon Dieu* saw fit to make half of the world so intriguingly different from women.

Perhaps that's the essence of appealing to men, whatever a

woman's age. To realize that, though we have many similarities, men and women do live in different worlds. The woman who is attractive to men is the one who steps into his world, on occasion, and allows herself to be impressed, beguiled, and fascinated as her tour guide shows her this masculine realm. And like sophisticated travelers everywhere, she doesn't criticize his world because it's different from the one she inhabits. Any more than one who lives in Paris would criticize London because it has no Place de Concorde, and because the stupid natives speak English rather than French. (Of course, they do *fry* everything, but then . . .)

What I'm saying, I guess, is *vive la difference!* I'm always aware of that difference, and I let a man know that I *enjoy* that difference between us. But here's a rather subtle point that too many women miss. All the time I'm acknowledging his sexual role, at the same time I make him aware that I'm interested in the *individual* within that sexual being. After all, this whole business of sexual roles is like a game. One should play with the amused knowledge that this *is* a game, played out by individuals. And so I seek to know each man as a unique individual, never just as Man—the meal ticket, escort, and automatic flattery machine.

I don't need to tell you that men respond to this approach. After all, we (men and women alike) are all individuals, each unique in our own way. We all bloom when our "specialness" is recognized and encouraged.

And so I give a man my full attention. I let him know that I think he's interesting and attractive. And if he isn't? Well, it's an amazing thing. Even the dullest fellow will "bloom" when this "specialness" is recognized and encouraged. He feels free to share those special aspects of his personality in this atmosphere of approval.

So that's the next step, to create an atmosphere of delighted acceptance and approval. Most women, I believe, don't realize how terrified a man is of being rejected—and that he never seems to get enough reassurance. Like a cat in the sun, he'll stretch and purr in the warmth of your positive, approving response to him. And is this wholehearted approval a bit dishonest sometimes? Perhaps. But what harm does it do? As Victor Hugo said, "There is in this world no function more important than that of being charming—to shed joy around, to cast light upon dark days. . . . Is not this to render a service?"

I think that a man is enormously attracted to a woman if he thinks, "She understands me—and therefore she appreciates what a fine fellow I am." On the other hand, a man can never remain interested in a woman that he thinks he understands completely. And this shouldn't be hard to analyze. To him, the very essence of femaleness is that women are unknowable, mysterious, different. He's delighted by a woman who wants to know all about him—he's bored by a woman if he knows everything about her.

The woman who would fascinate a man lets him know that, while she finds him tremendously interesting and attractive, she does have her own life, her own intriguing thoughts. She gives him her full attention—but not indefinitely. She's off into her own world, concerned with her own interesting life. And if he wants to enjoy that marvelous feeling of having her full attention, understanding, and approval—well, he'll just have to win it back.

Finally, I'm appalled at the foolishness of the American woman who strives to make "togetherness" a total way of life. Who finds it necessary to share the details of every thought, every uncertainty, and—*mon Dieu*—every amour, with the man in her life. That's what confidantes—girl friends—are for. And to the woman who says, "That isn't fair, why *isn't* he concerned about my innermost hopes, fears, problems? After all, I'm concerned about *his*." Well, the answer is devastatingly simple. He isn't, and that's that.

And so the woman who would be eternally successful with men accepts them *wholeheartedly* for what they are. She doesn't bemoan what they are not. And she never, never tries to change them.

> Adieu and fond good wishes,
> Marina

VIVE LA DIFFÉRENCE

We have just been talking about men as individuals, and now I am going to say, "Here are some characteristics common to all men." But it isn't really a contradiction. Although every man is indeed an individual, as are all human beings, there are certain personality traits that are common to almost all men in our society. Right now certain members of our society are creating considerable uproar over whether or not these characteristics are instinctual, physiological, or the result of social conditioning. And though most experts agree that there is a "male mystique," the battle of "why" still rages. But as far as we're concerned, who cares "why"?

The important fact to all women is this: these male personality traits are *there; and the older the man, the more pronounced these traits are likely to be*. The wise woman, the Ageless Woman, doesn't try to alter these characteristics. Nor does she bitterly complain about them. Rather, she acknowledges that these typical male traits exist, *she understands them,* and so she is able to deal with them in a positive way.

She considers the male differences to be as unchangeable as the law of gravity. Now it's true that the law of gravity may be inconvenient at times, but what wise person ignores it—particularly while standing near a cliff? The wise woman also remembers that the law of gravity has its good points—it helps hold wigs on, for instance.

There are some women on the fringe of the women's liberation movement who endlessly and tediously insist that there are no basic differences in the personalities, instincts, and emotional patterns of men and women. To them, the "unisex" concept seems to have become so compelling that they have almost lost track of what should be the vitally important and basic concern of the women's movement—equality. Equality before law and custom so that woman can work wherever and at whatever she chooses for equal pay. Equality with men before the flinty eye of a bank's lending officer. And so on. The list of such material goals has been well defined, and these are worth-while goals.

The liberation movement is also striving for equality on a subjective level—for a universal level of consciousness that will release women (and men) from rigidly stereotyped patterns of thought and emotion—patterns that have been ruthlessly imposed by centuries of paternalistic civilization. And in the long run this subjective line of effort is probably more important than the material goals, because it will ultimately allow the freed personalities of both women and men to develop fully. After all, why do women *have* to be afraid of mice and why do all men *have* to be "superstuds," perpetually in rut?

But, as so often happens in periods of social change, some groups have overreacted. In attempting to break women loose from restrictive patterns of the past, some splinter groups deny women their very femininity and are imposing other, opposite patterns that are equally restrictive. This denial of a woman's femininity has, at its extreme, resulted in varying degrees of the unisex concept. Ignoring hundreds of thousands of years of evolutionary history and thousands of scientific studies alike, the advocates of unisex deny that men and women are different. They insist, stridently and constantly, that *all* the personality differences between men and women are totally artificial, totally imposed by society.

These women are in a heap of trouble.

The unisex woman has painted herself into a corner. So did another smugly self-satisfied claque that trumpeted, "Never trust anyone over thirty." And where are *they* today? Well into their thirties —that's where.

The unisex woman's dream house also comes tumbling down sometime in her late thirties.

The young unisex couple shares every thought, every moment, every attitude, every emotion, and every sweat shirt or pair of jeans. All differences are ruthlessly suppressed as being sexist and therefore horrid. And at first everything is cheery. They are truly comrades.

But as the years go by the unisex woman becomes increasingly uneasy. Can it be that most of the suppressed sexual differences have been hers? Can it be that her faithful comrade, Gary, is paying more and more attention to that vapid little Wendy next door—the one whose consciousness level never climbed out of the basement rumpus room?

And when she complained about being deserted during the "happening" at their favorite art gallery—while Gary listened spellbound to that overly mammalian blonde—what did he mean when he said, "Don't go feminine on me"?

What he was really saying is, a woman can't win at the game of unisex. Unisex works for the very young woman during the years when she still has that powerful animal magnetism of youth. Even with her unisex make-up, hair styles, wardrobe, and high convictions, her animal magnetism surrounds her with a compelling female aura. Even when she is being "one of the boys," *they* know damn well she isn't.

But as she grows older the animal magnetism begins to fade. And without the youthful animal magnetism that misled her into thinking that unisex was working, she has nothing to fall back on. And, like it or not, she had better begin to make some adjustments—at least if she wants to keep a man in her life.

At this point the wise (and ageless) woman has already begun to develop a *conscious* feminine magnetism to replace the fading animal magnetism. She replaces glandular magnetism with mental magnetism.

And the essence of this mental magnetism lies in the fact that there *is* a difference between the sexes. No woman can really maintain a successful relationship with a man unless she is realistic enough to recognize that there are basic differences between the sexes.

Many unhappy women say, "I'll never understand men—my God! They drive me *crazy*." But generally their problem is that they think of men as peculiar and somewhat retarded women—not as *men*.

Remember, a woman's advantage is that she *can* understand men if she will just make the effort. And men, dear uncomplicated souls that they are, will never *really* understand women.

So let's talk about men. If it is true that there is a battle of the sexes, let's follow the basic military law that says, "Know thy enemy." But since this is really a friendly war (even cozy sometimes) let's rephrase the law—let's feminize it—"*Know thy friend.*"

WHAT EVERY AGELESS WOMAN KNOWS ABOUT MEN (AND SOME THINGS YOU MAY HAVE FORGOTTEN)

1. *Men Are Just Little Boys.* Good heavens! That old chestnut? But it's really true. According to Dr. Theodore Rubin, in his column in the *Ladies' Home Journal*, ". . . throughout life, men retain more of the 'little boy' in themselves than women do the 'little girl.' Men may transfer their interests from marbles to money, but they never rid themselves of the 'little boy' qualities of poor tolerance for frustration, inner conflict, responsibility, and anxiety." He goes on to add, "Women usually mature earlier in life than men do, and many remain more mature throughout life."

What does this knowledge mean to you? Simply that you will become more tolerant of those heretofore mysterious outbreaks of temper and frustration. That string of profanity and anger that accompanies the hunt for his misplaced tie clip. (Out of all proportion, you think.) The absolute turmoil that accompanies his preparations for a hunting trip. ("Where's the goddam sleeping bag? It was right here.") The angry blast of the car horn at that (expletive deleted) driver who won't move out of the fast lane. ("These pea-brained nitwits shouldn't be allowed on the highway.") These are all familiar examples of that male inability to handle frustration. And these outbursts may be a safety valve to let off even deeper feelings of anxiety and inner conflict.

Another example of this immaturity is that, like children, men don't recognize when they are tired and irritable. And this can lead to all kinds of negative, even destructive behavior.

Napoleon Hill and W. Clement Stone, in their book *Success Through a Positive Mental Attitude*, point out the need for recognizing fatigue and dealing with it. "The small child doesn't know when he is excessively tired. But he surely shows it in his behavior and actions. The adolescent may realize he is over-fatigued, but re-fuse to admit it—even to himself. Then [when overtired] sexual, family, scholastic, and social problems may seem unsolvable and un-bearable. They may motivate him to temporary or permanent destructive acts—acts that injure himself and others." And man—an adult adolescent in some ways—has the same problems. He can't admit that he is nervous and exhausted—machismo does not allow it.

You may ask, "What about us? After all, women get tired, Lord knows—and irritable, too." Yes, but we are trained from earliest childhood to recognize fatigue, nerves, illness. Whether this kind of sexist conditioning is good or bad doesn't concern us here. The point is, women in our age group have all been raised with this kind of training.

"You girls sit here in the shade and rest, while the boys go down to the stream and get some water." . . . "Alice is in tears again? Well, you know how girls can be in their teens. Why doesn't she take an aspirin and lie down before dinner?" . . . Miss Shultz, I have to be excused from P.E. today. I'm expecting my period and I have a headache. . . ."

And if you need any more proof that men push themselves, that they simply don't recognize fatigue and frazzled nerves when they appear in that indestructible male body, check the life expectancy tables. Women know how to take care of themselves better than men, and as a result they live longer.

The Ageless Woman, because she is more mature emotionally, is quick to recognize when her man is totally tired and suffering from nervous exhaustion. And at such times she would no more confront him with a serious problem and expect him to cope with it in an adult manner than she would expect a four-year-old to sit quietly through a chamber music concert—especially if he hadn't had his nap.

Does this mean that woman is never to lean on man, that she's doomed to go through life coddling that big, overgrown baby? Not at all. It simply means that the wise woman is, above all, a realist. *She knows that a sense of timing is everything.* If she wants to get the benefit of her man's strength, she'd better give him a chance to recharge his batteries. *Then* they can sit down quietly together and tackle that problem.

2. *Men Have Greater Conflicts About Their Sexual Identity.* While women today are concerned with becoming fulfilled human beings, with enlarging their choices, men are still locked into the impossible masculine ideal. Men are trapped in the cult of machismo, which sets such unrealistic and unreachable masculine ideals of courage, strength, independence, and sexual prowess that it would be almost impossible for any human being to fulfill them. But men *do* try to live up to this ideal, with varying degrees of success. And failure to live up to this masculine image results in inner conflicts, depression, and self-hatred.

Not only is man saddled with an impossibly idealistic role he has set for himself, but in our society, he has fewer and fewer opportunities to express that role. In his book *The Male in Crisis*, Karl Bednarik says that the very structure of modern industrial society makes it more and more difficult for man to express his masculinity. He adds, ". . . there is less opportunity for masculinity today. The ever more taxing demands upon men in professional life and the ruthless competition make it more and more difficult for men to assert their masculinity successfully. [Man] . . . can expect no comfort or support from women because he sees them as a threat; no consolation, because they expect him to be manly." And you think you've got troubles.

Bednarik continues, "Man's life appears to be on the way to becoming a sequence of minor and major crises—if not a chronic unbroken crisis—because he has lost the security and protection he used to derive from the old male role. Certainly the female role has changed along with the male role, but in her case the change tends to broaden her existence as a person. The old male role, by contrast, is diminished; indeed it seems to have become completely obsolete, with nothing new to take its place and furnish a guiding code of the same reliability and certainty. We have no serviceable, universally recognized image for the passive man . . . we have no image for the man who adjusts, who submits to circumstances without protest; for the man who is expected to display the one characteristic most contrary to his nature: submission."

Now this should explain the success of the woman who knows how to help her man feel like a man, who gives him every positive opportunity to express his masculinity. As Wolfgang Lederer says in *The Fear of Women*, "As to man, what he most wants of woman is that she should make him feel most like a man."

3. *Men Fear Sexual Inadequacy*. And this fear takes many forms. Men fear impotence. And in a complex way this basic sexual fear becomes related to a man's success, self-esteem, and adequacy in other areas of his life. Just to show you how messed up that man of yours can be, a business setback or other loss of face in the business world can cause temporary impotence in some men. That's because in our society man equates self-esteem in terms of power, money, and position.

This fear of sexual inadequacy takes another common form. Almost all men fear (if only subconsciously) that their sex organs are too small. In his book, *The Incompatibility of Men and Women*, Julius Fast explains, "From childhood on men feel in competition with other men about the size of their genitals. Their fantasies resolve around the conviction that women share this concern, though study after study indicates that they don't."

Now this doesn't mean that you're expected to take a quick glance below his belt, whistle loudly, and exclaim, "Oh, *wow!*" In fact, psychologists agree that a woman's reassurance seldom helps to alleviate these fears. (Though, interestingly enough, business success sometimes helps.) It does mean, however, that a wise woman realizes that the question of his sexual adequacy, in terms of either equipment or performance, is definitely not to be taken lightly. The woman with a sense of humor had better watch it.

I hear too many mature women saying things like this (and in front of their husbands, too)! "As I told Harry when we were in Hawaii, 'I don't mind if you look at all those gorgeous hula girls. A man your age wouldn't know what to do with one anyway.' " . . . or, "Good old Harry. I never worry about him and that young secretary of his. He may want to get into trouble, but he just isn't up to it." (Laughter all around.) . . . "Harry wanted to go on a second honeymoon to celebrate our twenty-fifth, but as I told him, 'At our age, what would we do on a honeymoon?' "

These funny, funny ladies are apt to find that these laughs can cost them more than they ever imagined.

4. *Men Fear Rejection by Women.* So what's new? Everyone fears rejection, in some degree. But to a man, rejection by a woman is especially important because it relates back to—you guessed it—his masculinity. I once conducted an informal survey among successful men whose careers ranged from advertising executive, personnel director, to television newsman; I was surprised to find that every one of them mentioned this fear of female rejection as a very important factor in their self-esteem.

And, of course, related to this is sexual rejection. Dr. Rubin says that sexual rejection by a man's wife ". . . is the most total rejection he can receive." As we have learned, men generally have a very low threshold of frustration, and sexual frustration is liable to throw a man into a rage . . . even though he may suppress that rage and have a peptic ulcer instead. Or he may overreact to dinner being late, or to a pair of mismatched socks, or to some other trifle.

So the moral of the story is, if you *really* have a headache, let him down gently. (And pounce on him as soon as you feel better.)

You didn't know that men were so fragile, did you?

5. *Men Don't Understand Women.* It's true. Of course some men will *claim* that they understand women, but if you question them closely you'll find their "insight" is made up of spicy clichés from *Playboy* or some such source, leavened with some bland "Betty Crockerisms" that they remember from Mom.

Now the reason that men don't understand women is this: they don't dare. Because if a man really understands a woman, is completely at home in her mental environment, what happens? He has allowed his precious masculinity to become threatened; and he has, therefore, become less of a man. Since men fear homosexuality, they must always be on guard against relating to things feminine. In other words, it's essential to their fragile masculine image that they actively reject anything that makes them feel at home in the female world. And the woman who remembers this will be able to solve many little mysteries that plague the man-woman relationship. For example:

"Why do we always do what he wants to do? Why can't we ever do what I want to do?" It all depends on what you want to do. If a night at the ballet is your idea of heaven, don't be surprised if he goes under protest—and spends the evening making ribald remarks (that you can't help giggling at) from behind his program. The simple explanation is that he feels like a fool, and an emasculated one at that. He may give some begrudging credit to the skill of the dancers, but the protection of his masculinity forces him to make fun of the entire affair.

You have every right to expect him to be a good sport and share your interests—up to a point. But if your interests and hobbies make him feel that he's out of his male milieu, the best you can hope for is a stolid and patient (or not so patient) determination to "get through this fandango somehow." Always remember, however, that when he gets that glazed look he isn't just bored—he feels threatened on a very elemental level.

The trick is to find activities that you can share that don't have this threatening quality. But this doesn't necessarily mean that you're doomed to spend your leisure time crouched in a duck blind. And yet, if you did, it's interesting, isn't it, that it wouldn't take away from your femininity one whit?

Of course, as I've pointed out, every man is essentially an individual, and what makes one man feel like Peter Pansie may reassure another man that he is the Master of His Fate. Tom and Ann Willoughby, for example, haunt the antique shops for additions to their collection of antique china. And with narrowed eyes, determined to give no quarter (or dime either) without a stout battle, Tom aggressively stalks each item with the single-minded concentration of a hunter. When he triumphantly buys a Limoges cup and saucer at a garage sale for $1.27, he has conquered the foe, by Jove! And when he recounts the details of his combat—how he had disarmed the enemy by pretending interest in a pressed glass pickle pot—Ann Willoughby listens to the great hunter admiringly. Which makes Tom feel *marvelous* in some mysterious way that he doesn't bother to analyze.

His friend Carl Hoffman, on the other hand, wouldn't be caught dead in an antique shop. Instead, he spends every moment he can spare charging through the countryside, bristling with a hundred pounds of camera equipment and taking exquisitely detailed pictures of tiny wildflowers. Like Tom, he feels no threat to his masculinity in this activity, since he is facing a challenge, pitting his ingenuity against the elements and emerging victorious, with a bad case of poison oak and a perfect picture of a rare phantom orchid. He has dared the elements and, though wounded grievously, returned to hearth and home laden with spoil. And his ageless wife wisely sounds the trumpets and prepares the fatted calf for the triumphal feast.

The important point to remember is this: these may not be traditionally masculine pursuits, but the payoffs in emotional satisfaction *are* masculine in that they provide a positive channel for aggression and an opportunity for conquest. You'll find that he'll love to join you in any activities that provide these payoffs to his masculine nature.

"Why does he expect me to talk endlessly about the things he's interested in, then yawn, change the subject, and just generally 'tune out' when I want to talk about what I'm interested in?" It all depends on what you are interested in at the moment. A discussion of the stock market or the situation in the Middle East is probably good for a spirited hour of conversation. But a detailed analysis of Jaynie's new hair style or the latest fashions will turn him off for obvious reasons. Not only is he not interested, but this kind of talk makes him feel less masculine and therefore uncomfortable. How can he possibly say, "And you say Yves has brought back the peplum? That's fascinating news"? Yet he sees no contradiction in the fact that he expects you to be enthralled by the idea that the new car he wants has a special turbo-frissed and cantilevered erknard. Why doesn't he see the contradiction? Because, in some ways, he's about seven years old, that's why.

This double standard in conversation can be much more subtle, however. Most men, whether through conditioning or an essential maleness in their thought processes, are *objective* in their thinking. They are interested in things, events, actions, and ideas outside of themselves. Women tend to be *subjective*, relating every thought and experience inward. As long as the conversation, whatever the subject, remains on a fairly active, abstract, and *objective* level, he's interested. And mentally, he'll pay you the ultimate M.C.P. compliment, "She thinks like a man." But when you turn the conversation inward, to a detailed analysis of motives and feelings, his eyes glaze, his mind wanders—and he's gone. Only in soap operas are men avidly interested in long discussions of other people's relationships, motives, and feelings.

This conversation, for example, overheard on the latest installment of "The World Flips," would never happen in real life.

"Yes, George, I know that Sandra is suffering from depression after the loss of her baby. If only Kurt would tell Laura that he feels threatened by her impending marriage to Steve, instead of bottling up his resentment and releasing it in hostile feelings toward Karen."

"You're absolutely right, Phillip, but I think we have to analyze Sara's reaction to the abortion—her feelings of despair, and her need for reassurance."

Now, to say that this kind of sappy mental hypochondria is the essence of women's talk would be the ultimate insult. Certainly the soap operas carry this female tendency to the extreme. But it is true that the bread and butter of most women's conversation is concerned with people, their motives, relationships, hopes, fears, and potential. A man who finds himself involved in this type of conversation feels as uncomfortable as if he were trapped in the ladies' powder room. Incidentally, this doesn't mean to imply that this awareness of people's feelings is an undesirable quality. On the contrary, this is exactly what we need more of in our plastic, impersonal, industrial society. Sensitivity training is helping men to develop these insights—but they have a long way to go. And, once again, understanding is the key to harmonizing this difference between the sexes.

6. *Men Need the Company of Other Men.* This is one of the most difficult truths that women will ever have to accept. Many a bride has cried herself to sleep because, "after just three months, he's out playing poker twice a week." And many a mature woman has wondered if there's something seriously wrong with her marriage, because her husband simply can't miss that monthly meeting with his buddies.

But this need to be with other men is one of the essential elements in the male mystique. Julius Fast explains, ". . . men form groups, clubs, teams, all-male gatherings of one sort or another because it is part of their heredity to do so." There is so much evidence that this male grouping is an essential activity that Lionel Tiger has written a fascinating book devoted entirely to the subject of *Men in Groups.* He explains that hunting was a way of life for primitive humans, a way of life that lasted for thousands of years. And this hunting activity, to be successful, depended upon the co-operative action of men in groups.

Julius Fast explains Tiger's theory. "He suggests that this male-to-male link for hunting purposes became programmed into man's life cycle. . . . It seems logical that natural selection would eventually seize on this bonding pattern and weave it into the chromosomes of men. When hunting was no longer necessary for survival, the bonding pattern would still persist." Whether it's a lodge meeting, a golf game, or simply a drink at the local pub, men crave the emotional security of this all-male atmosphere from time to time. Fast adds, "Scratch the surface of most men and you will find that often their happiest days were spent in the company of other men."

So let him go with good grace. Urge him to be one of the gang. If you do, two things will happen. (1) He will adore you; (2) he'll find that he doesn't want to retreat into that all-male atmosphere half as often as his buddies do.

And along this same line, a woman can justify encouraging her man to go hunting and fishing with the boys. I realize that it is unfashionable these days to approve of "blood" sports, but from a realistic viewpoint, hunting and fishing allow him a little relaxation away from the pressure of our urban society, while giving him an outlet for his aggression. And any woman who sees her hero returning from a deer camp—muddy, unshaven, smelling of strong drink, and desperately in need of a deodorant—can be certain that he hasn't spent the weekend with another woman. What woman would have him in that condition?

But even if you are a warm, knowledgeable, sympathetic paragon of female wisdom, you still may have problems to face.

THE MALE MENOPAUSE:
HE HAS HIS PROBLEMS TOO

If the man in your life is anywhere between thirty-eight and fifty-five, you may be asking yourself if you can be sure of *anything* about him. He's become so withdrawn, so irritable, that you don't know him at all. What's the trouble?

Although medical opinions vary on the existence of a physiological male menopause, almost everyone seems to agree that men go through a very traumatic period in their middle years. (Just ask the *real* experts—their wives.) These emotional problems are compounded by the fact that, as we have seen, men have a much lower level of introspection and self-awareness. They may be miserable and upset, but they don't know why.

Just what's happening to that man of yours? According to many psychologists, much of this strain is related to his business success. There is tremendous pressure on the American male to achieve. The man in his forties who has not fulfilled his highest goals in terms of success and power may feel that he is a total failure—that his life is meaningless. Adding to his problems is the fact that, in our society his business accomplishments seem to directly reflect his virility.

This mid-life crisis in a man's life can be likened to a "horizon." Mrs. Charlotte Darrow, a sociologist who is studying the phenomenon at Yale University, says, "It is a kind of crest in life, from which he can look back as well as ahead, and the vista can be troubling." Another conclusion of the Yale study is that during this mid-life period a man desperately needs to feel that, in his own eyes and in the opinion of society, he is fulfilling the roles he values most.

The Ageless Woman can help her man by a sympathetic realization that he, too, is going through a difficult period, by bolstering his ego in the many ways we've already discussed, and especially *by analyzing his ideal concepts of himself and helping him feel successful in those areas.*

But what if you're tired of catering to him, pampering him, in fact being concerned about him? What are the alternatives? According to Don Schanche in an article for *Family Weekly,* "Statistics have long shown that [for men] the years between thirty-five and forty-five are times of especially high risk for suicide, divorce, extramarital affairs, career dislocations, and accidents among other lamentable events."

And one of the most lamentable of these events, certainly the most devastating to the ego of the mature woman, is the phenomenon of the mature man and the younger woman.

WHY MATURE MEN ARE ATTRACTED TO YOUNGER WOMEN (AND WHAT YOU CAN DO ABOUT IT)

It happens every day. That "ideal" marriage of twenty-five years collapses because *he* has run off with a younger woman. We shrug our shoulders and accept this all too common event as "one of those things." But what does the younger woman have that the middle-aged woman doesn't? It's certainly an important question—one that every married woman mulls over from time to time (just in case). But it's essential that all women, regardless of their marital status, take a long, cold, analytical look at the problems presented by the younger woman. As Louise Athearn points out in her book *What Every Formerly Married Woman Should Know*, "There are over forty million women in this country today—single, married, divorced, or widowed. And the projection is for another three million by 1975. There are thirty-six million men over forty—single, married, divorced, or widowed. So the competition is very keen, not just because of the younger women but because of the shortage of men." The competition is even further intensified because today some mature women are looking toward the other end of the calendar, toward the younger man (an interesting new trend that we'll be discussing in the next chapter). But for the moment let's concentrate on the competition offered by the younger woman and see what we can learn from her.

1. *The Younger Woman Doesn't Remind a Man of His Mother.* Dr. Rubin explains, "Consciously, many men view their wives as sex partners, but unconsciously they regard them as mothers. This combination causes conflict and confusion. . . ." Oh boy, does it! And this conflict is increased if the mature wife "lets herself go" both mentally and physically and becomes the motherly, neuter figure that we see all too often in the over-forty group. This combination creates in her husband a Freudian battleground of repressed guilts and conflicts—which we needn't go into here. But this is one of the essential reasons for the appeal of the younger woman.

Dr. Daniel J. Levinson explains that during one period in a man's life he may welcome and enjoy "mothering." From about the age thirty-two to thirty-eight, the period that Dr. Levinson terms the "settling down" period, a man may welcome or even invite the nurturing, "mothering" attention of his wife.

But around forty there's a turnover point. From this time on he actively rejects this mothering, which reminds him of the restraints and dependencies of his "settling down" period. And, sadly, many married men choose this time to reassert their independence from Mama by having affairs with other women, usually young women who do not have the "maternal aura."

So the moral of the story is this: even though we know that men retain many "little boy" qualitites, it's a very foolish woman who plays "mama" to that over-forty husband of hers.

2. *The Younger Woman Is More Interested in His Work.* Not always, but often, that appealing younger woman in a mature man's life is a part of his working life. And naturally she will be aware of the details, the emergencies, and the triumphs of his work. By contrast, it's shocking how many wives have only the vaguest notion of what their husbands "do" all day at the office. As Dr. Hyman Spotnitz explains in his book *The Wandering Husband,* "Also ripe for affairs are those husbands whose wives do not understand how important it is for them to succeed in their work. A man staggers under the burden of proving himself in a career, usually against keen competition. If a wife does not realize how much he needs support, particularly when things do not go well, he will swiftly find some woman who is sympathetic."

And the chances are excellent that she will be a younger woman.

3. *The Younger Woman—"Makes Him Feel Younger Just to Look at You."* The clever ad man who created that slogan was expressing one of the great truths. As Dr. Joyce Brothers explains it, "Men frequently judge how they are aging by looking at their wives for a reflection rather than by looking in the mirror. This is one of the reasons men in this age bracket may be attracted to girls young enough to be their daughters."

Of course a man who's compulsively and constantly obsessed by much younger women has a real problem—and, if he's your man, so have you. Because if eighteen or twenty is his idea of heaven, he has problems that neither you nor anyone else can solve. And if it comes to that, why bother? You'll just have to rebuild your own life without that neurotic mess. But you might find some comfort in the fact that the man who is only attracted to young girls isn't such a helluva fella after all. According to Dr. Brothers, he may really be looking for his mommy. "Sometimes, a man who finds himself attracted to young girls is really running after the memory of his mother, who is forever young and beautiful in his childhood memories. In his middle years [his wife] may remind him of his mother at a period of his life he would like to forget."

But most well-adjusted men (and yes, there are some, in spite of all their problems and conflicts) will find that the mature woman who is the Ageless Woman, who follows all the guidelines that we've discussed, will make him feel all-man.

4. *The Younger Woman Doesn't Know Everything.* And unfortu-

nately the mature woman often gives the impression that *she* does. After years of managing her home and guiding her children, of coping with crises and problems, she may storm into every social situation with the obnoxious aura of a camp counselor "taking charge of Tent Number 3." When it comes to the man in her life, she knows everything too. She has an opinion about everything and always has the last word. She knows exactly where he should park the car and just *how* he should park the car—"No, no, Harry, back up about a foot." She reminds him to have his hair cut, reminds him that it's Election Day, and reminds him of how "they" had decided to vote.

In groups, this capable lady knows (and pre-empts) the punch line to every story that he tells, supervises his drink mixing ("For heaven's *sakes*, Harry, not so much gin . . ."), describes to the assembled company exactly how "they" felt about their recent vacation, and knows all the rules to every game.

The younger woman, by contrast, does not know everything. She's not dumb, mind you. (If she's stolen your man, how dumb can she be?) But because she's young she doesn't know *everything*. Even her serious and outspoken opinions can be taken with avuncular tolerance. And he can play one of his favorite roles—that of Pygmalion. He can teach her things—how to sail, how to buy stocks, how to make the perfect martini ("The secret, my dear, is to use *enough* gin . . ."), and of course, how to *really* experience love.

If you'll take a good look at the man in your life, you'll recognize the importance of this teaching role in the man-woman relationship. And you can think back to the many times he's wanted to play a proud Pygmalion to your Galatea. "Now look, hon', here's exactly how you bait the hook . . ." or, "Maybe I can give you a few pointers on that backhand. If you'll just move to a count of three . . ."

And perhaps you remember his proud reaction when he introduced you to something new. "Listen, it's her first backpacking trip, and she carried that pack without a murmur . . ." or, "Ellen's become a crackerjack bridge player since I've been working with her . . ."

And what about the "Sleeping Beauty" syndrome, the universal masculine desire to awaken those smoldering passions and teach a woman how to *really* experience love? Well, granted, no amount of magic is going to turn you into an innocent young virgin, aware for the first time of the unsuspected joys of love. But then, no amount of magic is going to turn very many of today's younger women into innocent young virgins either. So the competition isn't as great as you might imagine on *that* level. In fact, in some ways the mature woman who has retained her femininity may have more vulnerable appeal along this line than a jaded "your-place-or-mine" member of the "now" generation.

Before we leave this subject I have to say a word to those of you who are outraged at the idea of "catering to his ego." "Listen, if I know how to mix a better martini, I'm going to tell him about it!" or, "Why should I stand still for all this Pygmalion stuff? I'm as good a tennis player as he is, any day." I'm not suggesting that you pretend ignorance, that you "let him win." What I am suggesting is that you allow the man in your life the same consideration that you would extend to any friend.

If a girl friend of yours is explaining the details of her trip to New York, you let her tell her story. You don't jump in with your version of how she *should* have planned her trip. (At least I hope you don't. Or you have few friends.)

A friend who is sharing the details of her secret recipe for fondue won't appreciate it if you say, "Oh, but that's all wrong. You mustn't use just any white wine, but a touch of vermouth." It's *her* recipe and if you're a good friend you give her the ego satisfaction of sharing it with you. So why can't we treat the men in our lives with the same sort of consideration that we extend to our friends?

And why can't we see the "honesty" of these militant types for what it really is—a deep-seated hostility that seeks not equality but dominance; not recognition, but revenge?

5. *The Younger Woman Is More Fun.* ("Heh, heh . . . I'll bet!") Seriously, the prelude to a fun time in bed is a fun time out of bed. The younger woman is often more fun, more enthusiastic, more spontaneous than the mature woman. Admittedly, it doesn't always follow. Some younger women are as negative, inflexible, and downright *old* as the most confirmed Professional M.A.M. But of course this type isn't going to appeal to *any* man.

What does appeal to the mature man is the air of childlike spontaneity—and the willingness to be pleased. These two charming qualities can be present at any age, but unfortuntely the mature woman too often allows them to shrivel and die through lack of use.

Here are some examples of what I mean:

HE: "It's started to rain. Shall we call off the picnic?"
THE Y.W. "It might be fun to sit under that tree . . . and if we put the blanket over our heads, we shouldn't get too wet. . . ."

THE M.A.M. "I'm certainly not going to sit out here and ruin my hair. You go back and get the car, and here, take the basket while I gather up the dishes, and now don't forget to put the ice chest in the back seat on the plastic sheet, and remember to etc., etc."

HE: "I have the last two tickets in the world to that play we've been wanting to see. It's four o'clock now. Can you be ready by six? We'll go to dinner and then the show."

THE Y.W. "Wow, that's great news. It *is* short notice, and I've got a thousand things to do. But I can't pass up this chance to see Olivier, and you won't mind if my hair's a mess, will you? Hey, this'll be fun. See you at six."

THE M.A.M. "Oh *no*. I've got a roast in the oven. And the children said they might drop by tonight. And you promised to take the car in for its checkup tomorrow morning, and you know how exhausted you feel if you're out too late. Besides, I understand that Canby gave the play just so-so reviews, so maybe it's not worth the effort, etc., etc."

But such enthusiastic, positive attitudes are not the exclusive domain of youth. The Ageless Woman is also positive, fun-loving, and enthusiastic. Perhaps, to play it safe, the Ageless Woman should memorize the following set of contrasting attitudes that can help set her apart from the professional M.A.M.s

The A.W. says yes. The M.A.M. says no.
The A.W. is flexible. The M.A.M. is inflexible.
The A.W. welcomes change. The M.A.M. resists change.
The A.W. says "How can we . . . ?" The M.A.M. says, "We can't possibly . . ."
The Ageless Woman is positive. The Professional M.A.M. is negative.

WHO'S AFRAID OF HUGH HEFNER?

As I've said before, the mature woman who follows the guidelines in this book will have little to fear from the younger woman. As the Ageless Woman, she combines the best of two worlds, youth and maturity. Granted, there will always be some men whose S.Q. (sex quotient) never goes beyond Bunny Booby, the twenty-year-old with the forty-inch bust and I.Q. to match. But men, *real* men, will always be attracted to the Ageless Woman, because she is a unique person, indelible, impossible to forget. Being unique, she is a little unpredictable. She is fun. (There will be very few surprises with Bunny B.) And finally, because she possesses that rare quality among women—*she really understands men.*

"YES, BUT . . . WHY ME? WHY MUST I DO ALL THE UNDERSTANDING? WHY MUST I DO ALL THE ADJUSTING? WHY CAN'T MEN WORRY ABOUT FILLING MY NEEDS?"

You're right, of course. At first glance, it doesn't seem fair. In fact, it isn't fair. But the very concept of "fair" implies an equality between the sexes and, as everyone knows, the sexes certainly aren't equal. A quick review of all those typical masculine traits should convince you—*women are undeniably the superior sex.*

But to get back to your question, "Why me?" If not you, who else? Woman must take the initiative in establishing understanding between the sexes. As we have seen, men don't understand women: they don't even understand themselves. For all the reasons that I've discussed in the previous pages, men have little patience for unraveling the complex threads that make up their personal relationships. The very attitudes that define masculinity in our society make it difficult for a man to *initiate* changes in his relationships. However, because most men really are lovable, kind, good, and downright irresistible under that gruff exterior, they can, with our sympathetic guidance and encouragement, be freed from their narrow, stereotyped machismo conditioning so that the full spectrum of their human qualities and attitudes can flower.

Unfortunately the attitudes that breed misunderstanding and antagonism between the sexes are liable to be especially strong in mature men—and that probably means Your Man.

By contrast, women are natural experts in dealing with people on the "feeling" level. As Dr. Theodore Rubin points out, women are "more in touch with deep feelings, and more accepting of human limitations. . . ." The result of this natural tendency is this: women recognize interpersonal problems sooner than men do. And women don't have that horrendous masculine pride that prevents men from seeking help. That's why the offices of psychiatrists, psychologists, and counselors are filled with women. It's not that women are nuttier than men—but women are more likely to recognize personal problems and seek solutions. On the other hand, he's more likely to tell his troubles to Joe, the bartender—or that friendly redhead at the other end of the bar. Or he will bottle up his troubles inside himself, which makes him even more vulnerable to the "pressure" diseases—ulcers, high blood pressure, and heart attacks.

Women who don't get in-person help can turn to the newspaper, magazines, or books. These are filled with perceptive, practical articles that increase a woman's insight into the problems and motivations of the people in her life. (After all, you, and not your husband, are reading *this* book.)

But where does he go for help and advice? You can faithfully study the sports page and you'll never see an article like this: "How My No-hit Game Caused Psychological Problems in My Marriage." And men's magazines will just multiply his problems, because they accent the difference between his real life and the fantasy life of the super-male. You know, "How I Stapled 17 *Playboy* Centerfolds in One Erotic Night," or some such thing.

"YES, BUT . . . THIS IS REALLY TOO MUCH.
DO I HAVE TO GO THROUGH LIFE
ANALYZING A MAN, CATERING TO HIS COMPLEXES,
ADJUSTING TO HIS NEEDS?
I DON'T THINK IT'S WORTH IT."

Look, don't be mad at *me*. I didn't make up the rules, I'm just describing what they *are*. It's up to you to decide whether you want to play to win—or to lose. For that matter, it's up to you to decide what you consider winning and losing.

Every real woman clearly recognizes that we live in a world of women *and* men, and that we must all understand the world as it is today before we can begin to make meaningful and worth-while changes. How can we expect sympathy and understanding for our problems if we have no sympathy and understanding for the problems of men? How can we expect to live a happy, fulfilling life if we live in a constant state of conflict with our men?

The point is this: in an era when women are increasingly becoming aware of their own powers, and of the age-old prejudices and controls that men have used in their attempts to mask those powers, it's essential that women do not become embittered and twisted by feelings of hostility. Women must be careful not to make the same mistakes that men have been making throughout thousands of years.

It's essential that women learn to use their superior insights, intuition, and sensitivity to smooth out the rapidly evolving man-woman relationships—and to quiet men's fears about their changing role in the new relationships.

And believe me, those fears exist. Countless psychologists, psychiatrists, sociologists, and anthropologists have revealed that men have always suffered from an almost universal distrust, uncertainty, and above all fear in their relationship with women—fear that they may never fully understand.

And as women become more and more enlightened about their own shining destiny, the insecurities of men are likely to become intensified. It has happened before. Over two thousand years ago, the Roman senator Cato summed up the fears of men. Warning his fellow senators against the insurgent women of Rome, he said, "The moment they have arrived at an equality with you, they will become your masters and superiors." And to many modern men, that same moment of truth is clearly at hand.

But the Ageless Woman can make certain that the fears of men are unfounded. As every Ageless Woman knows, a world of masters and servants is no fun at all. Women have lived through enough aeons of this unequal social and emotional setup to realize that it's no good.

The Ageless Woman does not want another world of masters and servants. She wants instead a world where both men and women can be free to develop their own personalities and reach toward their own destinies without being shackled by outworn, medieval restrictions.

And if men find it difficult to adjust to the changing man-woman relationships, the Ageless Woman must be ready to help. She can do it.

The Ageless Woman, freed by self-knowledge and secure in the essential superiority of her female wisdom, can afford to be generous to the man in her life. She has developed enough emotional security to bolster his sagging ego without diminishing her own. She can allay his deep-seated fears. Why not?

It's clearly a case of *noblesse oblige*.

ELEVEN

Whatever Happened to Your Marriage?

"Nothing. Absolutely nothing." After fifteen, twenty, or thirty years of marriage, this can be a pretty common answer. But if you think nothing's been happening to your marriage, you just haven't been paying attention. Because, next to that crisis time popularly known as the Seven Year Itch, the middle years of a marriage are its most vulnerable, the time when the relationship is either irrevocably put away in moth balls, is canceled due to lack of interest, or, less often, blossoms out into a newer, more exciting version of its original self. In other words, at a time of life when both you and your husband are facing all the physical and emotional changes brought on by the advent of middle age, your marriage is in for a radical change too. But with a little knowledge, a little effort, a lot of wisdom, and a generous dash of humor, you can help your marriage change for the better.

Just what ails the middle-aged marriage? Balzac said it—"Mar-

riage must conquer the monster that devours . . . its name is Habit."
And that dull old monster, Habit, seems most at home in the bedroom.

BED AND BORED?

Habit in the bedroom can best be described as having three
characteristics—the same time, the same place, and the same position. As one friend described her sex life, "We're so predictable, we
could be listed in *TV Guide* as Wednesday Night Wrestling. The
same damned ritual every Wednesday, year in and year out—it's
driving me crazy!"

Of course, the most obvious solution to bedroom boredom is the
sex manual. And a quick glance at a list of best-selling books will
prove that millions of people are choosing this solution. But reputable experts in the field of marital relations are saying that, in many
cases, the cure can kill the patient.

Picture the bedrooms of America. Instead of a love scene, cozy
and intimate, we seem to see a shadowy C. B. DeMille mob scene.
Milling around the conjugal bed are Masters and Johnson, The Sensuous Man, The Sensuous Woman, Dr. Reuben, and even venerable
old Dr. Kinsey totters into view, all making judicious notations and
filling out IBM cards.

Thrust into this atmosphere of charts, graphs, and performance
levels, our lovers resemble nothing so much as a pair of Olympic con-
tenders on a segment of "Wide World of Sports." At the conclusion
of a most intimate moment, we half expect to see Masters, Johnson,
and Kinsey spring to their feet, each holding up a score card—89, 93,
97—to the sound of wild applause in the background.

And when they're not competing for points or grading each other
on performance, our tender lovers are practicing all those positions
with the dedicated solemnity of one striving to perfect a tennis
backhand. With a manual in one hand and a portion of anatomy in
the other, they go at it. "Position 210A: place leg A over torso B.
Now, in a lilting ¾ time . . ." One wonders if the next logical development will be something like this:

"Honey, I've signed up for a few lessons with the pro."

"Oh, great! That old 210A *is* tricky."

The point of the story is this. Although our enlightened attitudes
toward sex make it increasingly possible to take the doldrums out of

middle-aged marriage, we should be aware that some of the attitudes embodied in the technique books can have a very negative effect on any relationship. The old numbers game, the endurance contest, and the impersonal, push-button implications of "You do this to me, and then I'll do that to you" are appalling.

Where's the humanity? And where's the human fun? "The technique books shy away from only one four letter word—love. They overlook the fact that most people have sexual relations out of genuine feeling for each other . . . this doesn't enter the picture at all," says Dr. Walter Stewart, a New York-based psychoanalyst and specialist in sexual pathology. He adds, "You get smarter, but not wiser . . . technique is meaningful only when it leaves some area for spontaneity."

So don't be intimidated by the sex books. Use your own imagination. What's wrong with Thursday? How about a little love in the afternoon? A little lust for lunch? And unless you have a bad back or a trick knee, that king-size bed isn't the *only* possibility, you know. One of the great charms of illicit love (so I'm told) is the atmosphere of stolen moments in out-of-the-way places. That deserted boathouse, that double sleeping bag, that Las Vegas Hilton . . . but you get the idea.

TRY IT, YOU'LL LIKE IT

Of course, the same old routine performed at the top of the Empire State Building at high noon is still that same old routine. So experiment a bit. And though there's no shortage of sexperts to give you an in-depth picture of the range of possibilities, they all seem to concur on this basic point: if it feels good—do it.

Another area of mutual agreement is that communication is basic to success. All the experts in erotica say, "Talk it over—discuss your likes and dislikes, your sexual preferences." And that would be excellent advice if it didn't overlook one fact of supreme importance. The middle-aged marriage is almost always suffering from a total breakdown in communication—*all* communication. How can the overly married couple talk about their love life, when they haven't really talked *to* each other in years? There may be a spurt of desultory conversation now and then, but each partner has learned the trick of tuning out. The familiar voice of one's spouse drones on and on. But the adept tuner-outer can select a fall wardrobe, plan a safari to

Africa, decide what vegetables to serve for dinner, or even, if one is *really* good at it, live three days (and nights) as mistress of a Knight of the Round Table.

Think about it. How long has it been since you *really* listened to that man of yours? And how long has it been since he really listened to you? After a bit of soul searching, you may come to the same conclusion that hit many of my students. "Good heavens, we haven't actually communicated in years."

TÊTE-À-TÊTE

Here's a simple test that will tell you more about the state of your relationship than a trip to the local marriage counselor. Go out to dinner, alone with your husband. Of course you've no doubt been doing this regularly for years. But *this* time, pay close attention to the subjects of your conversation. What do you have to say to each other? Is your conversation totally enmeshed in domestic trivia? "When should we paint the house?" "Do we need a new water heater?" Or is your time together always related to problems? Where to get the money for Junior's next college tuition payment? Or a discussion of the rise in your insurance rates?

One student who tried this test was appalled to note that she and her husband segué-ed from a discussion of life insurance premiums during the salad to an analysis of the best place to purchase burial plots with the entree, and "seasoned" dessert with a spirited argument over whether they should rest in adjoining plots.

She later told me that she privately decided then and there on separate plots. "We're boring each other to death in this life," she said. "We should also bore each other throughout eternity?"

Well, there's never an excuse for being bored in this life. And we'll be discussing several techniques that will help you put some sparkle back into your marriage. But let's continue with our analysis for a moment.

A REMEMBRANCE OF THINGS PAST

What if you find that your dinner-table conversation is almost solely devoted to memories? If the theme of your time together is strictly a remembrance of things past, your relationship is surely floundering in the dangerous shoals of marriage boredom. If looking back is all you have in common, you're in trouble.

Of course memory is one of the miracles of the human mind, but nostalgia, like perfume, should not be overdone. In fact, memories should play a relatively small part in your life. And sometimes memories don't mean the same things to two people. You may be looking back to carefree times when the children were young, when you lived in a small house, and when life was simpler. But to him, these early years may bring back unpleasant thoughts of his beginning career struggles, his frustrations, and even to uncomfortable pictures of the man he used to be and would rather forget. He doesn't want to be reminded of those early years—and he doesn't thank you for constantly pulling him back to an unhappy time.

Or perhaps he's the one who's always looking back, with the bittersweet conviction that things will never be as satisfying as they were in "the good old days." If so, he needs your help. Blast him out of that rut. Remember, if memory plays too large a part in your life together, it reveals that the present and future are not meaningful and that you and your relationship are not growing. You have allowed your present and future to become so drab that you need to escape to the past—and probably to a romanticized version of the past that is more pleasant in wistful memory than it ever was in actuality. So whatever your age, be wary of overindulgence in memory trips. They're especially bad medicine for the ailing middle-aged marriage.

SOME PRESCRIPTIONS

Rebuilding those lines of communication can bring new and exhilarating levels of intimacy to your marriage relationship. "Getting to Know You" might be the theme song of your next evening out together. And a good way to start is to *listen*. Encourage *him* to talk. Do you find that this is difficult? Okay. You've learned a lot about your relationship already.

But with effort you can draw him out, and you'll inevitably be surprised at what has been simmering in his mind.

You'll probably be shocked enough to really go to work and try to learn something. What's going on inside his head? You may think you know all about his job, his hobbies, his hangups. But how does he *really* feel about his job? What is the basis of his satisfaction with his hobbies? And why the hangups? And how much does he know about what's been happening inside *your* head? Have you attempted to share your life with him? Does *he* think so?

Of course this kind of in-depth sharing shouldn't develop into a do-it-yourself psychoanalysis session over a plate of eggs foo yung. If you have to talk out serious problems, choose another time and place. The idea behind this getting-to-know-you session is that it should be a fun, positive time to get reacquainted with that partner whom you think you know so well. And a time that gives him a chance to realize all over again that you're a pretty fascinating woman—and he's lucky to have you.

And if you *really* listen, you will almost automatically become about 75 per cent more fascinating immediately. The rewards of actively listening to your husband are twofold. First, you will be astonished to find out what has happened to your man during the twenty years or so since you last paid attention. And second, if you show that much interest in him, you will inevitably get *his* attention. He will want to know more about the captivating woman who has suddenly become such a brilliant conversationalist.

Then it will be *your* turn. Communications must flow both ways. And once you have captured his full attention (perhaps for the first time in years), then you can finally begin to talk to *him*. Share with him that mysterious inner life that you have been developing. And if it seems that you are doing all the work, taking all the initiative in revitalizing this relationship—well, *you are*. If you don't, who will— or can, for that matter? Remember what we talked about in the last chapter?

One couple I know started some of my married students playing a version of twenty questions, but with a twist designed to make it even more intriguing for those who have been married for oh-so-long. A couple takes turns asking a key question. For instance, she may ask him, "What's your favorite color? But then *she* must answer it. After eighteen years, does she know what his favorite color is? And as the game progresses, can they answer such questions as "What's your favorite song?" "What's your pet peeve?" "What would be your dream vacation?" And, "How do you like your eggs prepared?" (Some startling revelations can materialize—after preparing seven thousand breakfasts, one woman found that her husband *loathed* eggs sunny side up. See? Love and learn.) Occasionally this little game can take on a rather bawdy touch. Question: "How many moles do you have?" Answer: "I can't remember, but let's go home and find out." Anyway, this is just one approach that can start couples talking again—and laughing together—and who knows what else?

Or you might take a tip from the Duchess of Windsor. She was explaining to an interviewer that the circumstances of her marriage to the duke made it imperative that they maintain a high level of romance and interest in their relationship. She explained that after ten or fifteen years of marriage the titled couple didn't dare go out to dinner alone and settle into that ruminative limbo that we see all too often at tables for two.

If they sat, staring off into space, two apparent strangers shackled together by marriage vows, rumors would immediately abound that their marriage was on the rocks and he'd given up the throne for nothing.

So the duchess would purposely save bits of news, gossip, a funny story or two, until they were out alone together. And then she'd have something new, amusing, and perhaps surprising to contribute to the conversation. The sight of the two of them, laughing and talking animatedly, kept the storybook picture alive. But obviously it had an even more important effect—that of maintaining their interest in each other, of keeping a sparkle and zest in their relationship.

You, too, can use this conversational gambit. When you've heard a new joke, discovered a new book, or know an amusing bit of gossip, *don't waste it.* Don't blurt it out before his first cup of morning coffee or during the half-time of Monday night football. Save these fun and juicy bits of conversation for a time when you are "alone at last." It will make that "alone" time more fun, more stimulating for both of you.

"YES, BUT . . . I THINK THIS IS THE MOST ARTIFICIAL IDEA I'VE EVER HEARD. WHAT'S MORE, IT SEEMS SOMEHOW DISHONEST."

Does it? Does it seem artificial to look at that man you've been living with all these years and really *see* him? Does it seem artificial to work at re-creating the interest, the intimacy, and the love that you once had in your relationship? (And if you've never had these things in your marriage, isn't it about time you did?)

The woman who considers this type of effort to be artificial is a woman we've met often in these pages. She's the one who wants to be totally natural, to be the "real me," who insists (from God knows what subconscious compulsion) that the only real, honest things in life are the ordinary things, the second-rate things, the dull things.

As writer Michael Drury says, "Some people insist that 'real life' inevitably comes down to dental bills and diapers and new tires for the car . . . [but] life consists of all the ways of living that there are, and every single one of them is real. . . . *It is inertia and distorted emphasis that flatten life out.*" (Emphasis added.)

Revitalizing the middle-aged marriage does take some thought and effort. But then, so does a passionate love affair. Love is not a game for the lazy, the dull, the unimaginative.

The woman who worries about the "honesty" of this kind of effort is usually the same woman whose marriage has degenerated into a numbing charade played by two strangers. Living with a man, making love to a man you don't even know, much less like—well, I think that's not only dishonest but downright degrading.

Remember, you can't have it both ways. You can't take the familiarity, the damned dailiness, out of the middle-aged marriage without a bit of seemingly artificial effort. And of course it will seem artificial at first if it's a completely new way of looking at things, a new attitude. It can't seem perfectly natural or comfortable or "old shoe" if it is brand new. And hurray for that! Something different is just what the doctor ordered.

And here's something else that the doctor ordered to revitalize the sex life of the middle-aged marriage.

THE CASE FOR SEDUCTION

One of the greatest problems in the sex life of the mature marriage is the different rate of sexual desire between mature men and women. As every expert from Kinsey to Masters and Johnson have noted, the sexual desires of mature women tend to increase with the passing years while mature men find that the hot-blooded, ready-anytime passions of their youth tend to cool somewhat, often to the consternation and chagrin of the man in question.

And this is where the importance of seduction comes in. The wife in a middle-aged marriage, who has been feeling hurt and neglected because of his seeming indifference, will find that a bit of seduction on her part can revitalize their relationship in some very satisfying ways. Sex expert Dr. Judith Antrobus, in an article in *McCall's*, reports that women's sexual advances, in the sense of invitations to love-making, are stimulating and potency-producing for most men. "In my practice," she says, "I find many men who report that they feel more, rather than less potent with women who make their sexual interest and enthusiasms known." Conversely, a wife's anti-seductive attitudes can so effectively turn off the mature husband that he may become panicky about implications of permanent impotence and frantically leap into bed with another woman—*any* woman—just to prove to himself that he can still do it.

What are some of these turn-offs? Not surprisingly, they're actions and attitudes that we've been deploring throughout this book. But hearing about their destructive effects on your sex life from a sex expert might just reinforce the point. Dr. Helen Kaplan, director of sexual therapy at a New York hospital, pinpoints them as attitudes that seem to insist, "Take me as I am, like it or not." And she enumerates them as "the anti-erotic things a woman is not always aware she is doing, like belittling her husband, or starting arguments just before bedtime, or saying, 'I'll come to bed after the late show,' or wearing curlers, cold cream, and an old flannel nightgown without considering his preferences."

Now such anti-erotic behavior might not have an adverse affect on a man's sexual prowess when he's vigorous and young (just look at your son's stringy-haired, whining girl friend), but Dr. Kaplan warns, "as a man gets older he becomes more sensitive to the love making technique and to any detrimental factors in the relationship."

And if you feel resentful that *you* must make the initial effort, remember that it all comes back to the inescapable superiority of women. As Dr. Martin Grotjahn says in his book *Beyond Laughter*, the mature woman "smiles tolerantly and pretends to accept the male's false claim of superiority over her, because every time the man approaches her sexually she can show her superiority. She is always ready, he must get ready. For the man, the sexual act is a test, an examination, a performance. If the woman so chooses, she may watch the performance and still perform. The man needs cooperation; so to speak, he needs a helping hand. The man is dependent: either he can do it or he cannot do it. The woman is always potentially potent. . . ."

So adding a good measure of seduction to your sex life is an ingredient that's guaranteed to bring some spice back into the middle-aged marriage.

"WHAT IS SEDUCTION AND HOW DO I DO IT?"

Oh, oh. The mature woman who has to ask this question definitely has a problem. She has become what I call overly married; and to find the answer to her question she must, first of all, look back past all those years of housewifery and childbearing and remember some of her attitudes and actions during the first years of her marriage. Then she should reread the section on sex appeal. And think about it. As columnist and Ageless Woman Suzy advises, "Seduction, darlings, springs from the brain, the imagination. . . ."

But if memory fails you and your imagination seems a bit uninspired, here are some suggestions from the Ageless Woman (not necessarily in the order of their effectiveness . . .):

1. Nibble his ear.

2. Listen to him. "When you really listen, love is what you'll find."

3. Wake him up in the morning with a kiss on the back of his neck.

4. Learn the difference between a pat and a caress.

5. Tell him that he's handsome. Tell him he's a marvelous lover. Tell him you love him. Tell him, tell him, tell him.

6. When you're together, don't let an hour go by without touching.

7. Look deep, deep into his eyes with a look that says, "You're the most wonderful man in the world." And mean it! (This is pretty potent, so don't overdo it. Even once a week is enough.)

8. Buy a good book on massage. Read it! (Honest. This was recommended by an outstanding marriage counselor whom I interviewed.)

9. Some Sunday morning, have strawberries and champagne for breakfast—in bed.

10. Remember the power of lace, chiffon, and the slinkiest material of all—your own perfumed skin.

FLOWER POWER: SCENTS—OR NONSENSE?

Can perfume drive him mad with desire? According to Dr. Ivan Popov, former physician to King Peter II of Yugoslavia and rejuvenation expert to the jet set, the effect of scent on the human body and mind is incalculable. Dr. Popov, who calls himself an aroma therapist, says that the effects of various aromas and scents on the human organism were well known to the ancients. In fact, aromatics were the foundation of Egyptian medicine. The ancients listed some 700 different substances that could be used to effectively treat various bodily conditions.

Dr. Popov, who uses aroma therapy to treat everything from heart trouble to insomnia, has compiled a chart which classifies 400 aromatics according to their effects. He lists fragrances that are tranquilizers, stimulants, narcotics, and exaltants (one thinks of the incense used in many religious ceremonies) and, of course, fragrances that are erogenous and anti-erogenous. And Dr. Popov maintains the erogenous scents can definitely stimulate desire.

Would you be at all interested in knowing what particular scents have the most profound effect on the male libido? I thought so. Surprisingly, they are jasmine and roses. But the doctor warns that they must be the natural substances in order to be sexually stimulating.

And what about those exotic, musky perfumes that are traditionally rumored to turn him into a tiger? Those perfumes that the salesperson is apt to caution you about? "Saks takes no responsibility whatever for anything that may happen to you when you wear 'Night in the Seraglio.'" Well, aroma therapists say these perfumes have a reputation for being sexy because they make *us* feel sexy and daring and a bit naughty. But they don't really do much to men.

So choose your poison, and splash a little perfume here and there. Could it hurt?

Subtle seduction and imaginative sex can definitely put some zip back into that middle-aged marriage—but we have to come out of the bedroom sometime, and that's when couples find, all too often, that they are playing marriage games that paralyze their relationship. Sometimes a satisfying sex life can exist in spite of these games, but more often than not couples will find that the destructive games that spoil their relationship in the living room also make it impossible to enjoy fun and games in the bedroom.

Of course an analysis of severe psychological problems isn't the province of this book. If you and your husband are truly driving each other crazy, you need professional help.

But often we find that a marriage collects a few barnacles over the years in the form of negative habits or attitudes. These barnacles may not sink the ship but they do prevent the smooth sailing that's possible when this debris is recognized and removed. So let's look at some games that can make you a loser in middle-aged marriage. And then we'll consider some winning tickets.

SURE LOSERS IN THE MARRIAGE GAME

1. *Mother Knows Best.* We've already discussed the negative vibes created by the woman who is aggressively maternal, but this role can be so destructive to the mature marriage that it bears repeating. Many women play this game innocently and unconsciously. They emphatically are not using it to express their basic antipathy toward men. They like their men. But they developed habitual "mama" patterns that have become ingrained during their years of mothering several small children. And if a woman doesn't watch it she may continue to play this role indefinitely, even after the children are gone.

We can observe "mother," at her very best, at almost any suburban party. "Harry dear"—see, she really loves him—"go out and bring in the drinks, would you? And be careful not to spill them." . . . "No, Harry darling. You're messing it up. It wasn't a salesman at all. It was an advertising man and a rabbi and a priest." . . . "Harry, don't forget to take the coats and put them in the bedroom. And don't let them trail along the floor." . . . "Be sure to remember and tell the Powells what a good time we had at their party. . . ." And on and on. We've all witnessed this somewhat uncomfortable scene, and it doesn't take much imagination to see where these destructive habit patterns came from. "Johnny, tell Mrs. Smith all about the good time you had at summer camp. . . . Get Mrs. Smith some tea. . . . Now don't spill it. . . . Did you thank Mrs. Smith for the cookies she sent you . . . ?"

Here is a woman whose children are all grown but she's still being "mother"—responsible for everything about her family's behavior and well-being. And there is no one left to "mother" but her husband.

The game goes on long after the party is over. "Harry, you shouldn't have that coffee. It'll keep you awake." . . . "Sweetheart, if you don't come to bed now, you'll only get six hours of sleep." . . . "Here, dear, don't forget your sweater, your galoshes, your muffler."

What this woman needs is a poodle. Some little thing she can fuss over and manage and mother. And then she'd better start playing the role of *woman* to her man. If she doesn't, he's liable to find someone who will.

2. *Daddy's Little Girl.* We all use the dodge, "I'll have to ask my husband," but if your whole life is hemmed in by this attitude, look out. Over the years you've become Daddy's Little Girl, unable to make a move without getting his approval or permission. This isn't good for you and it isn't good for him. And while some men may *seem* to enjoy this lord and master routine, on the subconscious level they are actually bored to death by this docile and dull little woman.

I've met so many D.L.G.s in my classes—women who are depressed, discouraged, and looking for something to blast them out of their rut. But when the opportunity comes to bring a tiny change into their lives—well, it's "I have to ask my husband" time. "Oh, I can't color my hair. My husband doesn't like it." . . . "I never wear bright colors, George won't let me." . . . "I can't come to classes at night. My husband doesn't like it if I'm out in the evening." . . . "Oh, I don't work. My husband won't let me. . . ." But I've observed that while Baby Mouse is sitting in a corner at our class party Daddy is chasing after a blonde career woman in a red dress—and finding her pretty exciting, too.

If you suspect that you have been playing this role, isn't it about time you grew up? After all, marriage is for grownups. And a carefully thought-out assertion of individuality on your part—a demonstration that you are an adult, a woman, and a person in your own right—can do wonders for a marriage in the ho-hum years. (Not to mention what it will do for *you.*)

Remember, it's better to be a headache than a bore, so shake him up a bit—there's nothing duller than that completely predictable, docile woman, Daddy's Little Girl.

3. *The Realist.* This is a game played to perfection by the Professional M.A.M. We've seen her in action with her girl friends. "Let's face it, Ethel, none of us are getting any younger. . . ." But when

she zeros in on her husband she surpasses herself. "Listen, Stanley, it's foolish to waste money on those hair preparations. Your father was bald and you'll be bald." . . . "A red sports car? Nonsense, we'll get a beige sedan, just like always. After all, we're both getting too old for that sort of foolishness" . . . and so on. But even the most loving Unwilling M.A.M. can drive her husband to desperate measures that will prove his youth and virility, just by being "realistic." "I don't care what the doctor said. You're too old for tennis. After all, I'm just trying to be realistic." Or, "What's the point of dreaming about retirement in Mexico? We'll both be too old to live in that environment. We'll need to be near a hospital, and the doctor. . . ." And finally, "I know you're tired, dear, but you have to face it. After a certain age, we all slow down."

The realist is so busy looking at "facts" that she hasn't faced the reality that her husband has just as many problems adjusting to the middle years as she does. With help, he can become the Ageless Man. But with the kind of help she's giving him, he'll desperately look around for some means of proclaiming that he's *not* old, that there's some life in the old boy yet. And to prove it, he'll go overboard—like taking up motorcycle racing, mountain climbing, or hang gliding. Or maybe he'll just take up with the girls at the office. Or he may join the next expedition in search of the Abominable Snowman. (And *that's* a sure way to get rid of the realist.)

If you really want to be a realist, remember that he needs the assurance that he is dynamic, exciting, and ageless, just as much as you do. So build him up, flatter him, *encourage* him. If you don't, someone else will.

4. *The Love Bird.* George and Mary never fought because Mary didn't believe in fighting. Year in and year out, she swallowed her irritations and angers. And to everyone, George and Mary were the perfect couple. Even George thought that they were the perfect couple. And then one day at lunch George said, "You know, hon, I think the stew could use a little more salt."

"That does it!" Mary screamed, throwing down her napkin as if it were a gauntlet. "I've had it up to here with your constant nagging and carping. I want a divorce."

Poor George. He still doesn't know what hit him. And Mary doesn't understand that her perennial tendency to swallow every irritation (with or without salt) had built up over the years into a solid hatred that eventually killed the deep feelings she once had for

George. They actually did go ahead with the divorce, after George had listened, with hurt surprise, to a seemingly endless list of justified angers and irritations that Mary had been nurturing through the years.

Now Mary, that sweet "love bird," is ready to start all over again with Paul. They'll be married soon, and so far there hasn't been a ripple on the placid surface of their relationship. Of course Paul does a few things that drive her crazy. Like bringing his children over to her apartment on Saturday afternoons while he goes to play golf. And never telling her where they're going when he's planned an evening out. But Mary just smiles sweetly and swallows her irritation. Yep. That'll be another "perfect" marriage, unless Mary learns from her past mistakes. Constantly giving in on every point, swallowing every tiny irritation, just to maintain "harmony," means that those tiny irritations grow and grow and eventually stifle love.

"A certain amount of 'combatability' is part of compatibility," according to Dr. Hyman Spotnitz in his book, *The Wandering Husband*. He adds, "Married life does not have to be complete harmony. Dissonance adds interest, just as in a musical composition."

Unfortunately, too many women have been conditioned to be "good little girls." "It isn't nice to fight, darling." . . . "Now let your cousin play with your doll, don't quarrel about it" . . . and so on. Women who are sweet love birds have never learned to let off a little steam. With them, it's the atomic bomb or nothing. But every marriage can benefit from these little safety valves of small quarrels and differences of opinion. It saves the marriage from that one gigantic explosion that could be a disaster.

And since life is full of frustrations and irritations that produce a kind of floating anger, anger that may have nothing to do with one's partner, it's a good idea to have a harmless outlet for these angry feelings. Otherwise we tend to hit out at the nearest object—and that object is usually one's spouse.

One marriage counselor I talked to had an interesting suggestion for dealing with this natural anger. He urges married couples to indulge in what might be called abstract criticism by actively and vehemently criticizing movies, books, plays—and of course, that perfect scapegoat, the government.

A couple whom he counseled regularly attend a current movie and then go out for coffee and ice cream afterward. Over the chocolate sauce they give the film an in-depth criticism. And movies being what they are today, more often than not they are able to have a satisfying hour ripping it up one side and down the other. A harmless way of releasing hostility.

Another couple regularly compose letters to the editor—clever, scathing letters—about any current events that are irritating them. They have a fine time ranting, raving, and desk-pounding. And after the letters are in the mail they serenely spend a pleasant cocktail hour together.

And this shared criticism has another advantage. It means that the overly married couple, who may have drifted apart, are doing something together—even if it's only damning the government.

The point is, we shouldn't expect marriage to be one long unbroken expanse of calm and peace. (Time enough for that in those adjoining plots.) A few fireworks add some spice to our lives together.

5. *The Homebodies.* Both husbands and wives contribute equally to the popularity of this losing gambit in the marriage game. Our overly married pair find that, as the years go by, they stay home more and more. A certain amount of natural fatigue is multiplied by boredom, and every year it seems just "too much trouble" to be up and out and doing. This couple is usually glued to the boob tube every night. They know more about Marshal Dillon and Miz Kitty than they do about each other. Weekends are *always* spent puttering around the house and doing errands. How dull. No wonder they have little to say to one another—and no wonder their marriage is drowning in boredom.

The homebodies need to be jarred out of that rut—and once again, it's the Ageless Woman who has to save the day. Why? Because, first of all, she's aware that there is a problem. He just knows that he's overly tired (a sure sign of boredom) and feeling increasingly depressed. Second, she's tuned in to the idea that she can bring change and growth into her life (and his) by using a little creative planning. And third, as we've noted so often before, women are the superior sex.

Of course, it's easy to advise, "Pack up and fly away to Acapulco for a stimulating weekend," or "dress up and go out to dinner at a good restaurant and then see a play or go out dancing." But these suggestions are not only expensive—providing the perfect "Yes, but we can't afford it" cop-out—they also can seem alarmingly drastic and complicated to entrenched homebodies. Instead, try some modest, easy outings to start with—a trip to the river to admire the fall color, a walk through the streets of a nearby historic town. Little by little, you'll become more daring. You'll get out of that rut—and then, Acapulco, here you come.

One of the most helpful bits of advice I can give you is to remember that you don't necessarily have to go out at night. As a working woman, I'm sympathetic to my husband's aversion to going out on a week night after a full day's work. But how about meeting for lunch at a special restaurant? One can almost always arrange for an extended lunch hour, if it's only once a month or so.

A working couple I know have a monthly lunch date and try every elegant restaurant in their city—restaurants whose dinner menus might be beyond the budget of this gourmet couple. They became so involved in this project, and the subsequent criticism and analysis of each luncheon menu, that they thought others might be interested. So they started writing a "What's for lunch?" column for their local paper. Believe me, this couple doesn't find any shortage of things to talk about these days. And they've found that this one little project has not only revitalized their relationship but, by banishing boredom, it has given them both a new charge of energy and enthusiasm.

Another couple is geared to the outdoors. They often plan a fun Sunday morning outing by packing eggs, bacon, a camp stove, and all the Sunday papers in the car. Early in the morning they leave their city apartment and drive along one of the many beautiful lanes in the nearby countryside. After preparing a leisurely breakfast at some attractive spot (and yes, he helps too), they read the papers. Then they set off on an exploring expedition. Sometimes for variety they take bicycles and ride along the country lanes. Thrilling? Exciting? Not terribly—but fun, yes. Especially when you consider that it's an effective contrast to their weekdays, which are spent in hectic people-oriented jobs.

Other couples may visit the local museum, haunt the art galleries in hopes of discovering a new, as yet unrecognized painter. Or they may be more athletic and take up square dancing, backpacking, bird watching, bike riding, skiing, or the like.

There are many fun projects that a husband and wife can share. For instance, my husband "discovered" Admiral Nelson, Britain's incomparable naval hero, and immersed himself in a study of Nelson's battles. I listened dutifully as he told about the audacity of Nelson's night attack at the Battle of the Nile. I was intrigued by his vivid descriptions of tall masts and sails lighted by the flash of broadsides or the red glow of burning ships. I was caught up by his enthusiasm, but Nelson himself didn't really mean much to me until my husband said, "And why in the world did Lord Hamilton put up with that *ménage à trois?* After all, it was *his* wife. Why didn't he pitch Nelson right out on his ear?"

Then *I* was hooked. I read every book I could find about the intriguing Lady Hamilton—an international beauty who carried on a torrid affair with Nelson over three continents, seven years, and in spite of *her* husband and *his* wife. Sort of the Elizabeth Taylor of her day.

This shared interest culminated in a trip to England where the fascination with the Nelson-Hamilton caper is almost a cult. We saw Nelson's flagship, the *Victory*, which is preserved at Portsmouth. We blinked respectfully at Nelson's tiny seaman's hammock and reluctantly decided (in spite of my husband's ribald suggestions) that they never could have shared it—not *nearly* enough room. At the naval museum we looked at gowns that Lady Hamilton had worn, china they had used, love letters, and a pair of her faded gloves. We saw a British teen-ager, his eyes brimming with tears as he stood before Nelson's death mask. We have been talking about the trip ever since and planning another.

Each couple must work out the patterns of companionship that suit them best. Once, for instance, we were introduced to a charming couple during the intermission of a play. Although they were nearing their seventies and seemed rather fragile, we were struck by their agelessness—their sense of fun. To our astonishment, we met them again a few weeks later while we were backpacking in the Sierra Nevada mountains. This "fragile" couple was four miles from the end of the road and still climbing briskly, even though they were burdened with binoculars and well-filled knapsacks. We learned that they had taken up bird watching when he retired and are now two of the most knowledgeable "birders" in the San Francisco area.

With a little imagination, couples can add a new dimension of fun to their lives by such shared activities. The important thing is that they make a definite point to get out of those two well-worn ruts and into some new and different experience that they both enjoy. This is a big, beautiful world, and the possibilities are endless. And growing from these shared interests are many conversations, private jokes, and ultimately a renewed intimacy.

6. *The Gadabouts.* On the surface, Ed and Elaine had it made. They had so much fun together that the term "middle-aged malaise" couldn't possibly apply to their marriage. Just consider a typical week. Tuesday they attended one dinner party and Thursday hosted another. Being avid golfers, they *always* spent Saturday morning at the club. Saturday nights usually meant a charity dinner dance (they didn't miss any of them—name your disease and they were supporting the charity that's battling it.) And Sunday would find them at, say, a wine tasting sponsored by the local art council. It was just one whirl of social events. Yes, they were always together at some fun and exciting affair—and they were growing further apart every day.

Of course the reason is obvious. Every single free moment of their time was taken up with social events that kept them in the company of others. After all, who can say more than four words ("It's time to go.") to one's spouse at any dinner party? And that golf game? Ed played with his cronies and Elaine had a standing date with her foursome. Dinner dances, cocktail parties, after-the-play suppers—all involved a whirl of people avidly avoiding any meaningful or in-depth contact.

Now if Ed and Elaine had disliked one another, this would have been the perfect solution to keeping the marriage going. Many a loveless marriage has limped along for years on this regimen of hors d'oeuvres and shallow chitchat. But in spite of a creeping sense of isolation and indifference, Ed and Elaine did *care*. And because Elaine is an Ageless Woman, she realized what they were doing before it was too late. So she and Ed sat down one evening (after canceling out on a concert) and talked it over.

They finally decided that they had to rearrange their leisure time, and they ruthlessly cut their former social life in half. But since they're still gadabouts at heart, they determined that the rest of the time would be devoted to a social whirl that involved just the two of them. So instead of attending the theater with a mob of acquaintances they go by themselves and have an intimate supper *à deux* afterward. Or they spend a weekend at a nearby resort, trying out a new golf course—just the two of them.

7. *The Grandparents.* Grandchildren are wonderful—as someone has said, "It's all the fun of having children with none of the headaches." But the mature couple who become what I call Professional Grandparents are putting their marriage into mothballs. Couples whose every leisure moment is devoted to "the children" are really

unwilling to face up to the empty nest syndrome. They're still clinging to the old family setup—Mama Bear, Papa Bear, and Baby Bear
—and haven't readjusted their lives to the reality that they are two
adults with grown children (who, incidentally, also have a right to a
life of their own).

The solution to this problem lies in applying the same medicine
that the gadabouts used on their social life. They should analyze the
time spent with the children—and cut it in half. (Mercifully, they'll
probably never know how relieved the children will be.) Then they
should concentrate on rebuilding that just-the-two-of-us relationship.

WINNING TICKETS IN THE MARRIAGE GAME

Live Alone and Like It. Shared activities are essential. But too
much togetherness can be just as bad for the middle-aged marriage as
spending all of our time apart, engrossed in our own activities. Child
psychologists keep telling us that it's the quality, not the quantity, of
time spent with our children that counts. The same could be said of
the time we spend with our spouses.

This idea of togetherness has been so overblown by the media that
many couples seem to think they must spend every single moment
together or their relationship is a flop. But ultimately this stifling
togetherness can be devastating to any relationship.

Shared interest and activities certainly add an important dimension to the mature marriage. But there must also be *understanding*
and a willingness to allow the other person to *be* a person, an individual with a life of his or her own. No married person can stay
happy as one half of a siamese twin act.

So don't overdo togetherness. Don't make a religion of it. Having
an opportunity to pursue our own interests is equally important. A
degree of individuality also helps to get us out of that middle-aged
rut, stimulate our over-all personalities, and just generally make us
more interesting people. And growing, expanding personalities will
add depth and meaning to any relationship. Two *interesting*, happy
people are going to have an interesting, happy relationship.

Having independent interests also creates a bit of mystery, a sense
of the unknown in even the most long-lived relationship. And each
partner retains a sense of identity—the morale-building knowledge
that he or she is a person in his own right. The key word is balance.

Each couple must strike some sensible degree of balance between the shared time and interests that mean companionship and another group of private interests that permit a healthy degree of individuality—individuality that will prevent one person from being a submissive (and, at the worst, parasitic) extension of the other.

But there is still another danger in too much togetherness. People need privacy.

Professor Alexander Kira is an outspoken advocate of the need in every individual's life for *privacy*. While so many psychologists and psychiatrists are urging us to share *everything*—every thought, every fear, every dream, and in some cases even the bathroom—Professor Kira champions the need of every human being to periods of solitude. He says, "*Being able to have secrets gives us a sense of security* . . . we need moments alone to reinforce our individual uniqueness, to feel free to be, to think what we want to think, to experiment, to dream."

Those who have been married for many years would do well to examine their attitudes toward the privacy of their spouses. Unfortunately, women are often the worse offenders in the destruction of individual privacy.

"What are you doing? What are you thinking? Where are you going? When will you be back?" These are all holdovers, I guess, from the years when "mother" felt responsible for *everything* pertaining to her children. (Though Dr. Kira points out that even children need to have their little secrets, their own private thoughts.)

But when the children are almost grown, it is healthy to rethink our attitudes toward privacy. Every adult needs some quiet time *alone*. Those in the middle-aged marriage will find that periods of privacy will only serve to enrich those times when they are together.

There are two ways you can bring more privacy into your married life. Mentally, you can re-examine your attitudes toward your husband. Have you been subtly demanding to know his every thought, his every feeling? Listen, that's the way secret police break down their captives. Truly, if carried to extremes, this need to know can drive one crazy. And what about you? Have you retained that intriguing mental "private life"? Or does your husband feel it's his right to quiz you on every opinion, every attitude? Or, worse yet, do you volunteer the information? Familiarity breeds, if not contempt, at least boredom. So keep your own counsel, and develop and protect your private life.

Another important aspect of privacy has to do with your surroundings. The modern house or apartment makes it difficult to have a
quiet place where we can be alone.

In fact, one of my pet theories is that modern architecture, with
its doorless rooms, see-through spaces, all-in-one "activity areas," contributes enormously to the nerves, neurosis, and mental inharmony
that are so common today. There's simply no place to be alone.

But it is *essential* for all human beings to have a place where they
can be alone. So, as the children move out, you can turn this otherwise melancholy phenomenon into positive actions that will revitalize your marriage—and you. Don't turn those newly empty rooms
into a family room or pristine guest room. Instead, set them aside so
that you and your husband can each have a room of your own.
(Aside from your bedroom.)

And if it isn't possible to have an entire room to yourself, at least
rearrange your house so that each of you has an area that is *yours
alone*. Respect the privacy of those areas and don't trespass! (Remember, often it's an accumulation of *little* annoyances that destroy
a relationship.)

So learn to live alone some of the time. You'll see. You'll like it—
and so will he. And since contrasts add that special zest to life—
those times when you *are* together will be more meaningful.

The Public Be Damned! So many marriages are afflicted by the
malaise of "outer direction." Everything from conversation to sexual
performance is measured against outer standards and norms. But one
of the most successful moves in the marriage game is made by those
couples who say, "The public be damned."

Some marriages have had this philosophy from the very beginning.
Many happy couples have been playing their own version of "open
marriage" for years. There's the couple who take separate vacations
every other year. No hanky-panky, mind you. But they're both strong
personalities with avid interests. His passion is fishing and hers is art.
So he goes fishing. And he revels in the feeling of being A Man
Alone Against the Elements. He goes to the darndest places, too . . .
remote villages in Alaska, a jewellike lake in Canada (not a town for
seventy-six miles in any direction), or a backward seaside village in
southern Mexico.

She would be utterly miserable in any of these out-of-the-way spots
—and they both know it. But that doesn't mean that he should miss

out on his fun. Nor should she. So while he's off in the wilds she pursues her interest in the arts.

One year she went to Europe by herself, on a guided tour that covered all the famous opera houses. Another time she took a theater tour to New York. Other vacations have included a study-travel tour set up by the local art museum. And then, every other year, they vacation together.

A bit unusual? Somewhat unconventional? Well, yes. And frankly, not a solution for most couples, who usually find that separate vacations are a prelude to going separate ways—permanently. The point is, while it's not for everyone, this very unusual life style works for *this* couple, and that's what counts. And while this unusual life style drives many of their friends and neighbors *crazy*, this couple has an unusually happy and enduring relationship because (1) they both feel fulfilled as people, being able to pursue activities which are important and meaningful to them; and (2) they have remained interesting, even fascinating people in their own right. Remember, you can't expect two dull people to produce a stimulating, exciting relationship.

I do believe we have the right to protect our marriages from undue stress ("Darling, I'm going to spend a weekend at the cottage with that beach boy we met in Honolulu. Okay?" Or, "I've joined an expedition that's sailing to Hong Kong on a raft"). But it's also important for each individual to have as much freedom as possible to *be*, to *do*, and to *act* in ways that are personally satisfying. The inner-directed marriage allows each partner the freedom to be himself, without the arbitrary norms set up by "the Joneses."

Another example of a couple that says, "The public be damned," is Art and Harriet. Harriet hates to cook. Harriet is a lousy cook. (Nothing new here. This happens in the best of families.) But instead of allowing their home life to limp along, overcome by bouts of indigestion and kitchen tantrums, Art and Harriet have made a very sensible adjustment. *He* does every bit of the cooking—and the shopping, too. He likes to cook and he's good at it. So why not? Yet such an obvious and simple solution would never occur to those couples who have allowed their marriages to be totally outer-directed.

In an era inundated with charts, graphs, public opinion polls, and instant experts, it's important to remind ourselves that marriage is not a group sport (in spite of what the swingers say). It's a very personal game for two. So if an unconventional solution works for your very personal, individual relationship, use it.

It's easy for a relationship of many years to become increasingly outer-directed. Two culprits contribute toward this trend. One is the ever present media. Television, magazines, and books overwhelm us with unrealistic pictures of "life among the beautiful people." The women's magazines are especially guilty in this area . . . doing picture stories of impossibly successful, totally elegant, superperfect women who have perfect children with straight teeth and naturally curly hair; spotless, smooth-running, superdecorated houses; and paragons for husbands. You know the scene. This couple is always photographed in an impeccably decorated room, wearing jodhpurs and matching turtleneck sweaters (vicuña, of course), and naturally they are lounging on an opulent sofa. And does that sofa have one single cat or dog hair on it? Of course not.

I spent years feeling totally inferior to these superwomen with their immaculate husbands. For years I remained vaguely dissatisfied with my real life and my less than perfect house (with cat hairs). And I'd find myself resentfully wondering why my endearingly human husband couldn't enjoy a candlelight dinner on the terrace ("I can't see a blasted thing and the food's cold").

And then several years ago I met and worked with one of these superwomen—and I was cured.

Superwoman was the creator of a well-known cosmetic line and was as glamorous as the perfume that bears her name. (You'd know it in a minute.) And she was a favorite subject for those "How does she do it?" articles. Interspersed with close-ups of Superwoman's antique-filled showrooms and long shots of her jetting here and there would be charming photos of our paragon at home in her exquisitely decorated house, surrounded by five perfect children and an adoring husband.

But I soon found that behind the scenes the picture was far from perfect. The magazines assured the gullible reader that "Mrs. S.W. manages to maintain a perfect balance between her exciting career and her perfect marriage—and the children adore her. . . ." But in reality the children were neurotic, whining monsters one and all. The husband was a high-stakes gambler and kept a bevy of playmates around to amuse him the moment she jumped on one of those jets. And finally, far from balancing this complicated house of cards with serenity, wit, and imagination, Superwoman was an emotional basket case, and her "beautiful" life was only an artificial veneer, hastily slapped on whenever someone "important" was there to admire it. What's more, 90 per cent of her business success was due to the efforts of a considerate father who left her a fortune and a stable, hard-working, and talented staff that the media never even noticed.

After this revealing glimpse behind the scenes, I was free forever from the subtle pressure of the media to live up to some impossible ideal, to try to fit my life into an unrealistic mold. I became slightly more tolerant when I found myself trying to serve dinner with my husband, two of his rather disreputable friends, and three large dogs gathered around the dining-room table, all six apparently trying to tie the same trout fly.

That's not to say that we shouldn't strive to make our lives exciting and creative, that we shouldn't indulge in the art of living, rather than just existing. My point is this: create your own picture—the one that suits you and your husband best. You may end up as "that slightly eccentric couple," but if you're true to yourself and to your individuality you won't have to worry about creating a beautiful, but artificial, picture for some magazine. You will instead be *living* a realistic, beautiful life of your own.

The opinion of our peer group is the other source of pressure that makes a marriage become outer-directed. After years of marriage, many couples find that they have allowed themselves to be in thrall to a group of old friends who exert subtle (or not so subtle) pressure for conformity to the group's ideas. Sort of a his-and-hers Professional M.A.M.ism. And I guess you know how I stand on this subject. And how can you tell when "that old gang of mine" is running your life? Well, when you reach the time when "what *they* will think" always overrides "what *we* feel," look out! You must examine what's real and true and important to you and your husband, and then go your own sweet way, and the public be damned.

I'm on Your Side. Which is another way of saying that the marriages that triumphantly overcome the middle-age crisis are the ones built on a strong supportive attitude. Each partner in the marriage knows that the other one is always there to provide support and encouragement. And in the middle years we both need plenty of this T.L.C.

As psychiatrist Pierre Mornell explains, "When we are helped, not hurt, in moments of vulnerability, feelings of warmth and affection for the other person grow. When we are supported at crucial moments, rather than undermined, we are more receptive to other levels of honesty at other times." This feeling of confidence, of emotional security, the "I'm on your side" attitude can add dimensions to your relationship not only during crisis times but at all times and on all levels.

Bill Hall, director of the Secretarial Development Program for the State of California, told me. "We find that this non-judgmental attitude is conducive to creative thinking and creative problem-solving. In the business world, we call it brainstorming. We get people into a relaxed atmosphere, present a project or problem, and then encourage people to 'open up,' to contribute any ideas they have on the subject—no matter how farfetched or original. When people feel free to express what they think and feel without fear of rejection, it brings out the best in them."

But how easy it is to turn off that creative train of thought. "You know, luv, I have kind of a crazy idea for our vacation this year—I wonder what you'll think of it?" "Well, if it's anything like that crackbrained scheme you had last year, I vote *no*."

If you want to work on establishing a non-judgmental creative relationship, banish two words from your intermarriage vocabulary— "always" and "never." "You always . . ." and "You never . . ." can stop a relationship, an idea, a confidence even before it gets started. These two phrases usually precede some subtle negative observation: "Sailing? But you *always* catch cold." . . . "You *never* understand." . . . "You're *always* late." . . . "You *never* make the reservations on time. . . ."

What's the reason for the negative reaction to "always" and "never?" Simple. It effectively puts the other person in a box— stifled, controlled, stultified. We instinctively rebel against this attitude. No one is completely predictable. And the very essence of the human state is one of change and the possibility of growth and improvement.

Listening is another important part of the "I'm on your side" attitude. I've talked about listening several times in this book, about how important creative listening is in developing charm, warmth, and magnetism. But listening is important to your relationships for a deeper reason. Dr. Carl Menninger, in discussing a general formula for a happy marriage, has said, "Marriages are contracts between human beings, and all human beings are fallible. We all disappoint one another in various ways, even with the best of intentions, and none of us has the best of intentions *all* the time. Fortunately, however, we all have some intelligence, and we can use it when frictions arise. We can listen to one another's version of the difficulties. *Just being listened to attentively has a magnetic, soothing, creative effect on people. Listening can be highly restorative. Listening is more important than talking but there has to be some of both.*" (Emphasis added.)

Michael Arlen, in his article "Saturday Father," expressed this idea a little differently, but his approach could well become the motto for a happy relationship: "I think, if I had to give a basic definition of Love, it would be this: the *noticing* of someone. Paying—really paying—attention."

Listen, pay attention, ask questions, communicate. This is almost the miracle cure for the middle-aged marriage doldrums.

He doesn't listen, pay attention, or communicate with you? Well, don't be a "love bird"—*tell him.*

IS IT TIME TO CHANGE PARTNERS?

When an interviewer asked Lynn Fontanne if she'd ever thought of divorce during her long and much-publicized marriage to Alfred Lunt, she replied, "Divorce? Never. Murder—often!"

Although most married women would probably say, "Them's my sentiments, exactly," the fact remains that divorce, not murder, is one of the favorite games of the over-forty. In fact, during this crisis time, statistics indicate that the divorce rate is almost as great as that among teen-age marriages, which were long considered the greatest risk area.

Well, is it time to change partners? Maybe he thinks so—and has come to you with an ultimatum. What to do? It all depends on you. If your first thoughts about losing him are practical—"Where will I live?" "Will I have to get a job?" "What will my friends say?"—baby, it's all over but the pouting. Retire from the field with grace, good humor, a minimum of wrinkles, and the most generous settlement that a clever lawyer can manage.

But if that ultimatum wrenches your heart, makes you think of a lonely bed without that familiar back to snuggle up to, makes you unaccountably remember a silly note he wrote to you, makes you wonder just how you'll live without that warm and wonderful guy—there's still *something* there—and it's worth trying to save. Hang in there and play a waiting game. Audrey Hepburn says, "People are too ready to give up when they should hold on. Take the love of a mother for her child. If it's real, it never dies, no matter what the child may do. I don't know why more people can't have that kind of relationship with a lover, a husband, a wife."

Still, in spite of all your efforts, divorce may be inevitable. And that's when you have to demonstrate that you're big enough to know that everyone, sometimes, has to be a loser. So face up to it. You'll live. Really! Take your lumps and get out. Physically and emotionally. Otherwise, you'll destroy yourself. You'll destroy any chance of rebuilding your life, too. And as the Ageless Woman that new life can be more fulfilling than you ever imagined.

Iris is a good example of the woman who can't let go. When she came to my studio, inquiring about classes in self-development, she said, "Now that I'm divorced, I need all the help I can get. You know, when Joe asked me for a divorce, I just cracked up. But now I want to get a job and get settled here, and I thought your course might give me a little more self-confidence."

I told her that the classes could, indeed, help her. And since many of my students came to class for exactly the same reasons, I was able to tell her many success stories of newly divorced women who had successfully made the adjustment to single life.

Iris was a delightful student. She had a warm personality and was eager to learn. Until she got on _that_ subject. "Of course, since my divorce, I don't go out much at night. I'm just not comfortable away from home after dark." Or, "I haven't knuckled down to finding a job yet. As soon as I've adjusted to my divorce I'll make some concrete plans. Now, I'm just hanging loose." And then we heard endless stories about her contacts with her ex-husband and how she still had to go over the settlement. Apparently there were endless phone calls, visits, long business lunches, and so on.

One afternoon, after class, I mentioned a receptionist job that I had heard about. "Iris, it sounds just right for you. Why don't you give them a call?" She answered that she didn't feel ready to commit herself to a steady job. She wasn't quite recovered from The Divorce. This time, for some reason, her defeatist attitude seemed exceptionally irritating and I was surprised to find myself blurting, "How long are you going to let that man haunt your life? How long ago _was_ that divorce, anyway?" Somehow, it had never occurred to me to ask her when the great separation had taken place. I naturally assumed, from what she'd said, that it had been six months or a year ago. I almost fell out of my chair when she answered, with a catch in her voice, "It's been six years now."

What a tragic waste. Poor Iris was still hanging on, still emotionally committed to a relationship that had been dead and buried years before. As far as her own life was concerned, Iris might just have been dead and buried too.

But suppose *you* want the divorce. Before you take that drastic step into the divorce court (would you really rather live alone in a studio apartment with a cat?), you had better make certain that your own head is on straight. If you build up some insights that tell why your present relationship deteriorated, perhaps you will learn how to save that relationship. And certainly those insights will help you create a more fulfilling life for yourself later if it develops that divorce is, indeed, the only solution.

Self-knowledge is doubly important if you've been married to a complete bastard. And let's face it. There are plenty of them lurking behind the façades of the seemingly happiest households. Maybe he drinks, gambles, or plays Don Juan. Or he's a subtle sadist with a thousand ways of destroying your ego. Why not "Wash That Man Right Out of Your Hair"? After all, could things be worse?

Yes, they could. If you don't have an honest insight into the workings of the relationship, the "whys" of what happened, there's an excellent chance that you'll make the same mistakes all over again. You've seen it happen again and again. So before you step out that door, and out of his life forever, study up on the problem.

Your first step may be into your friendly public library to get some books that deal with problems in personal relationships.

A good book to start on might be *I'm O.K., You're O.K.,* by Thomas Harris. This book is about Transactional Analysis (often called T.A.), a remarkable tool for giving us insight into our destructive behavioral patterns. As Dr. Harris says, "Transactional Analysis . . . has given patients a tool they can use. . . . Anybody can use it . . . people do not have to be 'sick' to benefit from it. . . . It has given a new answer to people who want to change rather than adjust, to people who want transformation rather than conformation. It is realistic in that it confronts the patient with the fact that *he is responsible for what happens in the future no matter what happened in the past.*" (Emphasis added.)

T.A. can give you an insight into your relationship. It's possible, just possible, that *you're* driving him to drink. Not consciously, of course. But perhaps you *need* that drunken, irresponsible husband because of some mental quirks of your own. And if he's a subtle sadist, could it be that you're a closet masochist—unconsciously asking for misery?

Well, this is pretty heavy going, it's true. But the point is, it usually takes two to create a destructive relationship. Dr. Murray Bowen, professor of psychiatry at Georgetown University Medical School in Washington, D.C., says that a problem never belongs to just one person. He feels that if a husband is demanding there is something in the wife's attitude that *invites* him to be demanding. And if a husband complains that his wife is a helpless, clinging vine, something in the husband encourages her to be weak and spineless. Most counselors would agree that a woman whose problems are centered around the phrase "my life would be perfect if only my husband wouldn't" usually has some gut-level problems of her own. The first step in solving her problems is not to change her husband but to change herself.

T.A. can help you see yourself and your actions in their real context—at the gut level—and can give you some of the insights that you need to help you make *constructive* changes.

Can all this be accomplished just by reading a book? Probably not. T.A. and similar types of counseling work on the basis of group therapy—a fast and proven way of getting insights into our habitual patterns. *But it's essential that you consider only those approved and bona fide groups.* Amateur encounter groups are psychological dynamite, as I'm sure you know.

So be sensible. Check out the group before checking in. A call to your local medical society is in order here, for a listing of professional counseling services.

You might also check with the marriage counselor associated with the Superior Court in your city. He will also have T.A.-type groups and counselors that he can recommend. And what about marriage counselors? Can they save that failing marriage?

They can often help, of course. But unfortunately, according to Brinkley Long, chief marriage counselor of Sacramento's Superior Court, most couples don't seek out the marriage counselor until it's too late. Usually one person in the marriage has already decided that "it's over" and sees the marriage counselor only to placate the spouse

—to be able to say, "See? I've done everything to save this marriage, but it's just no good. It's over."

Another drawback to the concept of marriage counseling is that, like the ark, one should go two by two into this kind of treatment if it is to be really effective. Many marriages limp along for years because "My husband (or wife) refuses to see a counselor."

But the partner who's most bothered by the marital situation can profit by going alone to seek professional advice. A competent professional can give those all-important insights into a person's own hang-ups.

If a woman is contemplating divorce, the more she understands about herself the more she'll understand about her husband's actions. Then she'll be better prepared to deal with those things that drive her crazy. And since "to understand is to forgive" she's taken a long step toward encouraging him in more positive behavior. She'll also learn to recognize her own automatic responses to his destructive behavior—responses that may perpetuate and encourage more of the same.

And if, in spite of all these efforts, divorce is the answer, the woman who has gained an in-depth understanding of whatever happened to her marriage has an excellent chance of developing positive, rewarding relationships in the future. She may even find herself playing a new and unaccustomed role.

THE AGELESS WOMAN AND THE YOUNGER MAN

Thanks to the Ageless Woman, a new equation in the love game is taking the place of the eternal triangle. The old script routinely contained the following cast of characters: the Older Man, his discarded Middle-aged Wife, and the Sweet Young Thing who was taking her place. But today we see a new kind of triangle forming, and the players are the Successful Young Man, the Ageless Woman whom he adores, and his former roommate, Bunny Booby, who's wondering, "Whatever happened to my love affair?"

The Ageless Woman happened, that's who. Increasing numbers of bright young men are discovering that, not only can you trust someone over thirty, but if she's the Ageless Woman you can have a helluva good time with her too.

No doubt about it, this is one of the most exciting changes that's come into the lives of today's mature women. They are free from those agist attitudes, those puritan prejudices that limited a woman's love life to the far side of the calendar. A man has always been free to pursue, to love, to marry a woman ten, fifteen, even twenty years his junior. And a slap on the back and a sly wink from his contemporaries told him just how clever he was to arrange such an alliance. "What a devil old Saxbe is. I understand that the new Mrs. Saxbe is young enough to be his daughter. Egad!"

But women have been locked into the unwritten code that said, "Listen, my girl, the only possible relationship that you can consider is one with a man who's *older* than you are. He's just your age? Welllll, all right. But not a smidge younger."

In fact, the picture of the older woman and the younger man has in the past conjured up images that are, if not downright depraved, at least distinctly seedy. Blanche DuBois for example—jaded, degraded, and definitely dotty as she languishes after her fragile and lilac-scented young men. Or neurotic Mrs. Robinson types, purposefully pursuing the grocery boy and demanding that he deliver. But sensible women, stable women, sane women, *nice* women would never even consider a relationship with a younger man.

The Ageless Woman has changed all that and for some darned good reasons. She's changed our concept of what the mature woman should be. She's no longer that nice little matron, that Helen Hokinson caricature. She's the Ageless Woman, and by now, we know all about her—we know that she's a pretty fabulous lady, downright irresistible if she chooses to be. Finally free of those age hangups, aware of her own infinite sexuality, wise and experienced, compassionate and secure in her own identity, she's a formidable adversary for Bunny Booby.

And he's changed too. The young man in his twenties and thirties has grown up in an iconoclastic era that rejects labels and categories. "Do your own thing" is his motto, and he's free to find love and companionship where it pleases him.

The Sweet Young Thing in his life has changed too. Oh boy, has she changed. With her unisex clothes, her unisex vocabulary ("Oh, gawd, I feel horny" is often her tender invitation to love-making), her aggressive self-centeredness, she's liberating herself right out of some of the most interesting beds in town. And the Ageless Woman is smugly taking her place.

The Ageless Woman and the Younger Man are a familiar combination in the celebrity register. Dinah Shore and Burt Reynolds, Sybil Burton and her young husband Jordan Christopher. Then there's Lucille Ball, who is six years older than husband Gary Morton. Faye Dunaway, thirty-three, recently married rock musician Peter Wolf, twenty-eight. And ageless Merle Oberon, fifty-seven, is now Mrs. Robert Wolders (he's thirty-eight).

Audrey Hepburn is nine years older than her husband, Dr. Andrea Dotti. She sums up the attitude of the Ageless Woman: "Yes, there is a big difference in our ages. It's as simple as that; there is. I was born nine years before him. Not that I am more mature. I just have seen nine years more of life. That's the only sense in which I am older. In other ways he is much older—intellectually, for example, though emotionally we are the same."

But celebrities aren't the only ones with this liberated attitude toward the pairing of younger man and Ageless Woman. More and more women are breaking down this archaic prejudice. In fact, statistics indicate that it is becoming increasingly commonplace for younger men to marry women who are older than they are.

In West Germany, for example, where approximately 450,000 marriages take place each year, 70,000 marriages have reversed the traditional pairing of the older husband and the younger wife. In Great Britain in recent years, the number of marriages in which the wife is older than the husband have increased tenfold. In Sweden it has increased twelvefold. And in the United States—no one seems to know.

But in the absence of statistics, the general acceptance of this kind of pairing shows that it is a growing trend. Mel Krantzler, in his book *Creative Divorce*, says, "A major eye-opener for me has been the number of women in their thirties and above who feel free to enjoy the company of younger men. . . ."

IS THERE A YOUNGER MAN IN YOUR FUTURE?

Who knows? But even the remotest possibility is bound to keep your present man on his toes.

Remember, just becoming and staying the Ageless Woman means that you can attract and hold a man, including a younger man, if you really want to. As we know, age is not a disadvantage to the mature woman as long as she becomes and stays the Ageless Woman. Because the Ageless Woman doesn't have to concede anything to the Bunny Boobys of this world. What the Ageless Woman already has, Bunny Booby will need about twenty years to learn.

So if, in spite of everything you can do, your marriage is over and you want out, don't despair. Don't walk away looking back: instead walk away looking forward. As the Ageless Woman, you have an exciting future ahead of you—one you don't have to spend alone.

TWELVE

Winning: It's All in Your Head

We have met many Ageless Women as we discussed Winning the Age Game—and we have met many Professional M.A.M.s, too. The differences between them seem numberless, at first. But actually there is only one *essential* difference between these two—*attitude*. In every case the Professional M.A.M. is victimized by a state of mind —a rigid, ingrained mental state that confines her to a limited, stagnating, negative, *old* way of life.

But many religious teachers, philosophers, and scientists, as well as countless Ageless Women, have clearly demonstrated that by changing her negative attitudes—replacing them with positive viewpoints —the Professional M.A.M. could change her entire way of life, her physical health, and even the rate at which she ages.

Will she ever change? I wouldn't bet on it. Her state of mind has become ingrained. If I were to bet, I would put my money on *you*. Because if you have read this far you have clearly proved that your attitudes are not set in concrete, that you already have many of those positive outlooks necessary for growth and change, and that you can become the winner—the Ageless Woman.

Now let us talk about the vital importance of attitude—or call it "spirit" if you will. We have discussed style, exercise, health, and many other things. Now let's see how attitudes can create or destroy —how they can keep you ageless or age you prematurely.

THE AGELESS WOMAN: A SCIENTIFIC REALITY

Countless experiments have proven that the body mechanisms respond to mental attitudes. When patients are given a placebo—a harmless sugar pill—that they *think* will make them well, their bodies often respond for the better, reacting to the positive thought rather than to any benefit from the sugar pill. Many doctors who are outwardly skeptical about the power of the mind over the body still use placebos in their daily practice.

We are all familiar with the eerie power of hypnotic suggestion. There have been many instances of hypnotized subjects who experienced an extreme physical reaction to a mental suggestion. For instance, when subjects under hypnosis were told that they had been burned, a blister actually formed.

There have also been many recorded examples of the destructive power that the mind can exert on the body. In primitive societies, the witch doctor can often kill by suggestion. Through ritual, myth, and magic that is accepted by the entire primitive society, the witch doctor convinces the victim that he is doomed. And he is doomed. At the appointed moment he just lies down and dies.

We too have our rituals, myths, and magic—our tribal convictions.

Remember the ritual litany of the Professional M.A.M.? "At our age" . . . "No fool like an old fool" . . . "When I was younger I used to" . . . "When we get older we slow down" . . . "It would be ridiculous at my age" . . . "Honestly! Why can't she(he) grow old gracefully" . . . "Of course at my age I don't" . . . And so on to her very last day, which such negative, devitalizing, destructive thoughts will certainly hasten.

On the other hand, a positive, dynamic attitude stimulates the mind and rejuvenates the body. The rejuvenating effect of mind has been observed by many people of many ages.

Dr. Maxwell Maltz explains in *Psychocybernetics* that there is a creative mechanism in the mind that influences our bodily functions and that, "in expecting to grow 'old' at a certain age, we may unconsciously set up a negative goal-image for our creative mechanism to accomplish." He also suggests that a positive goal-image can literally work to keep your body younger.

Many other doctors and scientists around the world are deeply aware of the relationship between aging and mental attitudes.

THE SECRET OF THE YOUTH DOCTORS

Scattered throughout the world are the rejuvenators, the mysterious medical magicians who keep the great and glamorous in the prime of life—regardless of what the calendar may say. These doctors cannot be theorists, they have to be realists; because their success or failure is brutally obvious in the mirrors of their patients. No scientific mumbo-jumbo will con an aging actress when her own mirror clearly proves that her doctor has failed.

These rejuvenators all have one factor in common that contributes to their success—*they work to build a positive attitude in the minds of their patients.*

Patrick McGrady, author of *The Youth Doctors*, spent two years in research and traveled twenty thousand miles in Europe and North America, interviewing the scientists, researchers, and physicians who are devoted to conquering age. He concluded, "Actually, quite impressive rejuvenation results can be gotten free, although many people do not appreciate or believe in anything that is not expensive. The first thing is to want—but *really want*—to be more youthful and to *believe* you can do it. Attitude alone, as any experienced youth doctor knows, can work miracles. Frequently, the only functional aspects of so-called rejuvenation regimens are do-it-yourself. . . ."

The physiologist Max Rubner observed, "Peasant women who work as cheap labor in the fields in some parts of the world are given to early withering of the face, but they suffer no loss of physical strength and endurance. Here is an example of specialization in aging. We can reason that these women have relinquished their competitive role as women. They have resigned themselves to the life of the working bee, which needs no beauty of the face but only physical competence."

Dr. Arnold A. Hutschnecker in *The Will to Live* also observed that widowhood has a similar effect on the aging rate of certain women. When a woman feels that, upon her husband's death, her life as a woman has come to an end, her mental attitude is reflected in her gradual withering and in her graying hair. Her negative attitude speeds up the aging processes.

But Hutschnecker also noted that other widows actually blossom. They may enter into competition for a new husband, start a new career, or busy themselves with a new interest. And such women, with a positive attitude toward their life and femininity, actually tend to change their physiological age for the better.

Positive attitudes have a rejuvenating effect on the body. And an expectation that you can be ageless will make agelessness a reality. This is why you must ruthlessly reject all those negative, limiting, age-making opinions and deep-seated, unconscious *attitudes* of the Professional M.A.M. If you can't get away from her, at least train yourself to tune her out. And most important, develop a gut-level sensitivity to her negative influence. The Ageless Woman develops a sensitive antenna that immediately recognizes and rejects these negative vibes. She protects herself from such destructive attitudes as carefully as if they were deadly atomic rays; because, in their effect on her, they can be just as dangerous.

Of course the knowledge that thought has the power to influence our bodies is nothing new, even though scientists are only now beginning to recognize this influence. Metaphysicians, on the other hand, have known this truth for centuries. Spiritual leaders of all creeds and ages have spoken of this universal truth, often in surprisingly similar words.

SOUL FOOD: THE MENTAL DIET
THAT KEEPS YOU YOUNG

The influence of the mind on the body has been noted by every religion and by every philosophy since the world began. The Bible tells us, "Be ye transformed by the renewing of your mind," and further advises, "As a man thinketh in his heart, so is he." And a quick look at our Ageless Woman will quickly prove that "As a woman thinketh in her heart, so is *she.*"

Charles Fillmore, the man who founded the Unity Church, is one of the many contemporary philosophers who stressed the importance of attitude in combating the inroads of age. When he was nearing fifty he wrote, "About three years ago, the belief in old age began to take hold of me. I began to get wrinkled and grey, my knees tottered, and a great weakness came over me. I did not discern the cause at once, but I found in my dreams I was associating with old people, and it gradually dawned on me that I was coming into this phase of race belief.

"I spent hours and hours silently affirming my unity with the infinite energy of the one true God. I associated with the young, danced with [them], sang folk songs with them. . . ."

And at ninety-three Charles Fillmore was still demonstrating the power of attitude over age. He was still at his desk daily, still conducting daily healing services, and still actively involved with the world around him.

Emmet Fox, in his classic book, *The Sermon on the Mount*, repeats this concept of mind over matter: "The great law of the Universe is just this—what you think in your mind you will produce in your experience. As within, so without."

The Indian sage Paramahansa Yogananda (who was guru to Mahatma Gandhi) said, "Mind is the chief factor governing the body. One should always avoid suggesting to the mind thoughts of human limitations such as sickness, old age, and death." He adds, "Will is [thus] a potent factor in maintaining youth and vigor. If you convince yourself you are old, the will becomes paralyzed and you do become old. Never say *you* are tired. Say 'My body needs rest.' The body must not be allowed to dictate its limitations to your soul."

Mary Baker Eddy, founder of Christian Science, is even more specific about the relationship between our thoughts and the age of our bodies, and more emphatic about the importance of denying the concept of old age.

In her book *Science and Health*, Mrs. Eddy said, "Never record ages. Chronological data are no part of the vast forever. Time-tables of birth and death are so many conspiracies against manhood and womanhood. Except for the error of measuring all that is good and beautiful, man would enjoy more than three score years and ten and still maintain his vigor, freshness and promise."

She went on to tell this story. "The error of thinking that we are growing old, and the benefits of destroying that illusion, are illustrated in a sketch from the history of an English woman, published in the London medical magazine called *The Lancet*.

"Disappointed in love in her early years, she became insane and lost all account of time. Believing that she was still living in the same hour which parted her from her lover, taking no note of years, she stood daily before the window watching for her lover's coming. In this mental state she remained young. *Having no consciousness of time, she literally grew no older.* [Emphasis added.] Some American travelers saw her when she was seventy-four, and supposed her to be a young woman. . . . Asked to guess her age, those unacquainted with her history conjectured that she must be under twenty."

Now, if you are thinking that losing all your marbles is a pretty steep price to pay for an unlined face, you are missing the point. The young woman in the story had remained young because she hadn't thought of herself as growing old. And she hadn't been aware of the passing of the years. Mrs. Eddy concluded, "She could not age while believing herself to be young, *for the mental state governed the physical.*" (Emphasis added.)

The power of the mind is enormous and this is why I am in favor of covering gray hair, having your face lifted if it needs it, exercising to keep your body slim and lithe, dressing in contemporary fashions, keeping your mind engrossed in the present and the future. All of these things help your mind to combat the idea of old age and reinforce the *truth* that you are ageless. And this is why I urge my students—

NEVER TELL YOUR AGE

That is, if you can help it. You'll have to come clean with traffic policemen, the Department of Motor Vehicles, the passport office, the marriage license bureau, and personnel departments. But once you have dealt with these unavoidable snoops, keep your age to yourself. There's a very sound reason for this advice. And it has nothing to do with vanity.

If you agree that the condition of your body is directly related to the mental image you have of yourself, you can see that telling your true *chronological* age creates needless obstacles. If you constantly talk about or brood about the passing years, you are setting in motion destructive mental forces that relentlessly remind your body to age. And dwelling upon your age also influences the attitudes of people around you.

If you tell your age indiscrimately, if you discuss your age, if you make it a habit to constantly refer to your age, other people immediately form a whole series of impressions and conclusions about you based on *their* concept of a person in your chronological age bracket. They immediately categorize you, and their concept of forty (which may be very negative and limited) becomes the basis of their relationship with you.

And think of the damage that their negative, confining, limiting attitudes—their negative vibes—may be doing to the positive "goal-image" in your mind that has been working so staunchly to keep you ageless. So why allow other people to pigeonhole you according to chronological age? Why be limited by *their* concepts?

You know that you're not getting older, you're getting better. You also know that as a mature woman in the modern world, with longer life spans and unlimited opportunity for growth, you are literally the youngest forty-, fifty-, or sixty-year-old woman the world has ever known. As the Ageless Woman, you reflect this truth—that age is not an absolute. It's relative.

If age were an absolute, like a mathematical equation or a chemical reaction, we would all age at exactly the same rate. But a quick glance at the Professional M.A.M., the Unwilling M.A.M., and the Ageless Woman clearly proves that age is a concept, not a reality. The woman whose concept of herself defies the stereotypes of calender years is literally able to rise above those stereotypes, both physically and mentally.

So, whenever possible, keep your age to yourself. Not because you're being coy, not because you're trying to be something that you're not (Would any of us want to be twenty again? Thirty? Not me.), but because you refuse to be *limited* by the conventional, negative, and restricting attitudes that most people have toward middle age.

Incidentally, this advice has nothing to do with "The Double Standard of Aging" as Susan Sontag calls it. Some feminists are urging women to stop lying about their age—to "tell the truth." But I'm advocating that mature *men* as well as women stop placing limitations on their lives and abilities by categorizing themselves according to calendar years.

Banish forever any stereotypes you may be harboring regarding the life style, the appearance, and the abilities of various ages. And we all tend to think in terms of stereotypes, whether we realize it or not. Let's look past the forties and fifties for a moment and think of the popular concept of a woman of eighty. What do we see? A dear little old lady with a vague expression on her face, a bundle of knitting in her lap, and a shawl around her shoulders. She's sweet, dull, and possibly a bit dotty.

But now let's look at some Ageless Women whose attitudes have freed them from these stereotypes.

ATTITUDES, NOT DIAMONDS, ARE A GIRL'S BEST FRIEND

Anita Loos is a sparkling example of the power of the mind. This enchanting sprite, creator of *Gentlemen Prefer Blondes* and hundreds of motion picture screen plays (remember *San Francisco* with Gable and MacDonald?), recently appeared on a TV talk show. Dressed in a svelte silk pajama outfit, the trademark bangs accenting her brown eyes, Anita Loos belies her years in both appearance and manner. She's still a tiny whirlwind of creative energy.

During the interview, she mentioned that she's only able to fulfill her extensive writing schedule by getting up every morning at 4 A.M. and writing until ten. Then it's off to lunch with some of her "young" friends—Helen Hayes, Joan Crawford, or the Gish sisters. Her latest project, slated for Broadway next season, is a musical version of one of her successful plays. The interviewer finally asked this busy and successful Ageless Woman her age. She answered, "I'm really not sure, since my birth certificate was burned in the San Francisco fire. But it's well over eighty."

Another Ageless Woman who defies agist stereotypes is dancer Martha Graham. She danced with her ballet company regularly until she was seventy-six, and now, at eighty, she heads her own twenty-five-member ballet troupe as its director. She says, "I don't like to be bored and I will not be bored. I like to be with people, meet with them, talk with them, and be on the stage with them. This is what I call appetite for life, the hunger for life that has kept me going."

Lily Pons is another Ageless Woman who refuses to fit into the stereotypes of age. In 1973 a concert in Palm Springs proved that the magic voice was "shining almost as brightly" as it was during the twenty-six years when she was the reigning coloratura at the Met— an amazing feat, since the operatic voice, as you no doubt know, is seldom so long-lived. Her voice, her manner, and her still exquisite appearance belied the facts in the reference books. They all agree that she was born in 1904 and made her operatic debut at the Metropolitan Opera in 1931. But Miss Pons refuses to be hemmed in by vital statistics.

"You are the age you look," she smiles slyly. "Let people guess, I say. I know it is in the encyclopedias, but who reads encyclopedias? *I never think of age at all.* [Emphasis added.] I just enjoy being in good health. I enjoy most the simple things of life."

Twenty-four-carat glamor isn't limited by years, either, as I've pointed out many times in this book. Gloria Swanson, somewhere in her seventies, was recently interviewed by a smitten Kevin Thomas. He described her this way: "In person, up close, Gloria Swanson does not disappoint. Dressed in a smart beige sport outfit she is chic and contemporary without seeming as if she were trying to look like a young woman. The face that has been called one of the greatest of the silent screen still is: large, piercing blue eyes, gleaming teeth, that famous mole on the left side of her chin and those bold, sculptured features. Barely five feet tall, she is a tiny dynamo, a lady of wit and wisdom, full of passion for life."

And may I add, she's the living proof that the Ageless Woman never stops being an exciting, female *woman*, that she never becomes the neuter matron, because she never stops thinking of herself as a woman.

Merle Oberon, a mere youngster in her fifties, also stresses the importance of avoiding the limiting stereotypes that we have toward age. "You know, it shocks me when people tell me how young I *look* (which really means 'how old you are!'), because inside I feel just exactly as I did twenty or thirty years ago! It's terribly important to 'think' young. Many women just give up at forty or forty-five, and then they tend to get bitter and sour. (One should also think *kind* . . . envy and greed take a toll on looks; you poison yourself with hating.) Don't let your mind get rigid—about fashion, morals, *anything*."

And that includes attitudes about age.

ATTITUDES THAT MAKE YOU OLD (LOSERS)

The recurring theme in the Professional M.A.M.'s personality is a negative one. We've seen her attitudes toward a variety of subjects—from make-up to men—but in every case she takes a "no" approach to life. Rigid, pessimistic, fault-finding, she fairly revels in the fact that "service, workmanship, morals, people—aren't what they used to be." She is inflexible and uncompromising, and what she fears most of all is change.

These pessimistic attitudes can actually create physical changes and bring on early aging. Dr. Maxwell Maltz points out that "indulging ourselves in the negative components of the 'Failure Mechanism' can literally make us old before our time." He is just one of many medical researchers who have concluded that pessimism is a major symptom of early fossilization. It usually goes hand in hand with the first subtle symptoms of physical decline.

Think about it. How often have you heard the M.A.M.s of your acquaintance having a wonderful time "viewing with alarm"? They bemoan the state of the world, the worthlessness of youth, the ungratefulness of children, the hopelessness of the future. But how old these attitudes are. And how they preclude any possibility of growth. By contrast, an interview I had with Joan Fontaine shows clearly that the Ageless Woman is optimistic, interested, and a part of today.

Miss Fontaine had just finished giving a lecture on "How to Stay Young," and she obviously had been practicing what she preached. Not only did she look ageless (the patrician beauty was as flawless as ever), but her vibrant facial expression and her enthusiasm fairly lit up the corner of the restaurant where we were having lunch. But the most significant point about our interview was that she was totally engrossed in *today*. She was very interested in young people and felt that they have a marvelous approach to life. When I asked her about Hollywood and the new movies, she commented that they are indeed different from the old fairy-tale formulas, but that they represent an evolution of the art form. "Everything has to change, in order to grow."

What a marvelous guideline for the Ageless Woman. This should be the cornerstone of her philosophy.

The Ageless Woman acknowledges the cosmic truth that nothing ever stays the same. Realizing that change is inevitable, she works to ensure that the changes will be in the direction she desires. She will grow.

And her decision to grow, to change, to live up to her greatest potential involves another essential quality. Above all, the Ageless Woman has courage. The courage to be a little different—and a bit more successful—than most of her contemporaries. She knows that—

"YOU ONLY GET IN LIFE WHAT YOU COMMAND"

Gloria Swanson tells about the time a young girl was introduced to her at a party—a young girl who rudely remained slumped on the couch throughout the introductions. Miss Swanson held out her hand to the young girl and then abruptly pulled her to her feet— "and my hostess applauded." And she adds the line that could be the motto of Ageless Women everywhere: "You only get in life what you command."

I've found that most of my students need to be reminded of this truth. After years of being wife, mother, chief bottle washer, and housekeeper—after years of being fed the idea that "Mother must sacrifice"—they have been beaten down to the point where they don't demand enough from life, from themselves, or from those around them.

How sad it is that so many women become servants in their own homes. They allow their position in the family to so deteriorate that they can't be the inspiring mother, the desirable wife, the fulfilled and respected adult—in fact, *the woman they want to be*—because they have allowed their families to restrict and thwart their personal growth. This is a tyranny that should never be tolerated from *anyone*.

If you have become a servant to your family, it's time that you gave your notice. This situation can be changed and it should be. It's good for you, good for your husband, and it's *essential* for your children. Leading psychologists have explained that the most valuable gift we can give our children is to demonstrate to them that the adult state has privileges and advantages—that it's a state they can look forward to because it offers many rewards.

Dr. John E. Eichenlaub suggests that we consciously demonstrate to our children that maturity is a desirable state, "This job demands that your own rewards genuinely exceed those of your children, *and that they know it*. [Emphasis added.] An unselfish desire to draw your children toward acceptance of maturity should often make you act a bit more selfish—at least to an extent which makes your children realize that adulthood involves a step up in life instead of the beginning of decline."

Young people must be made to see that, as the old army saying goes, "Rank has its privileges."

But in this country, sadly, the adults have abdicated and let their children rule. No wonder we have a youth cult. And no wonder many young people treat the middle-aged with a thinly veiled contempt. They're entitled. Because, by and large, we have betrayed them.

All too often we have presented them with a terrible picture of middle age—a dreary, gray, negative, depressing time of life typified by midriff bulge, denture breath, and overwhelming negativism.

And yet, what is *their* future? They know perfectly well that the calendar is leading them inexorably toward their own middle age. And if they despairingly reject that gloomy, negative future, who can blame them if they also sweepingly reject other mores, manners, morals, and customs of the adult world?

So becoming the Ageless Woman is not merely a vanity kick. The Ageless Woman can demonstrate to her children and to young people everywhere that life in this great, beautiful world is fun—that the mature years ahead can be a time of excitement, creativity, and fulfillment. She can, by example, instill in her children those positive attitudes that will allow them to look forward to maturity with optimism and anticipation.

So the Profesional M.A.M. must go. Who needs her rigid, limiting, destructive negativism? And what about the Unwilling M.A.M. —fearful, uncertain, self-effacing—who really needs *her*? Who needs either of them in these turbulant times?

What society needs now is Ageless Women—lots of them. They are a delight to their contemporaries *and an inspiration to the young*. And believe me, young people today need some heroines.

ENLIGHTENED SELF-INTEREST: THE WINNER'S ATTITUDE

But please don't misunderstand me. I am not suggesting that you once again martyr yourself on your family altar, this time by trying to become the Ageless Woman because "It's good for the children." Good grief! That won't work.

Become the Ageless Woman for *yourself*. Become that self-confident individual who radiates independence of ideas and interests—that special woman who has developed and encouraged her own unique personality—and who has the courage to let this personality shine. Become the Ageless Woman who has developed her mind so that she can have a rewarding inner life, and the wisdom and insight to sustain an exciting relationship with the man in her life. And finally become the Ageless Woman who has pride in the physical package that holds all these goodies.

Stop thinking of yourself in limiting terms—"Just a housewife"—"The Better Half"—"Debbie's mother." Use this book to help you build a fulfilling, rewarding life as the Ageless Woman—and have fun doing it.

And don't worry about the effect on your family. Or your friends. Or society in general. It will be good. Because the Ageless Woman is an inspiration to everyone. She's just what the world needs now.